VALIDATING PHARMACEUTICAL SYSTEMS

Good Computer Practice in Life Science Manufacturing

VALIDATING PHARMACEUTICAL SYSTEMS

Good Computer Practice in Life Science Manufacturing

EDITED BY
John Andrews

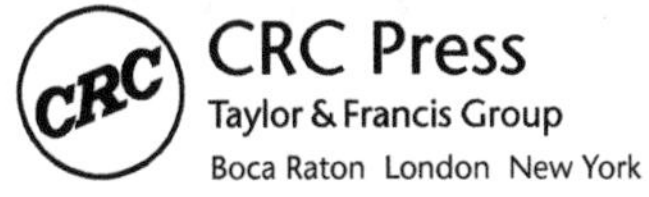

CRC Press
Taylor & Francis Group
Boca Raton London New York

CRC Press is an imprint of the
Taylor & Francis Group, an **informa** business
A TAYLOR & FRANCIS BOOK

CRC Press
Taylor & Francis Group
6000 Broken Sound Parkway NW, Suite 300
Boca Raton, FL 33487-2742

First issued in paperback 2019

ISBN-13: 978-0-8493-2324-9 (hbk)
ISBN-13: 978-0-367-39238-3 (pbk)
Library of Congress Card Number 2005050534

Library of Congress Cataloging-in-Publication Data

Validating pharmaceutical systems : good computer practice in life science manufacturing / edited by John Andrews.
p. cm.
Includes bibliographical references and index.
ISBN 0-8493-2324-X
1. Pharmaceutical technology--Data processing. 2. Pharmaceutical industry--Data processing. I. Andrews, John.

RS122.2.V35 2005
615'.19'00285--dc22 2005050534

Visit the Taylor & Francis Web site at
http://www.taylorandfrancis.com

and the CRC Press Web site at
http://www.crcpress.com

Contents

The Editor and His Contributors

John Andrews owns and operates Andrews Consulting Enterprises (ACE) Ltd from Worthing, West Sussex, U.K. Between 2001 and 2003, he managed the Information Technology (IT) Consulting Group of KMI, a division of PAREXEL International LLC (KMI). He is co-chairman of the GAMP 4 Special Interest Group on Process Control, which has produced a GAMP guide to Validation of Process Control Systems (VPCS). He also sat on the Editorial Board for GAMP 4, where his responsibilities included providing consultant services on computer systems validation, compliance and quality assurance activities within the pharmaceutical, biopharmaceutical, medical device, and other regulated healthcare industries.

Prior to KMI, Andrews held positions as a Computer System Validation Manager and Supply Chain Systems Project Manager with GlaxoSmithKline, U.K. Responsibilities there included all aspects of computer systems validation, from process control through to business and laboratory systems validation. He also managed teams with responsibilities for ensuring all computer system validation activities undertaken on site and within projects were delivered to an appropriate level to comply with the regulatory requirements.

Andrews worked for 15 years with SmithKline Beecham Pharmaceuticals, where he held positions as a Senior Engineering Standards Engineer, Secondary Manufacturing Electrical Engineer, Projects Engineer, and Electrical Supervisor. He attended Worthing College of Technology in West Sussex.

Mark Cherry is Systems Quality and Projects Group Manager for AstraZeneca with responsibility for the validation of computerized systems (laboratory, process control and information systems) used within U.K. manufacturing. Cherry is a member of the GAMP European Steering Group and has been an active member of both the IT Infrastructure and Process Control Special Interest Groups (SIGs) within GAMP. He is a Chartered Engineer and a member of the Institute of Measurement and Control. His previous experience includes 12 years with Glaxo (GlaxoWellcome and GlaxoSmithKline) where he held a number of roles ranging from engineering plant management through managing the design and implementation of a number of large distributed process control systems used within API manufacturing facilities.

Cherry became directly involved with quality management in 1999 when he was appointed Computer Systems Validation Manager for GlaxoWellcome's API manufacturing sites.

Tony de Claire and **Nichola Stevens** are both with Mi-Services Group based in the U.K. Stevens has been been the company's Senior Validation and Compliance

Consultant for the last 2 years, prior to which she worked for 10 years at SmithKline Beecham (as it was then) and 2 years each at Oxford Asymmetry International and Covance Laboratories.

de Claire joined Mi Services Group as Principal Consultant in 2001, after 6 years validation and compliance consultancy with APDC Consulting and Kemper-Masterson Inc. Prior to that he led the Manufacturing Automation and Information Systems Group for SmithKline Beecham's Corporate Engineering Department, responsible for computerized system application and validation across a wide-range of major capital projects, world-wide. de Claire has been active in number of GAMP Special Interest Groups over many years, and he also set up the Process Control and Automation Module for the MSc Pharmaceutical Engineering Advanced Training (PEAT) course offered by the University of Manchester/UMIST.

Chris Clark is Head of Quality Systems with Napp Pharmaceuticals Limited, located in the innovative Science Park in Cambridge, U.K. He holds a degree in biochemistry from Lancaster University, is a member of the Institute of Quality Assurance (IQA) in the U.K., and brings 26 years quality assurance experience with the pharmaceutical and healthcare industries to this book. A member of the GAMP Forum Council and European steering committee, Clark speaks regularly at conferences and training seminars on topics related to the implementation, qualification and validation of IT systems within those industries. He has contributed to the GAMP 4 guide and provides ongoing input to GAMP Forum publications.

Clark has worked in many automated equipment and computer related projects, ranging from manufacturing process equipment and tablet presses, to local implementation of ORACLE® Applications 11i, an enterprise document management (EDM) system, and an ORACLE® clinical data management system. He has a range of auditing experience gained from these and other projects, and assists international companies associated with Napp Pharmaceuticals on issues surrounding electronic records and signatures.

Sam Clark, a former Senior Consultant with the Information Technology (IT) Consulting Group of KMI, was an Investigator at the FDA for more than 21 years. He served as a General Investigator, a Medical Device Specialist Investigator, and an Investigator specializing in automated systems for the FDA's Atlanta District. Most recently, he was an FDA National Expert on Automated Systems.

Clark has conducted worldwide inspections in the entire range of the FDA-regulated industry and has extensive experience dealing with automated drug manufacturing and computer-controlled medical devices. He received his B.S. from the University of Georgia, Athens, Georgia and did graduate study in Computer Science at the Georgia Institute of Technology. Clark is a member of the Association for Computing Machinery, the Institute of Electrical and Electronic Engineers – Computer Society, and the American Society for Quality. He has published in *Pharmaceutical Technology*.

Peter Coady, BSc(Hons), CEng, FIMechE, FInstMC, is a consultant to the regulated industries sector (including GSK and its merged companies, Pfizer and

Wyeth), and runs his business (P J Coady & Associates) in Warsash, Southampton, U.K. He specializes in computer systems validation, electronic records and signatures, and system supplier auditing, having worked in these and related fields for more than 16 years.

Coady's career spans more than 25 years. Prior to becoming a consultant, he was employed at senior level by major British companies in the pharmaceutical, petrochemical, chemical and water sectors. He was appointed Manager of the Electrical, Instrumentation and Systems Group at AMEC Design & Management Limited, Southampton (formerly Matthew Hall Engineering Limited).

Coady is a GAMP Europe Forum and steering committee member. He represents GAMP on the BSI Disc TickIT Technical Committee, is a qualified IRCA Lead TickIT and QMS Auditor, and works internationally for LRQA as an independent lead assessor in these areas. He can be contacted via the publishers.

Since contributing to this book, Coady has joined Pfizer Ltd., Sandwich, U.K., as a Computer Validation QA Specialist.

Keith Collyer is a Principal Consultant in the Professional Services Group of Telelogic U.K. Limited, and **Jeremy Dick** is a Principal Analyst in the company's Products Division. Both have extensive experience in implementing successful requirements management and traceability solutions in organizations of all sizes across a wide range of industries, commercial organizations and government departments throughout the world. Dick is one of the authors of the book *Requirements Engineering*.

Paul Coombes was Head of Validation Europe for Washington Group International and is author of the successful book *Laboratory Systems Validation Testing and Practice* (PDA, 2003) and well-known papers on the design of compliant Excel spreadsheets, electronic signatures and other Part 11 issues. He worked for 10 years with Eli Lilly (U.K.) in analytical chemistry followed by positions with Hewlett-Packard, Tanvec and projects for major pharmaceutical firms as an independent consultant, a total of 25 years dedication to the industry. Equally experienced now in GMP, GLP, and GCP environments, Coombes works in computing, automation and IT as well as the science and chemistry disciplines that together create the special nature of the pharmaceutical and medical device industry.

Coombes contributed an excellent chapter on the effects of 21 CFR Part 11 on laboratories for *21 CFR Part 11 Electronic Records and Signatures in Practice* (Sue Horwood Publishing, 2003).

Wayne Duncan has been with PL Consultancy for 2 years. He focuses on Network and IT Infrastructure Compliance and Validation

David Forrest, Chief Executive of PL Consultancy was involved in the very early days of the GAMP Guide. His previous company, FJ Systems, was the initial editor of the GAMP guide. His experience spans a wide range of computer systems, from both an Implementation and Compliance and Validation perspective. Forrest has performed more than 50 audits of IT and Equipment suppliers and today manages

PL Consultancy a Specialist Computer Compliance and Validation Consultancy Company.

Mark Foss has been Head of Engineering for Boehringer Ingelheim in the U.K. for the last five years. He has worked since 1977 in both the nuclear and pharmaceutical industries. He was previously Engineering Manager for SmithKline Beecham for 11 years, and also worked for Roche Products and Glaxo. He is a member of the Industry Board and European Steering Committee of the GAMP Forum where he is the Chairman of the Process Control and the Calibration Special Interest Groups. The latter has developed an Industry Good Practice Guide for the management of calibration (issued by ISPE in February 2002). Foss has had articles on calibration published by ISPE and The Institute of Measurement and Control. He has also been a speaker on this topic at many ISPE and other industry conferences, seminars, and symposia.

Ben Gilkes is Head of Systems Validation with Exel Logistics with responsibility for their European Healthcare operations. Gilkes holds a Business degree from Nottingham University and has worked for Exel in the Logistics industry for 5 years, undertaking a variety of IT roles including site and project management.

Stewart Green is Director of Quality, Wyeth U.K. He has occupied senior positions in the pharmaceutical industry in a career spanning 30 years including production, validation, and QC. A microbiologist by training, he has maintained an abiding interest insterile area operations. He is author of two Executive Briefings for Sue Horwood Publishing Limited, on rapid microbiological methods and technology transfer.

David Hogg is a Systems Quality Group Manager with AstraZeneca. After receiving his MEng in Electrical and Electronic Engineering from Queen's University, Belfast, he joined ICI U.K. and has worked in project engineering, process control systems and systems validation over a period of 16 years. He has been an active member of the GAMP 4 Special Interest Group on Process Control. His co-author, **Fernando Pedeconi**, recently departed KMI Parexel to join CsOls plc, Runcorn, Cheshire, U.K., where he is deploying LIMS for Bristol-Myers Squibb in two countries across three manufacturing sites.

Paul Irving is Principal Consultant, PL Consultancy. He has been an active member of the U.S.-based GAMP Americas Manufacturing Executions Systems Special Interest Group (SiG) for the last 2 years. As a European representative, he has been a key contributor in the development of the GAMP MES Guidance Document. Irving has been involved in Compliance and Validation for over 10 years and has been involved in many European projects.

Orlando Lopez is Director of Information Management Compliance, with Cordis, a U.S.-based Johnson & Johnson Company. Formerly Executive Consultant to J&J Networking and Computer Services, and Senior Computer Systems Validation Consultant for McNeil Consumer Products, he has many years experience in validation, good manufacturing, and good automated manufacturing practice, with special interests in raw data, electronic records and systems, and SCADA systems. He has written many papers in his field of expertise, more than eight executive briefings for Sue Horwood Publishing, and *21 CFR Part 11 Complete Guide to International Compliance* (Interpharm/CRC/Sue Horwood Publishing, 2004).

Julian Peters is a Principal Consultant with the company's Business Consulting Division, responsible for the SAP practice, with chief responsibility for implementing ERP systems in regulated environments. With more than 10 years' ERP implementation experience, Peters has worked all over Europe and the U.S. validating and implementing ERP systems for some of the world's largest pharmaceutical companies. He specializes in 21 CFR Part 11 compliance, including implementing Electronic Records and Electronic Signatures.

Chris Randell is a Biological Group Leader at Wyeth Pharmaceuticals in the U.K. His career spans more than 15 years in the pharmaceutical industry, both as a bench microbiologist and manager. He has developed a keen interest in the application of rapid microbiological methods and has been active in promoting their use both in the U.K. and in Europe.

Dr. Siegfried Schmitt is a Member of the Royal Society of Chemistry, Chartered Chemist and Chartered Scientist. He started his career with F. Hoffmann-La Roche in Basel, Switzerland, where he worked as Senior Production Chemist in Active Pharmaceutical Ingredients and Vitamin production. Following a move to the U.K., he worked for several years as consultant and validation manager for Raytheon E&C on multiple projects for many blue-chip clients. This was followed by 2 years with ABB Eutech as Senior Lead Consultant, working mainly in Europe and the U.S.

In 2002 Dr. Schmitt joined Amersham Health as global Quality Assurance Director in Information Management, with responsibility for the IM Quality Management System and all IM Security. Amersham Health is now part of General Electric Healthcare, headquartered at Little Chalfont, U.K. Dr. Schmitt regularly publishes articles on a variety of topics, has written two books, is a member of several special interest groups and a member of the PDA publishing group advisory board. He is the editor of *21 CFR Part 11 Compliance in Practice* (Sue Horwood Publishing, 2003), which is an overview of first hand experience from industry professionals.

Steve Sharp is the Life Science Business Manager with Mi Services Group and has worked as a consultant delivering business solutions to regulated sectors for more than 10 years, working with Europe, North America and Malaysia. Sharp is responsible for definition of life science consulting services, delivery governance associated with all computer system validation programs and projects and specializes in validation of ERP business solutions. His previous industry employment includes SmithKline Beecham and Cyanamid, where he held positions within manufacturing management and logistics disciplines.

Dr. James Stafford is senior consultant at Mi Services Group Ltd., specializing in the specification, implementation and validation of LIMS, ERP, and Clinical Data Management systems subject to GxP regulations. These specialties are supported with expertise in auditing IT quality systems subject to GxP and ISO 9001 regulations and standards as a trained TickIT auditor. Prior to joining Mi Services, Dr. Stafford spent 6 years as pharmaceutical consultant to a major LIMS vendor with responsibilities for pharmaceutical domain and GxP knowledge transfer, specification and evaluation of pharmaceutical applications. Dr. Stafford spent his formative years at the bench applying new analytical chemistry techniques to investigate a range of problems in the fields of veterinary, clinical, pharmaceutical and bio-pharmaceutical sciences. Subsequently Dr. Stafford developed a specific interest in the use of computer systems for the capture, analysis and reporting of scientific data. Prior to leaving pharmaceutical R&D, Dr. Stafford was Head of Pharmacokinetics at Technologie Servier (France). He has also published and spoken widely on subjects as diverse as validation, Quality Systems, LIMS, veterinary biochemistry, analytical chemistry, pharmacokinetics, and robotics. He was editor of a book on *Advanced LIMS Technology: Case Studies and Business Opportunities* (1995).

David Stokes, who has contributed two chapters on the increasingly important topic of systems testing, is a Principal Validation Consultant and Industry Manager (Life Sciences) with Mi Services Group. He is an active member of the GAMP Forum, leading the GAMP Shared Interest Group on "Testing GxP Critical Systems." Having worked in the IT sector of the life science industries for many years, he is highly respected for his range of knowledge. He is the author of *Testing Computer Systems for FDA/MHRA Compliance* (Interpharm/CRC/Sue Horwood Publishing, 2004).

Carl Turner, Director and Principal Consultant, PL Consultancy, has been an active member of U.S.-based group Global Information Systems SiG since the start of GAMP Americas some 3 years ago. As a European representative, he has been a key contributor in the development of a global regulatory matrix and has presented on the subject matter many times. He has also been instrumental in developing a database tool that addresses global regulations.

Dr. Guy Wingate is an internationally recognized expert in the world of pharmaceutical systems validation. He speaks regularly at conferences and has published several books in computer systems validation with Interpharm/CRC and Sue Horwood Publishing Limited. Dr. Wingate is currently Director of Global Computer Validation at GlaxoSmithKline, responsible for standards, implementation, and inspection readiness of process control, laboratory, IT systems, and IT infrastructure across the company's worldwide pharmaceutical and consumer healthcare manufacturing operations. He has a B.Sc. in computing, an M.Sc. in advanced microelectronics, and a Ph.D. in engineering science (Durham University, U.K.). He has been associated with GAMP (good automated manufacturing practice) Forum for over 10 years, including key contributions to various GAMP publications (*GAMP4*, *Electronic Records and Signatures*, *Good Practice Guidelines*, etc.).

Dr. Wingate currently chairs the GAMP Forum governing council, which oversees the regional steering committees of GAMP Americas, GAMP Europe, and

GAMP Japan. He helps train various international regulatory authorities in computer systems validation, and lectures on the MSc Pharmaceutical Engineering Advanced Training (PEAT) course at Manchester University, U.K

Michael L. Wyrick, Senior Director of GMP Consulting and System Integration with Washington Group International, U.S. and has 30 years of pharmaceutical industry experience at Eli Lilly and Company in a variety of information technology and quality assurance leadership roles. He also has 3 years experience leading a Consulting Services Business Unit in the Life Science industry for KMI and is a globally recognized subject matter expert in the fields of computer validation, IT Infrastructure qualification, 21 CFR Part 11 compliance, quality management systems, internal auditing, and supplier management. He has been elected to three terms as chair of the PhRMA Computer System Validation Committee and has served as the founding chairman of the PDA Computer Validation Issues Task Group. He is an active member of Good Automated Manufacturing Practices (GAMP), International Society of Pharmaceutical Engineers, Institute of Validation Technology, and PDA. He is a PDA-certified Technical Report 32 Auditor. He serves on the GAMP Americas Industry Board, Pharmaceutical Technology Editorial Advisory Board, and the Sue Horwood Publications Editorial Advisory Board. Wyrick has been involved as an author, speaker, and instructor for more than 14 years and has written many articles for industry journals.

Foreword

Guy Wingate, Ph.D.

Validation has a key role to play in providing a high degree of assurance that computer systems supporting drug manufacture are fit for purpose. [1, 2] Those involved in computer validation tend to fall into one of two camps. One group believes in the inherent value of validation as a cost-effective means of quality assurance. The other group sees validation as an ineffective bureaucratic process whose only value is demonstrating regulatory compliance.

These two mind-sets can have a big impact on the practical implementation of computer validation. Those with a more positive attitude tend to be more pragmatic, looking at validation as flexible tool that can be tailored to address the individual needs of different computer systems. This group accepts and is willing to make judgment calls on how much validation is enough in different situations. Those with a more negative attitude tend to think of validation like an insurance policy against regulatory censure. They want validation to be an entirely standard process that can be applied without any ambiguity. This group often does not understand and does not want to understand validation; rather, it takes a "just tell me what to do and I'll do it" stance.

There are numerous horror stories of regulatory censure for lack of or insufficient validation. Consent decrees can cost pharmaceutical companies many hundreds millions dollars. Although computer validation has not yet triggered a consent decree, it has been a contributory factor. [3] And, of course, there are also horror stories concerning the cost of validation when implemented inappropriately. Not too surprisingly, the two are often connected as a drive to validate too quickly to remediate an adverse regulatory finding. Equally, short-cutting validation to reduce cost is likely to lead to an adverse regulatory finding. Such deficiencies may not be immediately found during initial regulatory inspections because of limited time to review systems. Indeed, it is not always the original validation that can cause problems; poor maintenance of the validated state currently accounts for about one third of adverse regulatory computer validation findings. [3] A sense of balance on how much validation is enough must prevail. While it is undeniable that potentially regulatory authorities have extensive powers to financially penalize companies that have critical validation failings, these powers are only executed in extreme circumstances. The expectations of regulatory authorities are founded on common sense and experience. Pharmaceutical companies need to recognize this. Regulatory censure tends to only occur when pharmaceutical companies are seen to take an unreasonable approach to published regulatory requirements.

Validation practices are becoming more effective and efficient as the discipline of computer validation matures. Validation costs exceeding 40% or more of project costs should be a distant memory. A survey of published best practices suggests that validation should now account for 10% or less of project budgets. [3] A key development in this maturing process is a much better understanding of the criticality and impact of data and systems supporting business processes and the application of risk management to focus validation activities.

The U.S. FDA has been particularly prominent in promoting a risk-based approach [4] although other regulatory authorities have allowed this approach for many years. [5] The ISPE GAMP Forum has published specific guidance on risk management within the context of computer validation [6] and is shortly to publish new guidance on applying a risk-based approach to electronic records and signatures. [7] The International Conference for Harmonisation (ICH) is further embedding a common approach to risk management between U.S., European, and Japanese regulatory authorities within the ICH Q9 initiative.

This book imparts some of the latest thinking on computer validation. GCP, GLP, and GMP regulatory requirements are explained with guidance from seasoned practitioners on how to fulfill them. GAMP guidance plays a central role. This book will be an key resource to IT staff, QA professionals, validation staff, control system engineers, suppliers, and consultants wanting to improve their validation capability. Invaluable suggestions are made throughout dealing with life cycle management, electronic records and signatures, risk management, and regulatory inspections. But, of course, it is not just about doing the right thing, but doing the right thing well, and several chapters deal with specific system examples.

REFERENCES

1. *Guide to Inspection of Computerised Systems in Drug Processing, Technical Report, Reference Materials and Training Aids for Investigators*, Rockville, MD: Food and Drug Administration, 1983.
2. Pharmaceutical Inspection Co-operation Scheme. *Good Practices for Computerised Systems in Regulated GxP Environments*, Pharmaceutical Inspection Convention, PI 011–1, Geneva, 2003.
3. Wingate, G.A.S. *Computer Systems Validation: Quality Assurance, Risk Management, and Regulatory Compliance for Pharmaceutical and Healthcare Companies*, CRC/Interpharm Press, 2003.
4. FDA. Pharmaceutical cGMP for the 21st Century: A Risk Based Approach, *FDA News*, August 21 2002, www.fda.gov.

5. ISPE GAMP Forum. Risk Assessment for Use of Automated Systems Supporting Manufacturing Processes: Part 1 — Functional Risk. *Pharmaceutical Engineering*, May/June Edition, pp 16–26, 2003.
7. ISPE GAMP Forum. *GAMP Guide for Validation of Automated Systems*, Fourth edition (known as GAMP 4), www.ispe.org, 2001.
8. ISPE GAMP Forum. *A Risk Management Approach to Compliant Electronic Records and Signatures*, www.ispe.org, 2004.

Editor's Introduction

John Andrews

Computer validation has come a long way since the early nineties. In those days the concept of a life cycle approach to manage the validation of a computer system was almost unheard of. The early practitioners of validation often had a major battle on their hands convincing project managers that the validation group should be involved from the beginning of a project and not as a bolt on activity at the project end. However, today, after years of regulatory interest in the subject and with the proliferation of related guidance on the subject, such as the Good Automated Manufacturing Practice (GAMP) guides, numerous expert papers, workshops/training events and books on the subject it is difficult to find someone who now questions these principles. It was with this in mind that I believe we must now move from principles to the application on how to complete computer system validation in a more focused, pragmatic, and cost effective manner.

Validation of Pharmaceutical Systems discusses practical advice on the validation of a range of different computer systems along with explaining what is expected from a regulatory perspective. Within the book there is a chapter from a former FDA national expert on computer validation, Sam Clark, where he explains what is expected from the regulator's perspective. Also discussed within this book is how to organize, plan, design, and test computerized systems in a way that ensures the whole exercise adds value to a project and delivers compliant systems along the way.

This book also includes a number of case studies in the Case Studies section to aid understanding of the principles discussed in the first chapters. These case studies have been carefully chosen because they reflect real life systems. These examples look at such diverse subjects such as System Control and Data Acquisition Systems (SCADA), systems used in distribution of pharmaceutical products, and the application of the GAMP 4 principles to Good Laboratory Practices (GLP) to name but a few.

I am indebted to all those who have given their personal time to capture their thoughts and experiences, without which this book would never have been produced. I would also like to thank Guy Wingate, Director of Global Computer Validation (GSK), who is a renowned industry expert and chairman of the GAMP Forum, for his Foreword. I hope you will find this valuable in applying GAMP principles in a pragmatic way ensuring that your systems meet both the high standards expected by the regulators, while at the same time meeting the business needs of your companies.

Chapter 1

Considerations for Computerized System Validation in the 21st Century Life Sciences Sector

Tony de Claire, Peter Coady, and Nichola Stevens

CONTENTS

INTRODUCTION

"What men really want is not knowledge but certainty."

— Bertrand Russell

As the U.S. Food and Drug Administration (FDA) embarks on its systems inspection and risk-based compliance approach for manufacturing systems, as we see worldwide recognition of GAMP guidance, and as new European inspection focus is identified in the new PIC/S Guide, this chapter focuses on some key considerations and issues that still surface to cause problems.

The prime objective of applying GxP regulations is to minimize the risk and potential danger of producing adulterous or ineffective life sciences products and releasing those products to the market. The GxP concept was instigated by the World Health Organization (WHO) in 1967. The FDA released the final good laboratory practice (GLP) rule in June 1979 with the current version of good manufacturing practice (GMP) dating back to 1992. Both the WHO GMP and GLP concepts require validation of critical processes and systems, and define validation as the documented act of proving that any procedure, process, equipment, material, activity, or system actually leads to the expected results. The major life sciences sector development, manufacturing, and user countries have defined their own sets of requirements, e.g., the U.S., European Community (EU), Australia, Japan, Switzerland, and Canada.

The regulations are the legal requirements of the country in which a life sciences sector product will be (or is already) marketed. Generally, by the nature of governmental due process in establishing each new law, regulations do not change significantly over time. Hence, the wording and terminology of earlier regulations are not always easy to follow when applying more recent technology. Where appropriate, the life sciences company must therefore consider and adopt current good practice as well as the more traditional interpretation of the regulations. To emphasize this responsibility and to indicate that good practice is continuously evolving, the U.S. FDA promotes the term current good manufacturing, laboratory, clinical practice (cGxP), which recognizes the availability and application of new process and technology developments.

Significant improvements were made in the validation of computerized systems in the latter part of the 20th century. The FDA Blue Book (1983) kick started the process by interpreting the GMP predicate rules for computerized systems and this, supported by industry sector guidance documents such as the STARTS (Software Tools for Application to Large Real-Time Systems) Guide from the National Computing Centre (1987) and the introduction of the TickIT scheme (1991), which provides a software interpretation of the international quality standards (latterly ISO 9000:2000), led to the publication of the GAMP Guide and its predecessors. Individual and collaborative efforts by the life sciences sector and its specialist consultants, the regulatory authorities, and system suppliers have, over the years, produced guidance on the activities and documentation that are needed to ensure successful validation. Table 1.1 compares the phases of the validation life cycle as defined by the PDA Technical Report 18 and the GAMP Guide. It is noticeable that the industry focus on guidance and methodologies devised to achieve validation of computerized systems has assisted validation programs in other areas of GxP compliance.

Table 1.1 Validation Life Cycle Phases [7, 14]

	PDA #18		GAMP	
1	Plan	1	Specification	Plan validation, define requirements and supplier audits
2	Define requirements			
3	Select supplier			
4	Design	2	Design	Prepare design specifications
5	Construct	3	Construction	Manufacture hardware and software modules
6	Integrate and install	4	Testing	Hardware testing, software module and integration testing
7	Qualify (installation, operational)	5	Installation	Installation qualification
8	Evaluate (performance qualification, operation, and maintenance)	6	Acceptance testing	Operational, performance qualification
		7	Operation	Operation, maintenance, change control

In the years following the publication of the FDA Blue Book the regulatory authorities issued some additions and changes in the regulations and guidance relating to GMP, most notably in the field of medical devices. Apart from upholding the concept of life cycle validation most of these did not have a significant effect on the general approach adopted by the life sciences sector for ensuring the compliance of computerized systems. However, all of this was to change with the publication of 21 CFR Part 11 in August 1997. The document introduced a step change in the level of compliance expected by the U.S. FDA, and this has carried forward into the current century.

As we enter the 21st century, the regulatory authorities have continued to introduce major changes. Good Manufacturing Practice Guidance for Active Pharmaceutical Ingredients (Q7A) was issued in August 2001. The FDA has now moved to a "systems inspection method" and adopted a new "risk-based" initiative (August 21 2002) for regulatory inspections. This has resulted in the life sciences sector having to reassess its approach for many of the regulatory processes, including those involving computerized systems. A risk-based approach is also promoted by the ISPE Baseline Guide, Commissioning and Qualification (March 2001) [12].

The risk-based approach has also impacted 21 CFR Part 11 with the publication by the FDA in August 2003 of a new guidance for industry entitled "Part 11, Electronic Records; Electronic Signatures – Scope and Application" [17]. This document represents the current thinking of the FDA regarding the scope and application of 21 CFR Part 11 and it announces the withdrawal of all previous draft 21 CFR Part 11 guidance documents and also the Compliance Policy Guide on enforcement (CPG 7153.17). Alongside all these regulatory changes there have also been changes in the quality sector. The quality management standards have undergone a facelift with the publication of the ISO9000:2000 series of standards in December 2000 which introduced a customer-focused process approach to quality, based upon the business objectives of the company. This has led to the publication of a new TickIT guide (now at Issue 5) and revision of the IEC/ISO9000-3:1997 guideline (to be renumbered as IEC/ISO 90003) which was published at the end of 2004.

Increased application of computer technology throughout the life sciences sector means increased attention from regulatory authorities. For the life sciences company it requires an understanding and interpretation of the regulations with regard to computer system implementation and operation, and also of the methods by which this can be best achieved.

Within the life sciences sector validation is frequently viewed as an extension of quality management systems based on the ISO series of quality standards and guidance documents. Even though the terminology used and the practices implemented can vary, many parallels can be identified, all with the shared aim of building quality into products and services in an effective and efficient manner. The pharmaceutical, biopharmaceutical, medical device, and *in vitro* diagnostic industries are required to take the quality goals a step further and achieve validation of all quality-related critical components.

At the time that this chapter was written it is expected that the FDA will revise 21 CFR Part 11 and that further guidance documents will be written to support it. Other regulatory activities expected are the revision of the FDA GMP regulations 21 CFR Parts 210 and 211, revision of the EU GMP (Orange Book) annex on computerized systems (Annex 11), and revision of the E.U. GMP section on GMP documentation (section 4 and specifically section 4.9 on electronic documentation), to name but a few.

As recently as September 2003, and by agreement to harmonize the rules of GMP applied under the pharmaceutical inspection convention (PIC) and the pharmaceutical inspection cooperation scheme (PIC/S) to those of the EU, the PIC/S *Guide to Good Manufacturing Practice for Medicinal Products* was issued. In the long term, the initiative to harmonize the various regulations in each country should introduce a consistent approach to computerized systems compliance. This, supported by future revisions of — or new guidance on — calibration, process control systems, legacy systems, IT infrastructure platform, manufacturing execution systems, building management systems, software testing, and document archiving, all as supplementary guidance to the GAMP Guide, ISPE Good Practice Guidelines and related documents from the PDA, should finally bring real and lasting benefits to the industry.

The outlook in the software sector is not so encouraging. Despite improvements in the development processes and the available regulations, guidance and certification processes, the sector still appears to be resistant to change and the adoption (seen in some areas as an imposition) of regulations and standards. There is still the feeling that the development of software should be unrestrained and that it should be allowed to evolve at the whim of the developer. It has been reported in recent software sector scheme meetings that some in academia consider that students who have been taught by them do not need to be "certified" by joining a professional body such as the British Computer Society (BCS). Hopefully this situation will improve with time, and with the imposition of more stringent regulations on the life sciences sector and other industries, pressure should continue to build on the software sector to improve its outlook and view the needs of its "regulated sector" customers as paramount.

This chapter will examine the current practices used to implement compliant computerized systems by means of a typical life cycle approach, the key issues and considerations at each stage, and the possible challenges which changes in the regulations could introduce. Where applicable, inherent problem areas will be highlighted at each stage. An overview of the life cycle processes discussed and their interaction is provided in Figure 1.5.

The computerized systems under consideration cover the broad spectrum of automated systems (including input and output devices, as applicable) utilized in life sciences including manufacturing automation, laboratory, and business information systems. These systems share the component make-up shown in Figure 1.1.

LIFE CYCLE PROCESSES

Validation is the governing process for the complete life cycle of a computerized system and must include the stages of planning, specification, programming, testing, commissioning, operation, monitoring, modification, and retirement [8§2]. Specific information on the validation of computerized systems which supports

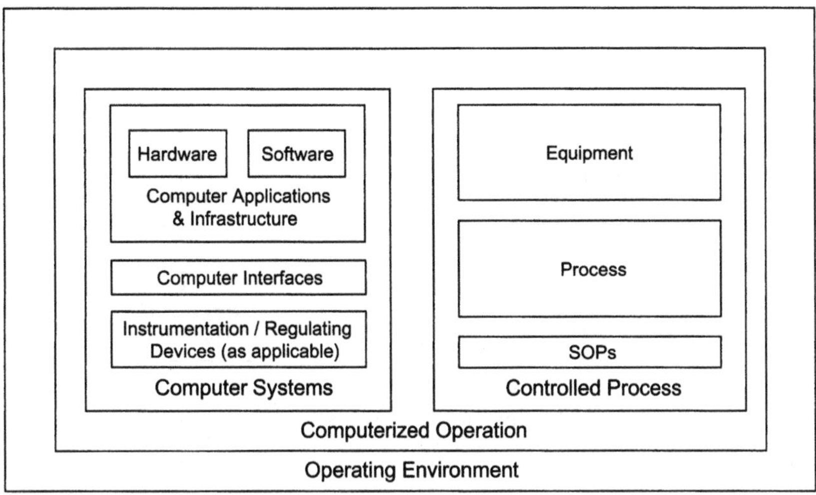

Figure 1.1 Elements of the computerized system [15].

regulatory requirements in the life sciences sector [1–3] can be found in the GAMP Guide [7] and PIC/S Guidance [14].

The implementation of a life cycle approach for computerized system validation is now an established process in life sciences, and is promoted in both the software sector (via the TickIT scheme) and in the life sciences sector guidance (via GAMP).

The V-Model became a recognized life cycle development model when used by the U.K. National Computing Centre and Department of Trade and Industry in the STARTS Guide in 1987. It also became a system and software standard for the German Federal Armed Forces in 1991–1992. It follows then that the model can be adapted and used for the validation of computer systems applied in the regulated life sciences industry [7].

The V-shaped model in Figure 1.2 illustrates in chronological order the life cycle activities for **prospective validation**. The user requirements and design specifications are the source of phase-specific test plans that enable formal qualifications to be conducted and reported. Each task on the life cycle, when successfully executed, results in documented evidence in support of the validation program.

For **IT infrastructure platforms** the focus is on separate risk-based qualification for the "standard" infrastructure hardware and software components, layers, or platforms. For infrastructure component functionality that is used solely when operating in conjunction with a business software application that shares the IT infrastructure, the qualification testing will be part of the OQ and PQ stages of the software application validation. This is depicted in the validation life cycle model in Figure 1.3.

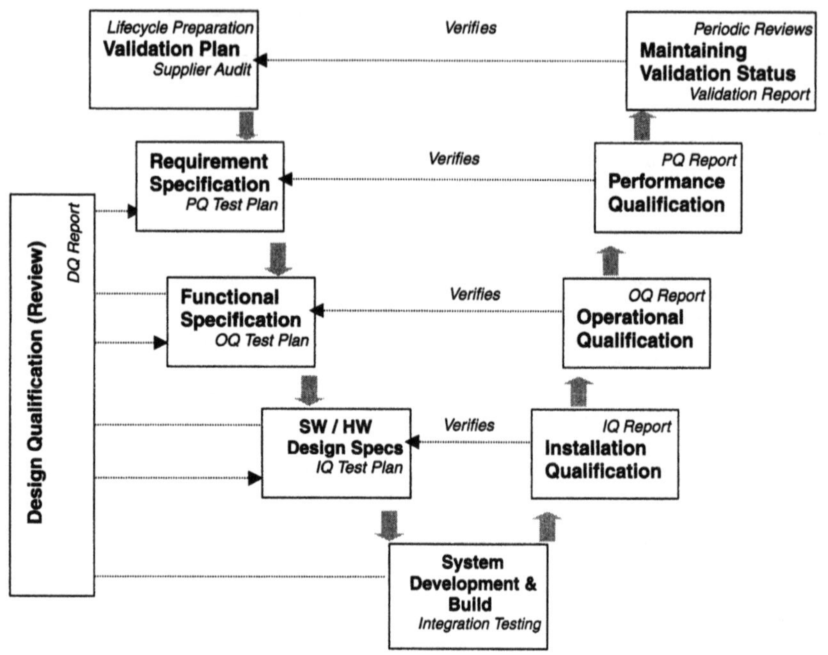

Figure 1.2 Prospective validation life cycle.

With this in mind, and recognizing the size and complexity of some infrastructure platforms, and for operations where GxP (and business) critical data, parameters, and functions are involved, there is a need to examine the type and level of "positive" and "negative" testing. This is necessary to demonstrate critical data integrity, security and availability, and operational reliability and repeatability.

For "retrospective validation" emphasis is put on the assembly of appropriate historical records for system definition, controls, and testing. Systems that are not well documented and do not demonstrate change control or do not have approved test records, cannot be considered as candidates for retrospective validation as defined by the regulatory authorities [14].

Hence, for existing (legacy) systems that are in operational use and do not meet the criteria for retrospective validation, the approach should be to establish documented evidence that the system does what it purports to do. The validation methodology to be followed for existing computer systems will therefore require elements of the prospective validation life cycle to facilitate the process of generating system specifications and qualification test records [14].

Difficulties that can arise include lack of up-to-date (or incomplete) documentation for critical parameter definitions, system specifications, operator

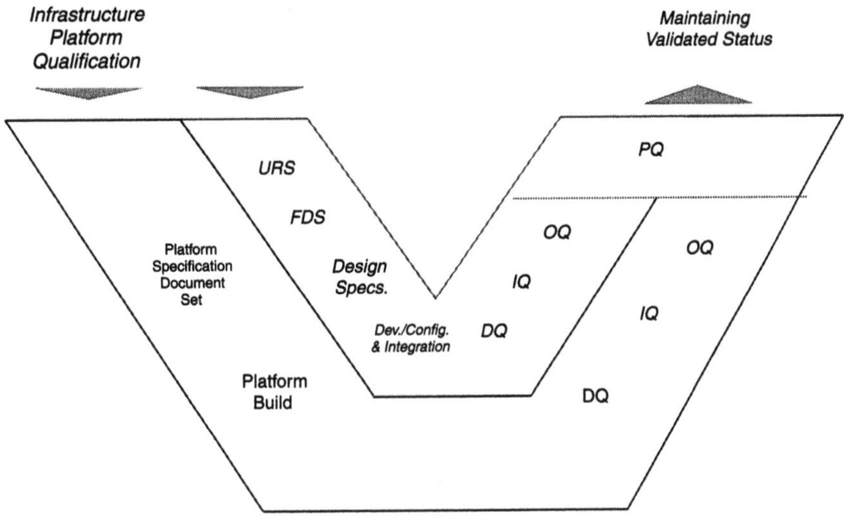

Figure 1.3 IT infrastructure life cycle model.

interfaces, definition of system or data logs, reports and records, and test and calibration records. Add to this the potential of compromise by the availability of a "live" system when qualification testing and the complications increase. In addition, quality and engineering procedures for ensuring controlled application and operation of the system may be nonexistent or may not focus on issues related to computer system or software application.

So, for **legacy systems**, determining the status and control of existing procedures and records will form the basis of the validation rationale, extent of redocumenting, degree of testing, and the validation life cycle entry level (see Figure 1.4). This approach is sometimes referred to as retroactive validation. When supported with an appropriate level of extended system performance monitoring and analysis, it can provide an effective method of accomplishing validation of existing (legacy) systems.

The issues raised are by no means insurmountable. However, with the complexity, duration and cost of validating existing systems, it would also be prudent to study the implications of replacing the computer system and starting afresh.

The validation process is itself a risk-limiting exercise and as such is the prime process for streamlining computer system applications, and controlling the life cycle phases through structured and documented procedures and records.

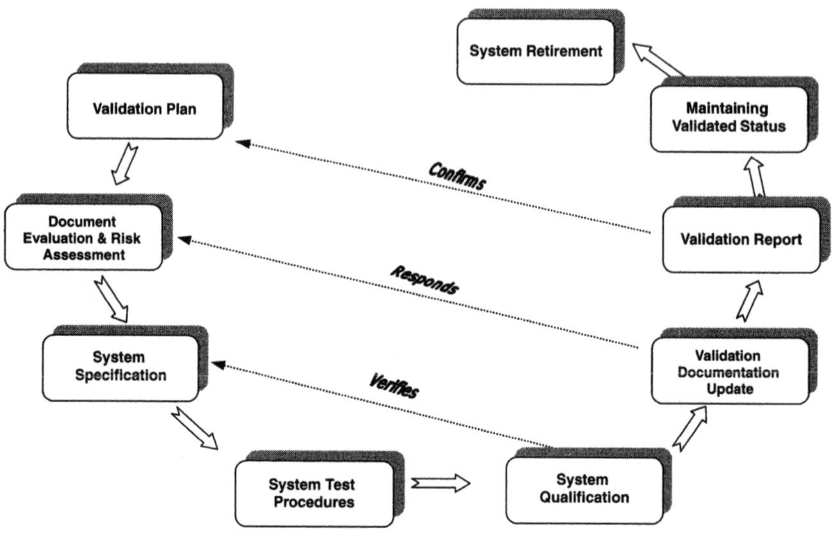

Figure 1.4 Typical legacy system life cycle.

Key Considerations

- Identify who has the necessary expertise and training for each validation activity [14]. Where nobody with the necessary experience is available, alternative arrangements must be employed (e.g., train existing staff, hire new experienced staff, or hire consultants). If these measures are employed there may be time or cost implications for the project which should be taken into account.
- The initial planning activities must be well defined, and for prospective systems, a documented gap-analysis of validation control or support procedures should be undertaken to establish readiness for validation planning. In the case of legacy systems, it is normal to undertake a compliance assessment to determine the validation status of the system. These preparatory examinations will identify any corrective actions that may be required, and allow inclusion of remediation considerations and the resulting validation rationale in the validation plan.
- For legacy systems, it can also be beneficial to compile a "history file," capturing all existing documentation and records as the baseline for adjudging the validation rationale and strategy. Further, changing regulations or their interpretation may have rendered the system's operational and technical control capabilities inappropriate or inadequate. Such issues need to be addressed to decide suitable risk-based remedial actions. Similarly, legacy systems should be examined to verify that data residing within the system are shown to have integrity and that data archived are secure and accessible.

- The life cycle steps align closely with the project stages for new computer system applications where, in general, structured project management methods are employed. These, together with good software engineering practice, can provide the platform for successful validation. With this in mind it is recognized that a large proportion of documentation required for validation can be generated from the controlled implementation of a well-planned project.

Current and Future Challenges

- Revision of SOPs to reflect a risk-based approach.
- Conduct appropriate levels of GxP impact and criticality risk assessment of systems and system functionality early in the planning stage and then throughout the validation life cycle as required.
- Map the stages and terminology of "information systems," e.g,. enterprise resource planning (ERP) and laboratory information management systems (LIMS) with the recognized validation life cycle model.
- Address the IT infrastructure platform with a view to documenting:
  - Hardware and software (operating system, utilities, tools) components.
  - Operating "boundaries" and "interfaces."
  - Business software applications that "share" the infrastructure platform, and the applicable predicate rules.
  - Data flow and ownership (the "responsibles" and "accountables").
  - "Controls" (both technical and procedural).
  - GxP data segregation by way of a dedicated server or partitioning within a server.
  - Risk assessment levels, with focus on data integrity and data security.
  - Qualification rationale or plan.
  - Testing strategy, to minimize qualification testing to components and functions directly impacting quality-related critical data and functions (ref. ISPE Baseline Guide, Commissioning and Qualification [12]).
  - Identify open and closed infrastructure systems.
  - IT groups that control the various elements of the infrastructure.
  - Adopt IT best practice.

COMPUTERIZED SYSTEMS VALIDATION

The determination of the extent of validation necessary for the computerized system must be based on:

- Its use in the GxP environment.
- The potential impact of the system upon product integrity or patient safety.

- The amount of satisfactory testing and documentation performed or supplied by the vendor.
- Whether the validation is performed prospectively (for new systems), or retrospectively for systems currently in use (legacy systems).
- Whether novel elements are incorporated into the system.
- Any other specified factors, as appropriate. [8 §2].

The revised 21 CFR Part 11 guidance [17] has reduced the number of systems that might be bound by the requirement of this regulation. However, even if a system no longer falls within the scope of 21 CFR Part 11, this does not mitigate the need to validate it appropriately in order to fulfill the requirements of the applicable predicate rules, for example, 21 CFR Part 211.68.

Key Considerations

- In addition to the usual objectives of validation the key requirements for data integrity, security, and auditability are paramount.
- To achieve and maintain validated computer systems a life sciences company must demonstrate commitment and should require that quality-related critical parameters, data, and functions must be the focus of each phase of a validation life cycle, including design and development.
- During the procurement of new computer systems, validation requirements and costs (including the cost of allocating or hiring suitable personnel) should be considered as part of the capital approval process.
- The FDA does not formally require a validation master plan (VMP), but inspectors will ask what your approach toward validation is and what steps you have taken to validate a specific system. However, the EU GMP Directive Annex 15 formally requires a VMP.
- The operational life of a system including its decommissioning or retirement must be under a documented and ongoing evaluation. This must include periodic reviews, performance monitoring, change control, configuration management, and any necessary or scheduled revalidation.
- The control and support procedures prerequisite to any validation program include document control, training, configuration management, change control, security access, training, incident management, contingency planning, decommissioning or retirement. These need to be established, (i.e., approved, signed, current, in-place, and in-use) [14].

Current and Future Challenges

- For large or complex systems such as an ERP applications the level and type of testing need to be considered. Generally, basic functional testing will be conducted, but for quality-related critical data and functions the degree of "negative or invalid" challenge testing to be carried out has to be determined. To best attain this, the business (software) modules operating in the GxP environment first need to be identified, along with the instances of electronic records and signatures required by the predicate rules. Thereafter, an assessment to determine the risk of inadvertent or deliberate action that can directly impact critical data [12] will provide direction as to the type of testing that can demonstrate that the system and its data are secure.

Validation SOPs

Computer systems validation must be conducted in accordance with predefined, established procedures that encompass the entire life cycle of the computerized system, from planning through development and implementation, operational use and maintenance support, to decommissioning. Thus, a comprehensive SOP program must be in place in a regulated organization to provide written and approved procedures that ensure that activities are conducted in the same way each time.

Key Considerations

- The early planning and definition of the validation life cycle processes.
- SOPs must contain clear and unambiguous instructions for each stage of the life cycle process.
- Identify who has the necessary expertise, with supporting documentary evidence.
- Restrict the number of persons who can sign SOPs to the absolute minimum. Include QA and a person proficient in the subject area.
- For up-front tasks in the planning phase, procedures will be required for the provision of approved validation guidelines and procedures, risk assessment, documenting the validation rationale and strategy, and for determining the quality-related critical parameters and data for each application.
- Suitable standards must be provided for accepting manufacturer-supplied documentation for specific life cycle stages (i.e., what should be included in the manufacturer's documentation for it to be accepted, what documentation should be produced to demonstrate that it has been accepted, and what to do if it does not fully meet the life science company's standards).
- Define the conditions under which external consultants may be used and the process for appointing them.

Current and Future Challenges

- Revision of SOPs to reflect a risk-based approach.
- Appropriate levels of GxP impact and criticality risk assessment of systems and system functionality early in the planning stage and throughout the validation life cycle as required.
- Produce SOPs and a VMP that define a consistent approach while accepting that "a one size fits all" approach will not work for every system (particularly in the light of the risk-based approach to be adopted).
- Prioritize the validation of systems based upon a documented risk assessment.

System and Application Evaluation

The requirement for validation and need for a formal assessment for electronic records and signatures must be determined through a documented impact and criticality assessment process that evaluates the regulatory context of the business processes and any data supported by the computerized system. All computerized systems used in support of regulatory requirements or regulated processes must be assessed. This assessment may either be a stand-alone document, i.e., a validation determination statement form (providing a high-level GxP criticality assessment) or may form part of a more detailed study conducted under methodologies that address applicable regulations or predicate rules, and GxP criticality.

Key Considerations

- Confirmation of the applicable regulations.
- Identification of the applicable "predicate rules" mandating records and signatures.
- Determination of the applicability of electronic records and electronic signatures produced or managed by the system.
- Determine if the system is widely used within the life science industry or if it is a highly customized or custom-built system.
- Ensure that the system size is adequate to cope with its intended function and number of users, etc., as required by 21CFR Part 211.63.

Current and Future Challenges

- Determine the GxP criticality of the software and hardware functionality.
- Identify the records and signatures mandated by predicate rules (and those determined as business critical).

- Determine the level of testing for quality-related critical system functions.
- Monitor expansion of the system (or system data) into other departments and the GxP implications of this.

System Register

A register (inventory) of computerized systems must be maintained either centrally or within each department as appropriate. The system register must identify whether a system is a GxP system requiring validation, as determined during the system evaluation process, and the current validation program status. Where it has been determined that a GxP system does not require validation, a justification for this decision should be documented or referenced. "If you do not know what you have got, then how can you claim to be in control," certainly applies.

Key Considerations

- Provide a complete and accurate register of computerized systems.
- The register must define GxP and nonGxP systems, with reference to the rationale that determined the categorization.
- The register can be used to trigger a scheduled periodic review of the computerized system.
- It is likely that a regulatory inspector will want to see the register.

Current and Future Challenges

- Ensure that the register is maintained up to date.

Validation Plan

A validation plan (VP) based on current industry practice [7], system criticality and business risk, and regulatory implications, must be produced. This defines the nature and extent of the validation life cycle activities to be performed (what will be done, and what will not be done and the reasons why). Subordinate VPs may be produced for large or complex systems. It is also permissible for the computerized system VP to be incorporated into the overall validation project plan for a manufacturing process or an item of equipment. Information on the content of VPs is provided in the GAMP Guide [7].

Key Considerations

- "Fail to plan, plan to fail."
- The VP is a live document and should be regularly reviewed and maintained.
- A clear, well-documented VP and associated validation report will provide confidence that the other validation life cycle stages have been adhered to, and that lower-level detailed validation documentation is under control.
- VPs should be supported by project and quality plans (combined or separate) to ensure that the system implementation tasks align with and support the validation life cycle activities.

Current and Future Challenges

- The VP can be the first instance where the compliance and validation training, and the system design, operation, maintenance training are formally identified and scheduled for review. This will ensure the computer system is specified, designed, implemented and operated by individuals who are trained (on a continuing basis) to a level commensurate with their work function.
- Identification of the validation activities following a risk-based approach.
- Preparation of an infrastructure qualification plan that takes into account applicable "predicate rules" and addresses the following:
  - Overview of business and compliance needs.
  - Identify control and support procedures to be adopted throughout implementation, operation, and training (both GxP and operational), e.g., change control, configuration management, backup–compare–restore, data migration, data archival or retention, problem management, performance monitoring, internal audits, periodic review, and service level agreements.
  - Identify where supplier specifications and procedures can be adopted.
  - Overview of main platform architecture and components, both hardware and software (operating systems, utilities, drivers, and tools).
  - Intended operating "boundaries" for hardware and software within the infrastructure platform.
  - Current view of all "application software" that uses (shares) the platform, i.e., both GxP and nonGxP, and identify intended use of electronic records and electronic signatures.
  - Overview all known intersystem, software, and hardware interfaces.
  - Overview data flow and ownership (the "responsibles" and "accountables").
  - Identify "controls" (both technical and procedural) for infrastructure platform and application software.
  - Identify risk assessments required and, with focus on "data integrity" and "data security," ensure an appropriate level of risk-based qualification testing.

- Identify validation rationale and life cycle for the platform infrastructure (prospective and existing (legacy) components).
- Outline testing strategy for platform components installation and operational qualification.
- Define platform implementation and qualification testing and verification of the application software implementation and validation program.

• There will be occasions when validation preparatory and support activities will be undertaken before the respective validation plans are finalized. This can be a common occurrence when reviewing existing system validation status. If there are no such activities prior to compiling the validation plan this should be clearly stated as: "No preplan activities have been identified." If preplan activities have been conducted these should be identified in the validation plan as such. Include detail and record references of all validation preparatory, support, or life cycle activities that were undertaken prior to issue of the validation plan. With regard to the impact on the system validation these earlier activities should be evaluated and resolved under the change control or risk assessment procedure. The result of each evaluation should be referenced in the validation plan (typically as an appendix). Examples of such preplan activities include:
- Review and prepare validation policy.
- Supplier or integrator audit rationale.
- Conduct supplier or integrator audits.
- Preordering of "standard" hardware and software system components.
- Gap-analysis of existing validation life cycle and support procedures complete with records and documentation where relevant, including high-level, quality system documentation and record and signature predicate rule requirements.
- Where implementation embraces an upgrade, and thus a significant change to software or hardware, this and the respective change control evaluation and any resulting rationale for a satisfactory level of redefinition, and any associated requalification testing or system revalidation referenced [14].
- Examination of any "interfaced" systems validation status with regard to data integrity, and data control and rationale for any redefinition or re-qualification testing or system revalidation.
- Preparation or review of prerequisite guidelines and procedures required to support and control the validation life cycle activities, e.g., change control, periodic review, performance monitoring, etc.
- Preparation of an overall computer systems registry (GxP, nonGxP, and new systems under way) including the identification of the validation rationale and status of each system.
- Conducting compliance and validation training [14].
- Conducting risk assessment training.

Qualification Protocols

The correct installation (installation qualification (IQ)), operation (operational qualification (OQ)) and performance (performance qualification (PQ)) of the computerized system must be documented using one or more of the protocols indicated. The protocols required (e.g., all three, just IQ and OQ, or a combined IQ and OQ protocol with clear demarcation, interstage signoffs, and justification for any carry-over actions) will depend on the type of computerized system and needs to be defined in the VP.

To provide the recognized level of documented evidence qualification protocols should be prepared in advance of qualification activities and typically describe:

- The objectives of the verifications or tests.
- How the qualification stage fits into the overall validation strategy for the project.
- Who is responsible for conducting the tests and authorized to sign off each level of the test record.
- What specific method is to be used for each test.
- How challenging the specific tests will be.
- Where specific functions are not going to be tested, provide a justification for this.
- How tests are cross-referenced to individual specified requirements.
- How data are to be collected and reported.
- Details of any tests which must be conducted in a specific order or in a specific group of tests.
- Details of any prerequisites that must be in place before testing commences.
- How to address deviations.
- Each test procedure (including acceptance criteria).
- What review and evaluation procedures will be used to determine whether the acceptance criteria are met.
- Qualification reporting.
- Formats for supplementary data sheets (test personnel signature identification list, test result data, additional test data, test incident reports, deviation reports, revision history).

Design Qualification

In addition to the scheduled design reviews carried out by the supplier as part of the system design and development process, the customer must also conduct and document its own design reviews to ensure that the system design meets its technical and quality needs as detailed in the user requirements specification (URS). These customer reviews also ensure that the URS, functional specification, detailed design specifications, drawings, manuals, and schedules have been produced, reviewed, revised, and managed in preparation for system testing.

Customer design reviews are often referred to as design qualifications (DQ) for new systems, and as design compliance reviews for existing systems. The reviews should be formally documented and are key validation deliverables. The term DQ will be used for the remainder of this section, in order to clearly identify the reviews conducted by the customer. The information contained herein will also apply to any design compliance reviews conducted by the customer.

DQ reviews need to consider all life cycle design and development documentation, and should establish that software design, development, and the related testing is conducted to written and approved procedures under the control of a software quality assurance plan. The DQ process should also embrace the technical, quality, and commercial reviews of the enquiry or tender package conducted and documented by the customer. This has the benefit of not only checking that the computer system requirements have been adequately defined and are complete, but also providing formal approval of the enquiry or tender package before it is issued to prospective suppliers.

Consequently, DQ is an ongoing process that comprises a series of reviews starting with the customer tender or enquiry stage and continuing into system design and development. These DQs and their associated reports can be referred to as DQ1, DQ2 ... DQn. An overall DQ summary report may be produced summarizing the DQ process, highlighting key findings and corrective actions, and managing any ongoing nonconformances.

Although DQ reviews are the responsibility of the customer they will normally require the involvement of the supplier during the system design and development phase. The following quality issues should be examined during each DQ review.

- All documentation has adequate revision control and an audit trail referring all the way back to an initiating document or instruction (see section on requirements traceability).
- All documentation has the required signatures.
- The documentation is presented in a form that will enable information to be easily found, and assist in ongoing system maintenance and future changes or modifications.
- The quality processes followed by the supplier are compliant with the supplier's quality management system for system design, testing, and documentation.
- The supplier has complied with any customer quality requirements and SOPs.

The following system design issues should be examined during each DQ review.

- The hardware and software meet the criteria defined in the URS and FS (see section on requirements traceability).
- Where applicable, the clauses in the hardware and software development

specifications have been written in a form which will enable a suitable test to be identified and specified.

- The test clauses in the hardware and software test specifications and system acceptance test specifications are traceable to the appropriate design clauses in the hardware and software development specifications. The individual tests are risk-based and sufficiently detailed, appropriate to the item under test, measurable and recordable, achievable and realistic.
- The hardware and software has been developed according to the predefined procedures or standards.
- Full, accurate, and current documentation of the hardware and software exists and is readily understandable by a suitably qualified person. Diagrams have been used, where applicable, to assist understanding (see section on requirements traceability).
- A risk analysis has been carried out on the computerized system to identify and resolve any potential risks to the public, personnel, plant, and the business (see section on risk assessment).
- All system functions that are directly related to GMP are identified in the documentation, and the implementation requirements for these functions have been examined and reported in the GMP risk assessment (see section on risk assessment).
- An electronic records and electronic signatures assessment has been carried out, where the need has been identified in the VP (see section on electronic records and electronic signatures).
- Adequate safeguards exist to protect software against loss, theft, and malicious intent.
- Adequate safeguards exist to protect hardware and software against loss, theft, and damage from environmental attack.

Installation Qualification

The purpose of the installation qualification (IQ) is to ensure that the computer platform and the application software are correctly installed at their operational site. The IQ typically includes (but is not limited to) the following items.

- Identification of hardware items and their interfaces.
- Verification of installed hardware.
- Verification of installed operating system, utility, driver, antivirus, etc., software.
- Verification of software applications.
- Verification of receipt of all expected vendor-supplied documentation (e.g., user manuals).
- Verification that all location requirements are met (e.g., correct environmental conditions, adequate electrical supply, etc.).

Operational Qualification

The operational qualification (OQ) demonstrates that the installed system works properly in its operational environment under both normal and abnormal operational conditions. The OQ may typically include (but is not limited to) the following.

- Access security tests.
- Input and output tests.
- Load and capacity testing.
- Boundary testing.
- Failure and recovery testing.
- Operator interface and screen display tests.
- Software logic and sequence operation (functional testing).
- Alarm handling and messages.
- Event handling and messages.
- System diagnostics.
- Data loading and reporting.
- Audit trail testing and security verification.
- Network tests.
- Data backup, storage, restoration, and compare verification.

Performance Qualification

The purpose of the performance qualification (PQ) phase is to verify that the complete system behaves as intended according to the user requirements under normal or expected operational conditions. The PQ may include (but is not limited to) the following.

- System access (including specific user permission configuration and testing).
- Expected system capacity tests.
- System diagnostic tests.
- System operational testing (typically three representative runs, batches, operations, etc.).
- Specific calculation verification.

Further information on the content of qualification protocols is provided in the GAMP Guide [7].

Key Considerations

- General recognition of DQ as a key tool for the life sciences company to review the design, development, and associated testing undertaken by the supplier during system build, and with a view to utilizing that work to support qualification testing.
- Where two or more similar qualification protocols are produced for a project it may be beneficial and more efficient to create a high level test strategy document that contains all of the information which is common to all qualification protocols in the validation project. Individual protocols will then only contain that information that is specific to that validation stage.
- The protocols must demonstrate that the computerized system meets the requirements of the user and can cope with the stresses that will be placed upon it (e.g., continues to function reliably when the maximum predicted number of users are connected, collects data at sufficient data transfer rates, etc.) through documentation and testing.
- Where the system will be rolled out to additional departments, ensuring that sufficient testing is performed to demonstrate that it meets the requirements of those departments while not needlessly repeating testing already conducted.
- Ensure that the testing is constructed such that any potential errors that may impact the use of the system are exposed and addressed.
- Ensure that the testing progresses as quickly and economically as possible by designing protocols that test more than one function simultaneously where possible.
- The protocols should be designed such that they can evolve and cope with changes to new versions of the software or changes in the user interface.
- The protocols must provide verifiable evidence that tests were completed and their outcome clearly stated with regard to the predetermined acceptance criteria.
- Each qualification must be formally reported to maintain an auditable system of documentation and to ensure an approved and controlled, fully documented transition to subsequent life cycle phases. The report must clearly reference its controlling protocol and should provide an overview of the results obtained during the testing, together with details of all problems encountered, including how the problems were resolved. If any problems are still outstanding, the report must provide suitable justification for progressing to the next testing stage. Approval of the report signifies the acceptance of the results and authorizes progress to the next stage of the validation project.
- The status of the traceability matrix should be recorded as part of each qualification summary report and documentation kept in a validation file.
- In the case of a computer system applied to a manufacturing process, with direct relationships to plant equipment and the process itself, the VP should specify whether separate or integrated qualification protocols and summary

qualification reports are to be prepared for IQ, OQ, and PQ. A similar situation applies to laboratory systems where the software is directly associated with a specific piece of equipment that must also be validated. The situation is further complicated where several applications are interfaced together and rely upon one another for successful operation.

- Conduct the appropriate level of calibration and provide documented calibration records to support the validation program. A methodical approach for conducting the calibration of control, monitoring and laboratory instrumentation is required. Calibration is to be undertaken with test instruments precalibrated against recognized national or international standards.
- The calibration periodicity should take into account the instrument supplier recommendations and the robustness, sensitivity, and duty of the instrument. Laboratory instrument calibrations may require running system suitability samples during each analysis to check the suitability of the system for use. Once a periodicity is established, the instrument should be added to a calibration program for call-off dates to be determined. Initial calibration periodicity should be reviewed against historical records. The current calibration status of critical instruments should be known and verifiable. It is advisable to schedule any recalibration to take place immediately after any scheduled maintenance of the system.

Current and Future Challenges

- The scope of the protocols should reflect a risk-based approach addressed under formal risk assessments.
- Align with the ISPE Baseline Guide, Commissioning and Qualification [12] and conducting qualification-level testing only where quality-related critical parameters, data, and functions can be "directly impacted."
- Control quality-related critical GxP data throughout supplier design, development, and build.
- Supplier software and hardware records should be available for or referenced by the DQ.
- Validation of self or remote calibration and test software.
- Qualification of network or fieldbus security and diagnostics.
- Performance monitoring during operational use can be viewed as an extension of the PQ process, because for most large systems it is not possible to operate and test or verify under all conditions. Consequently, there is a need to continually monitor the system performance under differing loads, and to review system self diagnostics and any self calibrations.

Validation Report

A validation report must be produced which provides a review of the results of the validation life cycle activities performed and documentation produced, as set out in the respective VPs, and clearly define the overall validation status of the computerized system. The validation report must include information on any deviations from the life cycle processes specified in the VP (e.g., additional activities, activities which could not be done, and the reasons why); information on any actions that remain open, their severity, who has responsibility for closure, and the expected date for closure (a place for the actual date of closure must also be provided). The computerized system validation report can also be incorporated into the overall validation summary report for a manufacturing process or an item of equipment. Information on the content of validation reports is provided in the GAMP Guide [7].

Key Considerations

- A clear, well-documented validation report will support the associated VP and provide a high level of confidence that life cycle activities have been satisfactorily completed. It is recommended that the report references the requirements traceability matrix (discussed later in this chapter) to demonstrate that the system meets all mandatory user, functional, and design requirements.
- The validation report serves as the approval document for all life cycle activities and the mechanism for releasing the computerized system for operational use. Recommendations may be made for any follow-up audit or additional testing.
- The validation report should refer to the subordinate qualification (summary) reports for each qualification stage where this approach is used. Alternatively, the qualification protocols themselves can provide a summary section for sign-off along with any justifications for proceeding to the next qualification stage if outstanding actions exist.
- The validation report may follow the same format as the validation plan to aid cross-reference and review of all the key validation life cycle documents. Any deviations and associated corrective actions should be reviewed, and any concessions on the acceptability of qualification test results examined and explained.
- The validation report should also reference the validation file documentation, control procedures, and support programs that are vital to the ongoing validation program and which will be used as the basis for maintaining the validation status of the computer system.
- The validation report should clearly outline the ongoing activities that are required to maintain and control the validation status achieved, provide the basis for periodic reviews, and enable preparation for internal audits and regulatory inspections.

- A review of respective GxP risk assessments should be undertaken and included as a section in the validation report.
- The validation report should not be approved and issued until all control procedures and support programs are in place.

Current and Future Challenges

- Timely closure of outstanding actions.
- Timely availability of validation life cycle documentation.
- The presentation of validation life cycle documentation to the regulatory authorities when it is stored in a document repository. The document repository may be used to store a far wider range of documents or data than the validation life cycle documents, and restriction of access by the regulatory authorities to some types of documents or data may need to be considered and implemented.

Periodic Review

The ongoing evaluation phase is usually the longest phase of the validation life cycle, covering the operational life of the computerized system. The earlier life cycle phases provided a comprehensive validation documentation set that is the mainstay of ongoing evaluation and the basis for regulatory inspection.

An important objective of ongoing evaluation is to uphold an auditable set of validation documentation and ensure a controlled, fully documented record of any activity that may affect the validation status of the computerized system throughout its operational use.

Periodic reviews are an important element of ongoing evaluation and may be undertaken as a scheduled or event-driven examination, e.g., a major upgrade to hardware or software. The frequency of the scheduled periodic reviews can vary depending on the application but are generally undertaken on an annual basis as a minimum. Detailed document reviews may be required more frequently and these, together with internal audits, will support the periodic review.

A periodic review will encompass the validation life cycle documentation and records, the associated control and support procedures and records, and ensure that these are established, i.e., approved, signed (including signatory function), dated, current, in place, and in use.

Periodic review meetings are held to document the review process, the documents reviewed, comments from attendees, and the collectively agreed course of action. The periodic review summary report records the findings of the review meeting and includes an action schedule, itemizing any documentation that requires updating, and those responsible for completing the work. The progress of updates should be monitored against agreed completion dates.

In the case of GLP, those study directors in charge of projects using the system, together with management, must be notified of any problems found, and the potential impact of those problems. The frequency of reviews must be in accordance with current company policy. Information on the periodic review process is provided in the GAMP Guide [7] and PIC/S Guide [14].

Following a successful periodic review, acceptance of the evaluation should be clearly stated in an approved periodic review report.

Key Considerations

- Obtain the necessary documentation in order to perform the review. This should be kept or referenced by a "validation file" which includes a detailed index to control and locate all validation documentation. Typically the file may be subdivided to align with life cycle stages or validation milestones.
- Training records must verify that persons affected by a control or support procedure have been satisfactorily instructed in its use. [14]
- A risk assessment should form part of each periodic review in order to verify the findings of the previous analysis, and to provide risk information for consideration when assessing the need for revalidation.

Current and Future Challenges

- It is vital that the validation status of the computerized system operation is not compromised.
- Ensure that periodic reviews are carried out according to a defined schedule (and maintaining the schedule up to date) or are event driven by significant changes to the system or its use or events impacting the system data integrity.
- Ensure that signed records of each inspection are maintained, showing the date of that inspection, as required by GLP.
- It is likely that a regulatory inspector will want to see evidence that the reviews are carried out.
- Typically, a periodic review will cover:
  - GxP, validation, operation training records.
  - Validation life cycle documents, records, and reports.
  - Operational or maintenance procedures and records.
  - Control and support procedures.
  - Impact of regulatory inspection findings and changes in the regulations.
  - Qualified resource availability.
  - Risk assessment review.
  - Health, safety, and environmental issues.
  - Periodic review summary reports.

- When reviews detect conditions or practices that deviate from predetermined criteria, then they must be investigated and approved corrective action documented and undertaken. If for whatever reason there is a need to redocument or retest the computerized system, then the level of revalidation needs to be determined, planned, approved, implemented, tested, and reported.

COMPUTERIZED SYSTEMS DEVELOPMENT

User Requirements Specification (URS)

A URS must be produced by, or on behalf of, the customer. The URS provides a clear, unambiguous description of what the system must do. It must be written in sufficient detail to enable prospective suppliers to provide a detailed quotation or tender for the work and its subsequent use for the production of system life cycle documentation. Information on the content of URS is provided in the GAMP Guide [7].

Key Considerations

- The life sciences company must ensure that sufficient and accurate information and quality criteria are available at an early stage.
- The URS is the base document (or in some cases, set of documents) for developing and testing the computer system, and it needs to provide clearly defined requirements that can be verified by means of inspection or testing.
- The required system functions should identify the features that must be satisfied and those that are desirable. Features that are necessary to uphold GxP and to validate a system should always be considered as firm requirements, not desirable features. The desired features should be prioritized as to their relative importance and GxP significance.
- In addition to required functions, the specification should include nonfunctional requirements, data requirements (e.g., access speed, data storage and retrieval), interface requirements, environmental requirements, and system constraints (e.g., compatibility, availability, procedural and maintenance constraints).
- Examine the feasibility of physically or technically segregating GxP data within a system database.
- A matrix can be prepared to identify both user and supplier responsibilities for the provision and management of documentation in the relevant validation project phases.
- The URS structure should be such as to facilitate traceability of each requirement, or group of related requirements, throughout the corresponding sections in the succeeding design specification documentation. In the case of customized and custom-built systems this helps ensure design decisions are auditable back to

source requirements. This will enable easy identification and audit of any design changes and technical compliance issues (along with associated cost issues). Traceability should also be carried forward to the qualification test procedures where it will link each test and the qualification acceptance criteria directly to the respective requirement. This can readily be achieved by employment of a "traceability matrix" that will identify the corresponding elements of the life cycle documents to ensure that all stated requirements are being provided and tested or verified throughout the system life cycle.

- The URS must contain clear, concise and unambiguous statements, and must be written in nontechnical language that can be understood by both the user and the supplier. Each statement should, where possible, only contain one requirement.
- To aid understanding of more complex requirements it may be helpful to include an example. Diagrams, simple flow charts, and more complex sequential flow charts are also beneficial for clarifying requirements and processing functions.
- The URS must be formally reviewed by all interested parties prior to issue for inquiry, and must be reviewed (and revised as required) during the project to reflect the system being purchased.

Current and Future Challenges

- Capture the users' requirements and express them in a suitable form that can be understood by both the users and supplier.
- Details of the quality-related critical data that must be "handled" and controlled by the computerized system is fundamental to upholding GxP compliance. The integrity and security of the quality critical data are the prime objective of computer system validation.
- The URS should identify all inputs and outputs to the computerized system (whether automatic or manual). These should be individually evaluated for their criticality to the operating or business process.
- Ensure that the user requirements properly match current GxP stipulations and current and future business needs.

Supplier Audit

A supplier audit is usually performed by, or on behalf of, the customer on suppliers of GxP critical or business critical computerized systems. The need for performing a supplier audit should be specified in the respective validation plan. Information on conducting a supplier audit and the areas to be covered are provided in the GAMP Guide [7].

A supplier audit can be used to provide objective evidence that a quality management system is in place and is followed. The supplier audit may be used as a preevaluation of a number of potential suppliers.

Depending on the criticality and available information of the vendor there are levels of assessment methods.

- Intelligence-based evaluation (industry track record).
- Mail-based assessment (questionnaire).
- On-site supplier audit.

Key Considerations

- Auditors must be trained and qualified in the audited areas.
- Audits should follow a systematic approach and utilize a checklist to ensure consistent coverage and reporting.
- Ask open questions and follow leads. Do not stick rigidly to the checklist – use it as a guide.
- Ensure that coding standards are used and that design and, where applicable, source code reviews are formally recorded.
- Be alert to the different issues impacting supplier capability and product suitability.
- A postal audit should focus on the system supplier's experience in providing a system that can be validated.

Current and Future Challenges

- Obtaining objective evidence to support any findings.
- Maintain awareness of changes in software development practices and languages.
- Be aware of other methods and considerations, e.g., recognize the role of the TickIT and forthcoming IEC/ISO 90003 guidance for auditing software quality systems to ISO9001:2000.
- Suppliers and contractors to the regulated life sciences sector must recognize the need for the life sciences company to successfully validate computerized systems used in the GxP environment.
- The life sciences company in-house technical support groups must also recognize the need to address and adopt recognized GxP compliance and support methodologies.

Supplier Quality Management System

All reasonable steps must be taken to ensure that the computerized system software will be produced in accordance with a quality management system [8 §5, 14].

Preference should be given to quality management systems which have been formally certified to an international quality standard [22] and any associated guidelines [24, 26], but objective evidence that an alternative quality management system (e.g., GAMP [7]) is implemented and in place is acceptable. Information on the structure and content of quality management systems is provided in the GAMP Guide [7] and international standards and guidelines [21, 22, 24, 26].

Key Considerations

- The implementation of a quality management system which provides the basis for business improvements.
- Certification of the quality management system to a recognized quality standard or the implementation of an alternative quality management system which is compliant with an industry-recognized guideline.
- The supplier's project and quality plan needs to define the quality management system used (including any deviations) and, in particular, the software quality assurance objectives that the supplier will use to support the life sciences company's GxP compliance and validation program.
- For customized and custom-built systems the supplier should apply a structured process to control the progress of the project from the initial requirement input to the delivery of a correctly functioning computer system.
- For established systems, the supplier should maintain a customer request or suggestion database (including documented evaluation of the requests or suggestions) that can be used to control the progress to delivery of a correctly functioning software upgrade. This should be based around an acceptable system development life cycle, and defined in terms of phases. Each individual phase may comprise a number of related tasks (e.g., a testing phase may include module testing and integration or package testing).
- Any special techniques or methodologies that have a bearing on software or hardware quality should be identified and their implementation documented. References should be made to appropriate standards or manuals.
- Software tools used for the production of project documentation, software development, or for project planning should be listed for agreement with the life sciences manufacturer.
- For customized and custom-built systems the project program should list all of the detailed tasks to be performed by the supplier on the project. For clarity, tasks that are not the direct responsibility of the supplier may be included on the task schedule if they are necessary to show critical dependencies and must be clearly identified as such. A method for monitoring progress (e.g., project review meetings) should be defined along with one for documenting progress and the decisions made regarding corrective actions. Strategies for resolving problems and project "holds" should be considered. All internal audits by the

supplier and any external audits required by the life sciences company should be scheduled to coincide with the phase activities, and their scope defined.
- Inclusion of a design and development activity schedule, complete with resource allocations, will document the structured approach to be used and will allow progress of key activities to be monitored. The schedule will also assist in identifying problem areas and identify tasks that require input from the life sciences company. Typically, the schedule will identify for each activity the procedures to be used and the acceptance criteria. Provision can be made for supplier and customer signatures against each activity to provide a record, and thus control, of the development phase of the validation life cycle in support of design qualification.

Current and Future Challenges

- Ensure that claims by suppliers that they use GAMP as their quality management system are verified.
- Ensure that supplier audits are conducted and evaluated prior to the purchase of the computerized system.
- Ensure that documented design and code reviews are conducted by the supplier during system design and development.

Requirements Traceability

A requirements traceability matrix (RTM) or similar mechanism should be developed, and maintained up to date. In the case of customized and custom-built systems it will normally be the responsibility of the supplier in conjunction with the user, to verify that each requirement of the URS has been covered by the supplier's life cycle design, production, development testing, and qualification and acceptance testing processes. For established, commercially available systems the user will maintain the RTM to demonstrate that the system meets each of the mandatory requirements set out in the URS. The RTM may be included within the appropriate life cycle documents. Information on the production of an RTM is provided in the GAMP Guide [7].

Key Considerations

- The RTM can either be a stand-alone document or can be broken up and included in each individual design and test document.
- If the RTM is a stand-alone document, then it should provide traceability from individual clauses in the URS to corresponding clauses in the subsequent design and associated test documentation.

- If the RTM is divided up and included in each individual design and test document, then it should provide clause level traceability from each document to the preceding document used to generate it. This will enable design reviews to take place.
- The RTM is a key support document for reference and consideration in the validation report.
- A number of software solutions are available for maintaining traceability information and may be particularly useful for larger, more complex systems, where a large number of requirements must be maintained.

Current and Future Challenges

- Extend the RTM to encompass the qualification protocol testing activities.
- Provide adequate coverage through all of the life cycle phases.
- Manage updates to the RTM when document changes occur.

System Development Lifecycle

The supplier must follow a documented system development life cycle methodology for the design, production, testing, release, and documentation of the computerized system. The life cycle processes must be supported by quality framework processes that encompass:

- Documented reviews for key activities.
  - User and regulatory requirements.
  - Development and production activities.
  - Clause traceability between life cycle documents.
  - Source code.
  - Testing.
  - Documentation.
- Change and configuration management.
- Coding and production standards and practices.
- Document control.
- System support, maintenance, and help desk facilities (as appropriate).
- Backup, archiving, and disaster recovery.
- System security.

Information on the system development life cycle and support processes is provided in the GAMP Guide [7] and International Standards and Guidelines [24–26].

Key Considerations

- Ensure that the user requirements are adequately broken down in a systematic and documented way to the level where coding can take place, and that the design can be verified though adequate testing at each level.
- Implement formal, documented design and code and configuration reviews.
- Adhere to life cycle and coding standards.
- Manage documentation and code under formal change control and configuration management processes.

Current and Future Challenges

- Ensure that the supplier maintains awareness of, and produces systems that comply with regulatory requirements.
- The influence of a risk-based approach on system design.

System Description

A description of the computerized system must be produced (including diagrams as appropriate) and maintained up to date. The description must include the principles, objectives, security measures and scope of the computerized system, and the main features which govern the way in which it will be used and how it interacts with other computerized systems, equipment and procedures [12 §4]. The system description may be provided in a dedicated document or incorporated into an appropriate system life cycle document (e.g., the functional specification) as indicated by the GAMP Guide [7]. The system description can also be incorporated into the VP for the computerized system to provide an overview of the system and its capabilities.

Key Considerations

- The diagram or description should convey sufficient information to enable the principles of operation of the system, the data transfer and storage attributes of the system and any interfaces to be understood. For example, data buffers used for the temporary storage of data obtained from laboratory instrumentation where the server has become unavailable after a run has commenced.
- The hardware and operating system upon which the application is installed should be described. Where the application will be installed on more than one operating platform (e.g., in a client server situation), consideration should be given to the effects those platforms may have on each other, and testing planned accordingly, to ensure that each platform is sufficiently validated.

Current and Future Challenges

- Maintain the system description up to date for complex and evolving systems.
- For information systems in particular, address the general reluctance to produce data flows, network infrastructure diagrams, and reference installation specifications, even though this information is invariably available.

Development Methodologies

Although the responsibility for validation remains with the life sciences company, the supplier can play a key role in life cycle activities, and should contribute a full set of auditable design and development documentation to support the validation. The entire system development process should be carried out to written and approved procedures and all development, testing, and verification activities documented, reviewed, and approved. The life sciences user cannot afford this key and usually intense phase to become invisible.

For large or complex systems, the functional design specification on its own may not enable the prospective user to fully understand how the system will be applied and used. One method of overcoming this problem is to develop a system prototype.

Techniques such as prototyping and rapid application development (RAD) are acceptable for use when developing computerized systems providing that the use of these techniques is planned, controlled, and documented. These techniques must not be used as a means of circumventing life cycle controls and documentation, and must be implemented in line with logical life cycle stages [14]. Information on system development methodologies is provided in the GAMP Guide [7].

Prototyping can provide the following benefits:

- Misunderstandings, missing functions, and inconsistencies may be detected earlier.
- A limited working system may be used to demonstrate feasibility to other parties.
- Users can gain early exposure to the operating principles of the system.

The purpose of a software prototyping exercise is to examine and present the feasibility of the software proposed for a specific requirement.

Examples of the use of system prototyping include:

- Checking the ergonomics and acceptability of a user interface.
- Checking the overall characteristics of a critical algorithm.
- Checking the outline performance and size of an overall system.

The examination should be treated as a "sample demonstration" in support of the functional design and considered under the ongoing GxP risk assessment. However, the prototype should not be retained. The ideas demonstrated should be incorporated into the life cycle design of the system.

Key Considerations

- Although the responsibility for validation remains with the life sciences company, the supplier will be involved in life cycle activities and must contribute a full set of auditable design and development documentation to support the validation.
- Computer system development and acceptance test procedures and records, when documented in line with life sciences validation practice, can be used to support qualification testing, and thus must be a prime focus for DQ.
- Align terminology and design or development and the associated development testing (whether it be manufacturing automation, laboratory or information systems) with a life cycle that is recognizable to the regulatory authorities. This in turn demonstrates an understanding of the validation life cycle.
- Prototypes must only be used to determine a design approach. They must not be released as the final product and no data produced on a prototype system can be used in support of a GxP study or manufacturing program.
- Development processes must be well controlled and regularly baselined. Each baselined deliverable should provide a usable solution that can be formally released.

Current and Future Challenges

- Align the "extended" system definition processes (i.e., conference room pilots, planning of large or complex systems with recognized life cycle controls and deliverables).
- New methodologies may require radical changes in approach.
- Evaluate the availability, use, and impact of development tools.

System Development Testing

The computerized system must be thoroughly tested and confirmed as capable of achieving the desired results before it is brought into use [8 §7, 14]. Development testing is a process of challenging the system at various levels of development based on predefined written test procedures. The tests must be derived from, and traceable back to, statements in the appropriate design specification which can be audited.

The design specifications for software and hardware provide definition of the component parts and the system integration from which corresponding tests can be developed. Tests for each requirement should be developed on completion of the respective specification to help to ensure all matters are addressed. For large systems test plans are usually developed soon after a design specification is approved in order to capture the overall test requirements and any particular issues identified at that time. The test plan will then evolve into a detailed test procedure that will address the more detailed criteria that become apparent as development proceeds.

The test planning process must identify the necessary scope and extent of testing, as well as the predetermined acceptance criteria. Tests and their acceptance criteria must be defined and documented prior to execution. Evidence of testing must be documented (e.g., individual tests completed, signed, and checked, and screen shots, reports or other evidence generated wherever possible and appropriate). Each individual test must have a pass or fail result.

Test reporting must conclude on the overall outcome of testing, and summarize how outstanding issues (including corrective actions to address test failures) are managed. If the computerized system is replacing a manual one, the two must be run in parallel for a time as a part of this testing and validation process [8 §7].

Testing may include software module, software integration, and package configuration testing. Where the system is based upon custom-built hardware, hardware acceptance testing will also be necessary.

Key Considerations

- Tests must be formally documented and verified by authorized and qualified individuals.
- Each test must be traceable to the clauses in the design specification that it verifies.
- Changes and deviations during testing must be formally documented and managed.
- Incorporate the traditional development testing, FAT, SATs, and acceptance testing into IQ and OQ as supplementary records where appropriate and practicable.
- If the computerized system is built in a place other than its final operating environment, a repeat IQ must be performed to prove that it has been properly installed, and a repeat of some of the OQ/PQ tests to demonstrate that it functions correctly in its operational environment.
- For quality-related GxP critical system data [13, Appendix A], functions and parameters, the test procedures should align with qualification test requirements and document the test and calibration results against expected results and acceptance criteria. This will support validation requirements and allow records of the supplier development testing to be considered in support of qualification testing. It will also minimize duplication of test effort.

- Appropriate validation, qualification, calibration or verification of any equipment, processes or alternative software used to perform or support the testing.

Current and Future Challenges

- New and evolving technologies may prove difficult to test conventionally. New approaches to testing may be required.
- Evaluate the availability, use, and impact of automatic testing tools.
- Consider rationalization of testing stage terminology, e.g., decide whether to adopt IQ, OQ, PQ "speak."
- Determine how much testing is enough during the system development. This may include a combination of functional and structural testing.
- Demonstrate the reliability of the system. It may also be necessary to perform advanced software testing using statistical testing. Using this technique, specific areas of concern are targeted and large amounts of data generated, thereby increasing the probability of encountering rare unanticipated operating conditions.

Data Migration

For new systems replacing existing one, data migration must preserve the integrity and security of the original data. Processes and methods used to load data (manual and automatic) must be defined and validated with supporting documentation before they are accepted for use [14].

Key Considerations

- Tight management of the migration process at all stages including:
  - Definition of responsibilities.
  - Security issues.
  - Definition of prerequisites, dependencies, and constraints.
  - Data sourcing.
  - Data mapping.
  - Data purging.
  - Archiving of legacy data.
  - Data collection.
  - Data cleansing.
  - Data creation.
  - Data aggregation.
  - Data verification.

- Formal verification of the data received on completion of each stage.
- Data sampling techniques must be defined for large databases.
- The choice of the final data repository supplier and application should be based on an established database technology which will facilitate any future migrations.
- Establish contingency plans to address potential problems.
- Mark or tag migrated data where that data does not include all information supported by the new system (e.g., where a full audit trail is not associated with the migrated data).

Current and Future Challenges

- Awareness of the risks associated with data migration which include:
  - Technical failures.
  - Quality of source data.
  - Access to and availability of source data.
  - Its effects on target systems.
  - Access to and availability of target systems.
  - Definition of the level of data checks required and their documentation.
  - Actions required on process failure.
  - Insufficient knowledge of source data or documentation.
- Manage the migration of data from dissimilar systems.

System Documentation

The user documentation must include, as a minimum, those items of the supplier's system development life cycle documentation necessary to provide evidence of validation in order to support a regulatory inspection (e.g., system specification and description, diagrams, test specifications or scripts, test results). The extent of the supplier's system development life cycle documentation to be provided to the customer will depend on the complexity, product and business criticality of the computerized system and will be defined in the URS and any contract agreements. Where the supplier's documentation will be used to support the validated state of the system, it must have been properly assessed and accepted by the user organization. Such review and acceptance must be formally documented. Information on system documentation for the user is provided in the GAMP Guide [7].

Key Considerations

- The documentation should be sufficient to enable the operation and maintenance of the system in a validated state.

- The documentation set should be stored in a managed repository under a controlled index with appropriate environmental control.
- The media for the documentation should be defined in the respective validation plan.
- The life sciences company is responsible for maintaining a validation document set or file, and for ensuring that the computerized system suppliers update their related document sets. The validation file document set must be under document control at all times, and is typically kept in the quality document archives to ensure control and access when required.
- Consideration should be given to structuring the computerized system validation set or file so as to reflect the validation life cycle activities.
- Information which cannot easily fit into a validation file (e.g., standard system manuals, etc.) may be filed elsewhere. This should be identified on the document schedule stating where it can be found. All documentation provided by the supplier must be clearly marked so as to be easily cross-referenced to its location in the validation document set or file.
- It is acceptable to have the system development records archived by the supplier. If the life sciences company requires the supplier to store and maintain the documents a formal agreement on the retention period is needed.

Current and Future Challenges

- Maintain the user and support documentation set up to date following changes to the system.

COMPUTERIZED SYSTEMS OPERATION

System Location

The computerized system must be located and maintained in a suitable environment to prevent damage and extraneous interference [8 §3].

Key Considerations

- Electromagnetic (EMI) and radio frequency (RFI) interference from other equipment should be prevented.

Current and Future Challenges

- Legislation changes could impact the location of the system.

System Changes

Alterations to a computerized system (e.g., changes, replacement parts, calibration) or to a computer program must be made in accordance with a defined change control procedure. This includes provisions for investigating (determining the nature and extent of the change), authorizing, implementing, checking, validating and approving the change, and for documenting each stage. Alterations must only be implemented, tested, and verified with the agreement of the persons responsible for the part of the computerized system concerned, and the alteration must be recorded. Every significant modification must be validated [8 §11, 14].

Key Considerations

- The extent or impact of each change must be fully investigated and documented. Where changes are routine (e.g., the automatic update of a parameter in the software following the routine calibration of an analytical instrument) the change control SOP may allow that change to occur without the need for investigation, providing the change is appropriately logged.
- Site changes by the supplier must follow the same procedures or processes as those used by the customer.
- System documentation must be updated where applicable.
- All items impacted by the change must be examined to ensure that the change audit trail and change history is complete.
- Software configuration management records must be updated.

Current and Future Challenges

- Replacement of broken or obsolete equipment with an item considered equivalent or similar requires careful investigation.

Error and Problem Reporting

A procedure must be established to record and analyze errors found in the computerized system and to enable corrective action to be taken [8 §17, 14]. Corrective action should be identified, evaluated, planned, and implemented.

Errors and corrective actions should be assessed as part of the periodic review to ensure that the system is still suitable for use in a regulated environment. Periodic review of errors encountered may also help to identify specific training needs.

Key Considerations

- The corrective action process should be linked to the change management process.
- The root cause of any errors should be established and a solution found which will prevent a recurrence.
- Corrective action plans must encompass all documentation (specifications, records, procedures, report updates).

Current and Future Challenges

- Measurement and trending of corrective actions must be maintained to determine common causes.

Backup and Archiving

Software, system configuration, data, and any associated documentation must be protected by backing-up at regular intervals. Backup media and documentation must be retained at a separate and secure location for a defined period, which is at least as long as that required by the applicable GxP predicate rule or EC directive, and must be readily available within predefined timescales throughout the period of retention [8 §14, 14]. Storage media must be protected against willful or accidental damage, and be periodically checked for durability and restoration. A procedure for backup and archiving must be established, appropriately tested, and implemented.

Key Considerations

- Protection of data and records.
- Frequency of the backups and the retention period in the archive.
- Backup and archiving media.
- Verification of successful backup.
- Verification of the restoration process.
- Consideration of whether to use electronic or nonelectronic media for the long-term archive of electronic records.

Current and Future Challenges

- Obsolescence of the archive media is possible.
- Changes in regulatory requirements could affect archive duration and access times.

Disaster Recovery and Business Contingency Planning

The procedures to be followed if the computerized system fails or breaks down must be defined and validated. Adequate alternative arrangements must be made available for systems which need to be operated in the event of a breakdown. The time required to bring the alternative arrangements into use must be related to the possible urgency of the need to use them (e.g., any information which is required to effect a recall or to maintain an animal study must be available at short notice). All failures and the remedial actions taken must be recorded [8 §15, §16, 14].

Key Considerations

- Alternative arrangements must be based on the risk of failure and business impact.
- Security and integrity of both quality and business critical data.
- Appropriate methodology transfer to an alternative system, equipment, or personnel to ensure consistency and accuracy of data.

Current and Future Challenges

- Changes in regulatory requirements may affect the approach taken.

System Maintenance and Support

The arrangements for computerized system maintenance and support by the supplier or by another support agency (e.g., a company, organization, group or person) which is either internal or external to the life science company, must be formally documented. This document must take the form of an agreement which clearly defines the scope of the support service, response measures and the responsibilities of the supplier or support agency [8 §18, 14]. Where support is split between different companies, groups or people, the precise responsibilities of each must be fully documented. If the supplier or support agency is external to the life science company the appropriate rules concerning contract manufacture and analysis [A1: Part 4, Chapter 7] will apply. These rules will also be used as guidance for determining an appropriate support agreement when the supplier or support agency is internal to the life science company.

Key Considerations

- A service level agreement (SLA) should be provided.

- Maintenance and support activities should link into customer procedures and processes.

Current and Future Challenges

- In house and outsourced maintenance and support should be managed in the same way.

System Decommissioning and Retirement

Computerized systems taken out of operational use must be decommissioned so that the archiving and retrieval of system configuration, data and any associated documentation is assured for a predefined period [14]. The principles for long term archiving are the same as those described for backup and archiving. Access agreements must be maintained for information and media held by suppliers or other third parties. Archived materials must not be destroyed until their retention period has expired. The decision to destroy the records must be documented.

Key Considerations

- Archiving of existing data and records.
- Possible data migration to a new system.
- Accessibility of legacy data which needs to be retained in archive.

Future Challenges

- Changes in regulatory requirements may affect the approach taken.

Inspection Readiness

Sites, facilities, and organizations using and supporting validated computerized systems must maintain a state of internal and external (regulatory authority) inspection readiness [14].

Key Considerations

- Accessibility and availability of controlled records and data.
- Maintenance and management of records and data.

Current and Future Challenges

- Changes in regulatory requirements may affect the approach taken.

ELECTRONIC RECORDS AND ELECTRONIC SIGNATURES

The FDA issued the 21 CFR Part 11 Electronic Records; Electronic Signatures, Final Rule in March 1997 [16] and this was followed over the next few years by a Compliance Policy Guide on Enforcement Policy (CPG 7153 – 21 CFR Part 11; Electronic Records; Electronic Signatures, July 1999), and a series of draft Part 11 guidance documents covering Validation (August 2001), Glossary of Terms (August 2001), Time Stamps (February 2002), Maintenance of Electronic Records (July 2002), and Electronic Copies of Electronic Records (August 2002) which represented the agency's current thinking on each topic. However, in February 2003 the FDA issued an announcement in which it withdrew the CPG and all of the guidance documents and announced that Part 11 was to be reexamined.

FDA Guidance for Industry, Part 11, ERES – Scope and Application

Subsequent to this announcement a new document was issued by the FDA in August 2003 entitled *Guidance for Industry, Part 11, Electronic Records; Electronic Signatures – Scope and Application.* [17] This document provides clarification of the FDAs' current thinking on Part 11 and focuses on the following.

- A narrower scope for Part 11.
- The agency will exercise enforcement discretion for *some* Part 11 requirements, namely validation, audit trails, record retention, and record copying. However, records must still be maintained or submitted in accordance with the underlying predicate rules which apply to the operation.
- The agency will exercise enforcement discretion for *all* Part 11 requirements relating to prerule legacy systems *if* certain conditions are upheld.

The next step is for the FDA to reexamine the Part 11 rulemaking process as part of the cGMP initiative *Pharmaceutical CGMPs for the 21st Century: A Risk-Based Approach; A Science and Risk-Based Approach to Quality Product Regulation Incorporating an Integrated Quality Systems Approach.**

In response to the publication, the life sciences industry must recognize and act accordingly to embrace the following key indicators.

---

* www.fda.gov.oc.guidance.gmp.html.

Predicate Rules and Part 11

- FDA will enforce all predicate rule record and record keeping requirements.
- Records must still be maintained or submitted in accordance with the underlying predicate rules, and the Agency can take regulatory action for non-compliance with such predicate rules.
- Part 11 remains in effect.
- Part 11 is intended to permit the widest possible use of electronic technology, compatible with the FDAs responsibility to protect public health.
- The predicate rules define:
  - What records must be maintained.
  - The contents of the record.
  - Whether signatures are required.
  - How long records must be retained.
- Records and signatures that meet the criteria:
  - Will be considered equivalent to paper records and signatures.
  - May be used in lieu of paper, unless otherwise started in other regulations.

Narrow Interpretation of Scope

- Part 11 applies to maintenance of records required under the applicable predicate rules or which are submitted to the FDA.
- Part 11 applies when persons choose to use records in electronic format in place of paper format.
- Part 11 applies to records which are submitted to the FDA in electronic format, even if such records are not specifically identified in FDA regulations, and assumes that the records have been identified as the types of submissions the Agency accepts in electronic format.
- Any other records and signatures maintained electronically are outside the scope of Part 11.
- Time stamps should be implemented with a clear understanding of the time zone reference used, and system documentation should explain the time zone references and conventions.

What the FDA Still Intends to Enforce When Part 11 Applies

- System access control.
- Operational system checks.
- Authority checks.
- Device checks.
- Education, training, and experience.

- Policies that hold individuals accountable.
- System documentation controls.
- Controls for open systems.
- Electronic signature requirements.
- Signature manifestations.
- Signature or record linking.
- Electronic signature uniqueness.
- Verification of individuals' identities.
- Certification to the FDA.
- Electronic signature components and controls.
- Controls for identification codes and passwords.

The Life Sciences Industry's Responsibilities

- To understand the implications of the final guidance on the scope and application of Part 11.
- Establish clear policies and procedures.
- Implement a reasonable risk-based approach.
  - The risk assessment approach may vary from case to case. Methodologies ranging from a simple impact assessment methodology to a full failure modes and effects analysis (FMEA) or impact and criticality analyses and may be used as appropriate [7, Appendix M3, 12 §3 and Appendix 2, 13 §9].
  - Establish priorities by focusing on the predicate rule requirements, the impact and value of specific records, and risks to those records.
  - Risk is a key decider in examining the need for specific controls for specific records, i.e., controls commensurate with documented risk.
  - Within user organizations different circumstances may call for varying levels of controls for each record, i.e., there may not be a single level of controls across the organization and covering all records.
  - It should be remembered that whatever the assessed risk, Part 11 applies to all Part 11 records.
- Apply appropriate controls.
- Understand their regulated processes and determine and document where they have records and signatures and, based on predicate rules, whether specific records are Part 11 records.
- Recognize that some records are directly identified by predicate rules, but in the case where a record is implied rather than specifically stated, then the company should consider whether the record is required for them to fulfil the requirements of the predicate rule or required to provide evidence, document their decision and rationale.

Validation

- Computer systems must be validated if they have impact on product quality, product safety, and record integrity.
- If there are no predicate rule requirements for validation, it may still be important to validate the systems to maintain control.
- Controls should take into account risks to product quality, public safety, and record integrity.
- Basic requirements for risk-based computer validation and record controls required by other applicable regulations must still be satisfied.

Hybrid Systems (Paper and Electronic Records)

- If a record is required to be maintained and paper printout of the electronic record is generated for business purposes, if it is the electronic record that is used to perform regulatory activities then Part 11 will apply.

Electronic Signatures

- Part 11 signatures include electronic signatures that are intended to be the equivalent of handwritten signatures, initials, and other general signings required by predicate rules.
- Part 11 signatures include electronic signatures that are used to document that certain events or actions occurred in accordance with a predicate rule, e.g., approved, reviewed, and verified.
- Recognize that in some instances business practices may require using electronic records and that the Agency may take the business practices into account in determining whether Part 11 is applicable.

Audit Trails

- Must still comply with predicate rule requirements related to documentation.
- Apply appropriate controls based on a risk assessment.
- Should be considered when users are expected to create, modify, or delete regulated records during normal operation.
- Even if there are no predicate rule requirements, it may be important to have controls such as audit trails or other physical, logical, or procedural security measures in place to ensure trustworthiness and reliability of records.

Copies of Records

- Must provide an inspector with reasonable and useful access to records.
- Allow inspection, review, and copying in human readable form at the user site using user hardware and following established user procedures and techniques for accessing records.
- Copies of records should be held in common portable formats (e.g., PDF, XML, SGML), and use established automated conversion or export methods where available.
- Ensure copies preserve the content and meaning of the record.
- Provide search, sort, and trend capability if technologically feasible.

Retention of Records

- Must meet predicate rule requirements.
- Unless specifically stated, record retention time should be based on predicate rule requirements, a justified and documented risk assessment, and determination of the value of the record over time.
- Coexistence of paper and electronic record and signature components, i.e., hybrid solutions, are acceptable as long as predicate rule stipulations are met, and the content and meaning of the records is preserved. Dependencies on electronic or paper records to carry out regulated activities must be documented.

Legacy Systems

- A computer system in use before August 20, 1997, i.e., when Part 11 came into effect, that has met, and continues to meet, all applicable predicate rule requirements throughout the system's operational life, is outside the scope of Part 11.
- There is documented evidence and justification that the system is fit for its intended use and has an acceptable level of record security and data integrity.
- Any changes to the legacy system must be controlled and the changes assessed. If the changes prevent the system from meeting predicate rules, Part 11 controls must be applied to Part 11 records and signatures.

Key Considerations

- 21 CFR Part 11 is "simply" a record-keeping regulation that tells us how records are to be dealt with.
- Electronic records and electronic signature requirements are also addressed in the EU [8, 14].

Electronic Records Compliance

In the context of this section, any text, graphics, data, audio, pictorial, or other information represented in digital form that is used for regulatory submission or to support a regulatory submission, or that is required by local laws and relevant regulations, and is stored electronically, is considered to be an electronic record; and the requirements of the regulatory agencies will apply [1, 8, 16]. The information provided here should be used for guidance in the application of the appropriate regulations for a "closed" system, but in all cases the requirements of the FDA [16] and the associated life sciences company corporate interpretation [28] will take precedence.

Validation Requirements

Computerized systems supporting the regulated use of electronic records or electronic signatures must be validated in line with the governing predicate rules or EU directives. Validation must cover both technical solutions and the implementation of any procedural controls for electronic records and electronic signatures [8 §2, 16 §11.10(a)].

Key Considerations

- Validation is a requirement of the FDA GxP predicate rules and EU GxP regulations.
- Validation of computerized systems forms the foundation and bedrock of the FDA electronic record and electronic signature rule. However, it should be understood that this rule does not itself impose any additional validation requirements upon the system.
- It is not uncommon for user companies to consider key business requirements important enough for inclusion in the validation program. This is particularly so in the large systems that monitor and direct the supply chain, e.g., ERP, MES.

Current and Future Challenges

- Recent surveys have shown that lack of validation is still the most prominent finding by the regulatory authorities.
- Instilling a validation culture in both the life science companies and their suppliers.
- Identification of the records to be generated to satisfy the appropriate "predicate rules" and held within the system. In the case of larger control and information

systems e.g., ERP, MES, LIMS, the instances of records required by the predicate rules are to be determined throughout the software functionality.

System Access

The computerized system must only be used and data must only be entered or altered by authorized persons [16 §11.10(d), 16 §11.10(g)]. Suitable methods for deterring unauthorized access to the system and its data must be used including the use of keys, pass cards, and personal codes, and by restricting access to networked computers and terminals, and interfaces to other computer systems which can provide access to the system. A procedure must be established for the issue, cancellation, and alteration of authorization to enter and amend data, including the changing of personal passwords. Unsuccessful attempts to access the system by unauthorized persons must be recorded [8 §8, 16 §11.10(d), §11.10(g), §11.300(d)].

Key Considerations

- Systems must be tightly managed and unauthorized access prohibited.
- Periodic review of system access attempts should be made to ensure that any unusual login attempts are identified and appropriate action taken if necessary.
- Careful consideration and planning should be undertaken if allowing Internet access to remote users or customers to access or view specific data.
- Definition of user roles. Users should only be granted sufficient access to allow them to perform their job properly. If a user no longer needs access to a particular function or data, that access permission should be retired.

Current and Future Challenges

- Globally distributed and accessed systems may present access administration problems.

Data Entry Checks

The computerized system must have built-in checks, where appropriate, for the correct entry and processing of data, verification of the data source, and the correct sequencing of steps and events [8 §6, 16 §11.10(f), §11.10(h)]. Additional checks must be carried out on the accuracy of the records generated when critical data are entered manually (e.g., the weight and batch number of an ingredient during dispensing). This check can be carried out by a second operator or by a validated electronic method [8 §9].

Key Considerations

- Incorrect data entry, such as out-of-range limits and inappropriate characters, should be rejected.

Current and Future Challenges

- Data verification.
- Transfer of electronic approval (signatures) from one system to another.

Audit Trails

The computerized system should generate secure, time-stamped audit trails which record the identity of operators entering, confirming, altering or deleting critical electronic data and the action taken [8 §10, 16 §11.10(e)]. Any alteration made to a critical data entry must be authorized and recorded with the reason for the alteration and the date and time the alteration was made [8 §10]. A complete record of all entries and amendments made by the operator to electronic records should be generated and retained by the system throughout the records retention time [8 §10, 16 §11.10(e)]. Where this is not technologically possible, appropriate alternative measures must be implemented to ensure the integrity and accuracy of the electronic record. Changes to records must not obscure previously recorded information [16 §11.10(e)].

Key Considerations

- Definition of what must be logged.
- Definition of the time clock used, particularly if the system is used over several different time zones.

Current and Future Challenges

- The ease with which changes to records can be detected.

Copies of Data

It must be possible to obtain accurate and complete copies of electronically stored data for quality auditing purposes and for regulatory inspection [8 §12, 16 §11.10(b)].

Key Considerations

- This requirement has now been "toned down" by the FDA. However, the FDA still requires "useful and reasonable access" to records. They recommend using established automated conversion and export methods to produce copies in common data formats. The copy should preserve the meaning and content of the record and where technically feasible, should provide sorting and trending facilities.

Current and Future Challenges

- Objectively assessing potential data formats to ensure they are appropriate for the storage of data and are acceptable to the relevant regulatory authorities.

Data Security

Data must be secured by physical or electronic means against wilful or accidental damage. Stored data must be checked for accessibility, durability, and accuracy throughout the records retention period. [16 §11.10(c)] If changes are proposed to the computer equipment or its programs, these checks must be performed at a frequency appropriate to the storage medium being used [8 §13].

Key Considerations

- A data backup, archiving, and restoration process is required appropriate for the computerized system.
- Where possible, data should have a checksum or cyclic redundancy check associated with it to confirm integrity.

Current and Future Challenges

- Use of an appropriate storage medium.

Batch Release and Qualified Persons

Computerized systems used to release batches for sale or supply, must only allow a qualified person to perform the release. The identity of the qualified person must be clearly identified and recorded by the system [8 ß§9, 16 §11.10(d), §11.10(j)].

Key Considerations

- The concept of a qualified person is currently peculiar to countries regulated by EU GMPs. However, other non-EU countries who want to supply product to the EU are increasingly recognizing the concept, and global regulatory harmonization initiatives may see an extension of the role.
- Similar restrictions should be applied to GLP environments where it is the responsibility of the study director to approve various functions [5 §58.33].
- Management representative responsible for ensuring that the quality system requirements are effectively established and maintained and for reporting on the performance of the quality system as required by 21 CFR Part 820 [6 §20 (3i, 3ii)].
- Individual companies may have policies that require specific individuals to approve various functions within the computerized system.

Current and Future Challenges

- Changes in regulatory requirements due to global harmonization initiatives.

Documentation Control

Appropriate controls must be provided for the distribution, use, and access of documentation for system operation and maintenance. Change control processes must ensure that change history (audit trail) information is maintained for the development and alteration of system documentation [16 §11.10(k1, k2)].

Key Considerations

- Documentation must be properly managed and accessible.
- Documentation should be in a language that is easily and clearly understood by the users. For global systems this may require that documentation is translated into the relevant local language.

Current and Future Challenges

- Access to the documentation for global systems can be problematic.

Open Systems

In addition to the requirements described here for closed systems, open systems must have additional measures, such as document encryption and the use of appropriate digital signature standards, to ensure the authenticity, integrity, and confidentiality of electronic records [16 §11.30].

Key Considerations

- Choice of technologies needs careful consideration.

Current and Future Challenges

- Detection of unauthorized access.

Electronic Signatures Compliance

In the context of this section, any legally admissible electronic signing applied by an individual to an electronic record that is used for regulatory submission or to support a regulatory submission, or that is required by local laws and relevant regulations, is considered to be an electronic signature; and the requirements of the regulatory agencies will apply [1, 7, 16]. The information provided below should be used for guidance in the application of the appropriate regulations, but in all cases the requirements of the FDA [16] and the associated life sciences company corporate interpretation [28] will take precedence.

Association with Electronic Records

The appropriate requirements for electronic records must also apply to electronic signatures [16 §11.50]. Electronic signatures, and handwritten signatures applied to electronic records, must be permanently and unambiguously linked to their corresponding electronic records [16 §11.70].

Key Considerations

- The linking of the user name or password combination to specific records and events.
- Technology used for applying handwritten signatures to electronic records e.g., validation of pattern recognition software to ensure correct signature is applied.

Current and Future Challenges

- The updating of computerized systems with appropriate technology to maintain their security features at a level necessary to ensure that "reasonable" measures have been taken to prevent changes to electronic records.
- Assessment of evolving computer applications, architectures, and technologies.

Accountability

Business areas must ensure that individuals understand that they are accountable and responsible for actions initiated under their electronic signatures, as if it were a handwritten signature [16 §11.10(j), §11.100(c)]. This responsibility and accountability has been certified by the pharmaceutical company in a letter sent to the U.S. FDA [16 §11.100(c, c1), 20].

Key Considerations

- Appropriate training must be supplied so that each individual is fully aware of the implications and responsibility he undertakes when applying an electronic signature. This training must be documented in the user's training record.

Current and Future Challenges

- Provision of refresher training.
- Maintenance of system access records for new starters, transferred staff, and staff who leave the company.

Meaning and Timestamps

The purpose of an electronic signature must be apparent. The application of an electronic signature must include the date and time of the signature and the unique identification of the signatory [8 §10, 16 §11.50].

Key Considerations

- The operator should be made aware of what is signed and the implication of that signing (e.g., review, approval, release, etc.).

Current and Future Challenges

- Definition of when and where an electronic signature should be applied.
- Identification of the "predicate rules" for the applicable signatures to be applied to a record should be held within the system.
- When identifying where signatures are applied, consideration must also be given to where signatures are implied in the "predicate rules" (e.g., where words such as reviewed, approved, and verified are used).
- In the case of larger control and information systems e.g., ERP, MES, the instances of signatures required by predicate rules will be determined throughout the software functionality. This should also include the identification of points where the user ID and password are used as an acknowledgement rather than a signature for regulatory purposes. This may also be considered for instances requiring acknowledgement by a key business signatory.

Security – Personnel

Electronic signatures must be unique to an individual [16 §11.100(a, b), §11.200(b), §11.300(a)]. Nonbiometrics signatures must use a unique combination of at least two distinct identification components (e.g., an identification code and password) [16 §11.200(a1)]. Procedures and controls must be maintained to ensure that electronic signatures cannot be falsified by ordinary means [16 §11.200(a3)]. The disclosure of confidential electronic signature components between personnel and the use of another person's electronic signature is unacceptable and will be considered as falsification of records [16 §11.200(a2,b)]. The ability to apply electronic signatures must be withdrawn for individuals whose status means that this is no longer applicable (e.g., new company role or termination of employment) [16 §11.300(b)].

Key Considerations

- Personnel must be provided with IT security training that explains their responsibility to protect their electronic signatures against misuse and possible consequences.

Current and Future Challenges

- Provision of refresher training.
- Maintenance of system access records for new starters, transferred staff, and staff who leave the company.

Security – Equipment

The initial and periodic testing of any identification devices must be carried out and documented [16 §11.300(e)]. Identification codes and passwords must be periodically checked, recalled or changed, and their unauthorized use recorded and reported to the appropriate company authorities [16 §11.300(b, d)]. Arrangements must be made for the issue of replacement identification components which have been lost, stolen, or otherwise compromised, and the generation of appropriate documentation [16 §11.300(c)].

Key Considerations

- Passwords must be periodically changed and should always be changed if it is believed they may have become compromised.
- Passwords should comply with corporate policy and have a defined minimum length and complexity.
- Reuse of a previous password must be subject to time or number of renewal restrictions.
- Expired user ID and password combinations, including those of company leavers, must be retained in order to identify an individual and prevent reuse.
- Password issuance and voiding must be managed.

Current and Future Challenges

- The updating of computerized systems with appropriate technology in order to maintain their security features at a level necessary to ensure that "reasonable" measures have been taken to prevent changes to electronic records.
- Assessment of evolving computer applications, architectures, and technologies.

Security – Continuous and Interrupted Access

The computerized system must detect periods of interrupted attendance by the operator and terminate the operator's work session by performing a log off operation. The nonattendance period must be adjustable. During periods of interrupted attendance, the operator must perform any signings using all of the electronic signature components. During periods of continuous attendance, the operator must perform the first signing using all of the electronic signature components and subsequent signings using at least one electronic signature component that is only executable by, and designed to be used only by, the operator [16 §11.200(a1i, a1ii)].

Key Considerations

- There should be a corporate definition of what constitutes a continuous signing session and what nonattendance period is acceptable before log off or session lock.
- Session lock-out times must be appropriate to the task at hand. For instance, if a computer system is used to monitor the end point of a reaction in the plant, it may be necessary to have a longer lockout time associated with the system than a system which is being used by a qualified person to release batches to the market.

Current and Future Challenges

- The use of network access security features (e.g., user ID or password combination; user lock-out controls) to control access to an application running on a local PC.

PERSONNEL

Internal and external personnel who specify, develop (design, implement and test), install, validate, operate, manage, support, and decommission computerized systems must have the education, training, and experience commensurate with the tasks concerned. Training must be documented [8 §1, 16 §ß11.10(i)] [B8].

Key Considerations

- Use personnel who are competent to perform the work supported by appropriate documentary evidence.
- Inspect education certificates for new personnel where necessary.
- Periodic reviews of personnel competence supported by the identification of training needs and a schedule for their implementation, and any necessary re-training.
- Multidisciplinary teams may be required for certain types of computerized systems.

Current and Future Challenges

- Establish and maintain training programs.
- Maintain competence with changing technologies.

Roles and Responsibilities

The validation of a computerized system and its assessment for compliance with the appropriate GxP regulations and electronic records and signatures regulations must be performed by personnel who are competent in the areas for which they are responsible. These include the process, system or technology, application, appropriate regulatory requirements, and appropriate life science company local and corporate requirements [14]. This section identifies the key job roles and responsibilities relating to the validation of computerized systems, for ensuring that they comply with the appropriate GxP regulations, including the regulations relating to electronic records and electronic signatures. The job roles and responsibilities will be governed by the size and type of computerized system and will be described in detail in the validation master plan (or VP), and if appropriate, any associated project documentation.

Executive Sponsor

Executive management responsibility for the successful implementation and validation of a system; commits and empowers resources to ensure adherence to all relevant GxP regulatory requirements.

Senior Quality Management

Commits the quality management group to providing the system owner with the procedures and agreed resources to ensure all quality-related activities are satisfactorily conducted and documented to meet the respective regulations, and to applying all relevant quality system procedures to ensure and monitor the computer registry, document control, change control, training programs or records, and internal audits. Also, to support the system owner during regulatory inspections.

Senior IT Management

Commits the IT group to controlling system configuration, maintaining system security and data integrity, providing qualified technical support, conducting regulatory compliance, validation and system technical training, supporting the System Owner in the utilization of respective validation and support procedures, and provision of validation documentation.

Senior Supply Chain, Manufacturing Management, Study Management

Commits the candidate site or facility to providing or verifying the data required for records under "predicate rules," enabling the system owner to approve system functionality and any change requirements, supporting the system owner with the procedures and agreed resources to ensure that all quality-related data and records are derived from validated computer systems, controlling life cycle validation programs during implementation and throughout the operational life of the GxP systems, and conducting GxP validation and operating training programs for study or manufacturing and support personnel.

Site or Facility Director

Commits the site/facility to identifying the applicable GxP regulations and the data required for records under the "predicate rules" applicable to the computerized system. Also, provides timely resource for controlling and monitoring the life cycle validation program throughout implementation and operational use of a computerized system, and resources to fulfill ongoing training programs for GxP, validation and system operation.

Quality Assurance Subject Matter Expert

Responsible for reviewing and approving validation life cycle documentation, high-level computerized system life cycle documentation, and system change control documentation to ensure that they comply with accepted industry computer systems validation practice, the appropriate GxP regulations, including the regulations relating to electronic records and electronic signatures, and that the activities and document sign-offs have been carried out by trained and authorized personnel. The quality assurance subject matter expert is also responsible for:

- Providing guidance to the life science company and associated groups on the regulatory requirements and industry guidelines for computerized systems validation and electronic records and signatures.
- Performing quality and technical audits on internal and external suppliers of computerized systems.
- The production of the life science company computer systems validation policies and SOPs.

System and Data Owner

Responsible for ensuring that the computerized system is validated and that it meets the appropriate regulatory requirements in terms of the technical solution provided (e.g., equipment, hardware, software), the validation and computerized system life cycle documentation generated, and supporting SOPs and any equipment protocols. The system owner can also be the system administrator or the project manager.

System Administrator

Responsible for providing support during the validation of the computerized system, and for ongoing system administration (e.g., control of user access accounts, system backup and recovery, etc.) and system maintenance (via an internal life science company group or by an external company).

Project Manager

Directly or indirectly responsible for the specification (URS), selection, design and regulatory compliance review, acceptance testing and validation of the computerized system, and the supply of its associated validation life cycle documentation. The validation work or project management may be performed by an internal life science company group or on their behalf by an external company.

System Supplier

Responsible for the design, production, testing, delivery, installation and operational verification (commissioning) of the computerized system and provision of its associated life cycle documentation. The system supplier may be an internal life science company group or an external company.

SUMMARY

This chapter has explored the impact of the current GxP and supporting regulations on computerized systems compliance and validation and the challenges imposed on industry practices in order to ensure and streamline the compliance process.

As this chapter is being written the use of new technologies is again being encouraged, with process analytical technology (PAT) recognized by regulatory authorities as encompassing strategic new technologies that will impact the way the industry operates. This will lead to significant changes in the regulation of product and service quality and will demand compliance and validation enabling methodologies.

PAT encompasses technologies such as optronics, computer technology and methods of abstracting information from complex data matrices (chemometrics), that will afford direct measurements with manufacturing processes (online and at-line analysis) and inside chemical and physical processes (in-line analysis). PAT will afford opportunities for design of advanced real time analysis and control of manufacturing processes to assure product quality at the completion of the process. Similarly, through the advent of combinatorial chemistry, the number of potential drug candidates entering development is increasing. This has led to the use of high throughput drug metabolism, pharmacokinetic and drug fate analyses and the need for improved and "real time" toxicology and safety assessment techniques. This has resulted in a large increase in data volume and increased employment of advanced data processing and data deconvolution techniques.

These new technologies, in turn, provide more in depth process knowledge from development to manufacturing and require reliable tools and systems for non-invasive (in some cases) and speedy measurements (e.g., spectroscopic techniques such as liquid chromatography–mass spectrometry/Sciex, near infrared, infrared, raman, fluorescence, UV–Vis absorption and advanced nuclear magnetic resonance and magnetic resonance imaging).

The new technologies that will surface in the coming years will be well served by the FDAs risk-based approach and evolving industry guidance and practices, so as to ensure the right level of controls and validation are in place to achieve and maintain regulatory compliance, and hence safeguard product and service quality attributes.

DEFINITIONS

Computer System. A computer system is a group of hardware components and associated software designed and assembled to perform a specific function or group of functions.

Computerized System. A computerized system is a combination of business process, hardware, software, documentation, and surrounding infrastructure.

Customer. The customer is the life science company organization, group or person who will be purchasing or acquiring, and utilizing the computer system or computerized system. The customer can comprise the system owner, end users, support personnel, validation, and QA personnel, technical specialists and consultants, as defined in the VMP.

Electronic Records and Electronic Signatures. The definitions relating to electronic records and electronic signatures in [16 §11.3] are accepted.

GxP. A generic expression used to represent one or more of the following: good manufacturing practice (GMP), good laboratory practice (GLP), good clinical practice (GCP), good distribution practice (GDP).

Supplier (Vendor). A supplier of a computer system, or of a computerized system, may be either a company or person external to the life science company, or an organization, group or person internal to the life science company.

REFERENCES

The documents identified below aim to establish the controls that will ensure that all appropriate computerized systems are validated and, where applicable, are compliant with the current regulations relating to electronic records and electronic signatures. The compliance of computerized systems will be assessed using the regulations, directives, guidelines, and life science company documentation listed below.

GxP Compliance and General Validation

1. MCA (now MHRA) Rules and Guidance for Pharmaceutical Manufacturers and Distributors (Orange Guide), 1997. Incorporates the EC Guides to GMP and GDP, EC Directives on GMP (medicinal products for human use 91/356/EEC, 13 Jun 1991, and veterinary medicinal products 91/412/EEC, 23 Jul 1991), and EC Directives on Wholesale Distribution and GDP (92/25/EEC, 31 Mar 1992).
2. FDA 21 CFR Part 210 – Current Good Manufacturing Practice in Manufacturing, Processing, Packing or Holding of Drugs.
3. FDA 21 CFR Part 211 – Current Good Manufacturing Practice for Finished Pharmaceuticals.
4. FDA Guideline on General Principles of Process Validation, May 1987.
5. FDA 21 CFR Part 58 – Good Laboratory Practice for Nonclinical Laboratory Studies.
6. FDA 21 CFR Part 820 – Quality System Regulation – as related to medical devices.

Computer Systems Validation

7. ISPE/GAMP Forum. GAMP4 Guide for Validation of Automated Systems, December 2001.
8. Annex 11 – Computerized Systems (subsection of [A1]).
9. FDA Guide to Inspection of Computerized Systems in Drug Processing (Blue Book), 1983.
10. FDA Technical Reference on Software Development Activities, July 1987.
11. FDA Compliance Policy Guides on Computerized Drug Processing:
    - CPG 7132a.07 Input/Output Checking, 01 Oct 1982.
    - CPG 7132a.08 Identification of "Persons" on Batch Production and Control Records, 01 Dec 1982.
    - CPG 7132a.11 CGMP Applicability to Hardware and Software, 01 Dec 1984.
    - CPG 7132a.12 Vendor Responsibility, 18 Jan 1985.

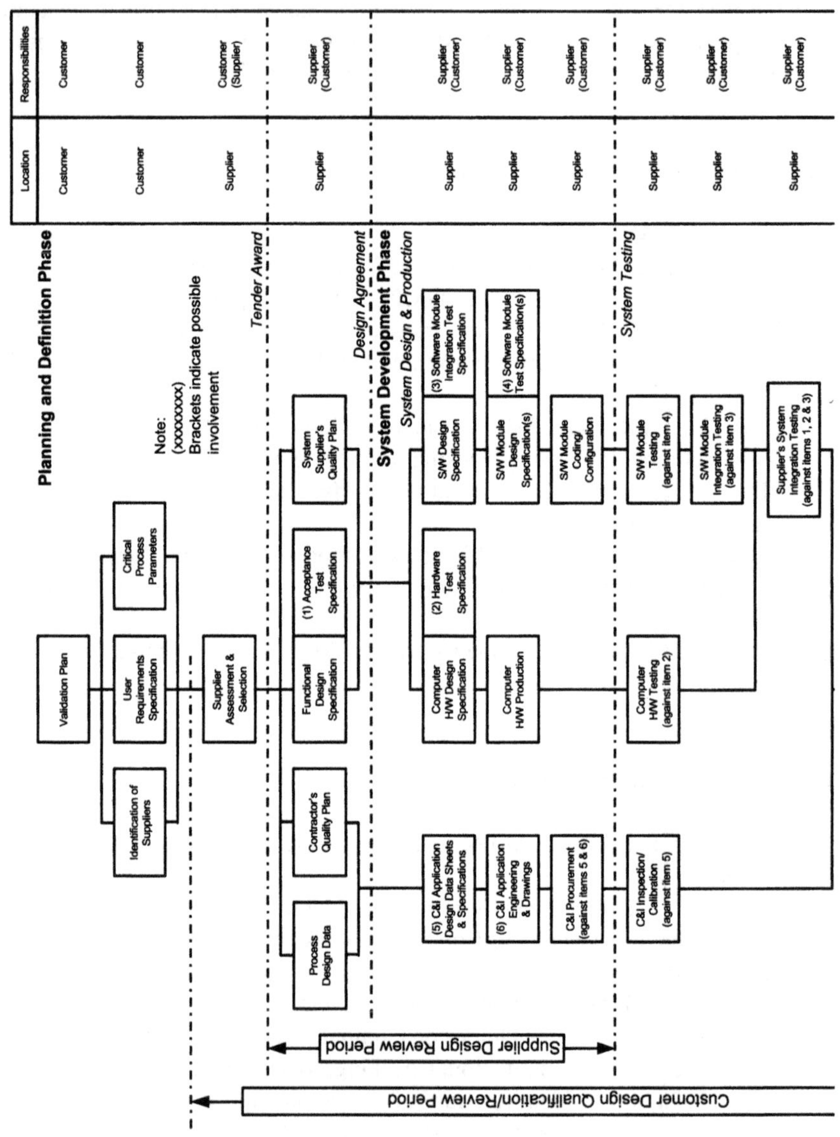
Location
Responsibilities
Customer
Customer
Customer
Customer
Supplier
Customer (Supplier)
Supplier
Supplier (Customer)
Supplier
Supplier (Customer)
Supplier
Supplier (Customer)
Supplier
Supplier (Customer)
Supplier
Supplier (Customer)
Supplier
Supplier (Customer)
Supplier
Supplier (Customer)
Planning and Definition Phase
Validation Plan
Identification of Suppliers
User Requirements Specification
Critical Process Parameters
Note: (xxxxxxxx) Brackets indicate possible involvement
Supplier Assessment & Selection
Tender Award
Process Design Data
Contractor's Quality Plan
Functional Design Specification
(1) Acceptance Test Specification
System Supplier's Quality Plan
Design Agreement
System Development Phase
System Design & Production
(5) C&I Application Design Data Sheets & Specifications
Computer H/W Design Specification
(2) Hardware Test Specification
S/W Design Specification
(3) Software Module Integration Test Specification
(6) C&I Application Engineering & Drawings
Computer H/W Production
S/W Module Design Specification(s)
(4) Software Module Test Specification(s)
C&I Procurement (against items 5 & 6)
S/W Module Coding/ Configuration
System Testing
C&I Inspection/ Calibration (against item 5)
Computer H/W Testing (against item 2)
S/W Module Testing (against item 4)
S/W Module Integration Testing (against item 3)
Supplier's System Integration Testing (against items 1, 2 & 3)
Supplier Design Review Period
Customer Design Qualification/Review Period

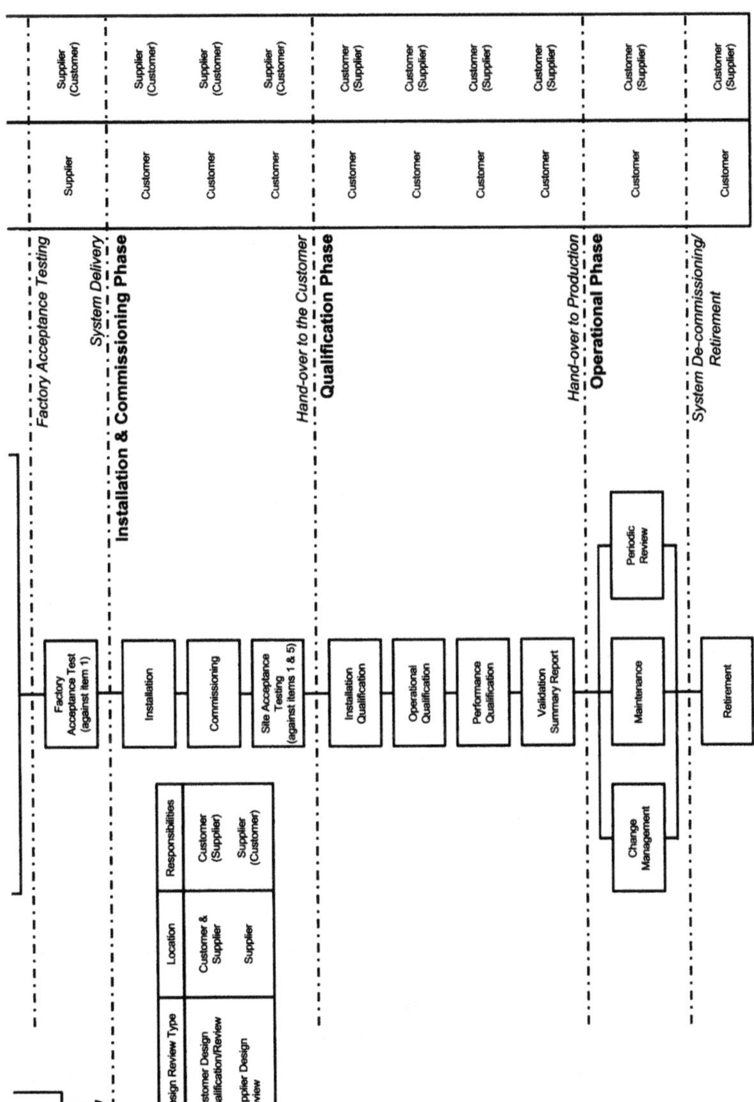

Figure 1.5 Computerized Systems Validation Lifecycle Activities and Documentation

CPG 7132a.12 Source Code for Process Control Application Programs, 16 Apr 1987.

12. ISPE Baseline Guide, Volume 5, Commissioning and Qualification, First Edition, March 2001.
13. GAMP Good Practice Guide, Validation of Process Control Systems, December 2004.
14. PIC/S Guidance – Good Practices for Computerized Systems in Regulated GxP Environments.
15. PDA Technical Report No. 18, Validation of Computer-Related Systems, 1995.

Electronic Records and Electronic Signatures Compliance

16. FDA 21 CFR Part 11 – Electronic Records; Electronic Signatures, 20 March 1997.
17. Guidance for Industry. Part 11, Electronic Records; Electronic Signatures – Scope and Application, August 2003.
18. EC Directive 1999/93/EC – Community framework for electronic signatures, 13 December 1999.
19. ISPE/PDA Guideline. Good Practice and Compliance for Electronic Records and Signatures, Part 2 – Complying with 21 CFR Part 11, Electronic Records and Electronic Signatures, September 2001.
20. Letter sent by a senior official of the Pharmaceutical Company to the Office of Regional Operations (HFC-100), U.S. Food and Drug Administration, 5600 Fishers Lane, Rockville, MD 20857; dated 20 August 1997.

National and International Standards and Guidelines

21. ISO 9000:2000 Quality Management Systems – Fundamentals and Vocabulary.
22. ISO 9001:2000 Quality Management Systems – Requirements.
23. ISO 9004:2000 Quality Management Systems – Guidelines for Process Improvement.
24. ISO 9000-3:1997 Guidelines for the Application of ISO9001:1994 to the Development, Supply and Maintenance of Computer Software. [Currently undergoing revision to align with ISO 9001:2000].
25. ISO 12207:1995 Information Technology – Software Lifecycle Processes.
26. The TickIT Guide issue 5. Using ISO 9001:2000 for Software Quality Management System Construction, Certification, and Continual Improvement.

Related Life Science Company SOPs

The following SOPs are intended to highlight key subject areas. These would need to be supplemented by lower level SOPs, in some cases, to cover specific topics.

27. Computerized Systems Validation SOP.
28. Electronic Records and Electronic Signatures Compliance SOP.
29. Personnel Training and Competency Reviews.
30. Documentation Control SOP.
31. Change Control SOP.
32. Data Back-Up, Archiving and Recovery SOP.
33. Disaster Recovery SOP.

Further Reading

34. de Claire, T. Computer System Validation: Controlling the Manufacturing Process, in *Pharmaceutical Process Validation, International Third Edition*, R.A. Nash and A.H. Wachter, eds. Marcel Dekker, New York, 2003.
35. Coady, P.J. The Validation of SCADA Systems. Measurement + Control, *Journal of the Institute of Measurement and Control*, February 1998, Vol. 31, No. 1.
36. Coady, P.J., de Claire, A.P. Best Practice Engineering for Validation of Process Control Systems, *Pharmaceutical Engineering*, Vol. 15, No. 4, July/August 1995.
37. de Claire, T., Coady, P. Case Study 5: Control Instrumentation, in *Computer Systems Validation*, G. Wingate, ed., CRC Press, Boca Raton, FL, 2004.

Chapter 2

An Inspector's Viewpoint

Sam Clark

CONTENTS

INTRODUCTION

Control of any systems that impact the safety, quality, identity, purity, or potency of pharmaceutical products has long been expected under good manufacturing practice regulations (GMPs). This expectation extends to computer systems used in the pharmaceutical industry. Control of a computer system means:

- Thorough understanding of what functions the system is intended to perform.
- Ensuring that the system performs as intended.
- Monitoring the system performance within prescribed parameters.
- Recognizing when the system has exceeded the parameters.
- Taking appropriate corrective action when the system does not work as intended.

In other words, the basic expectation is the same for computer systems as for any other regulated system or process. The difference between computer systems and other systems is that computers are inherently more complex and thus control is more difficult to establish and maintain. This is especially true of the software component of computer systems.

Three critical activities for achieving and maintaining control of computer systems are quality design practices, well-planned hardware qualification and software validation, and effective change control. Quality design means carefully analyzing the solution to the problem by the computer system; determining the requirements the system must meet to solve the problem; and designing the system to meet those predefined requirements. Well-planned hardware qualification and software validation means carefully planning and executing the reviews, verifications, and testing needed to demonstrate to a high degree of confidence that:

- The computer performs according to the predefined requirements.
- The computer does not perform unintended functions.
- The computer system has been installed properly in its operating environment.

Effective change control means a planned process to ensure that the impact of any changes to the system is thoroughly evaluated before the changes are implemented, and that the system is appropriately revalidated to show the changes did not have an adverse impact.

This chapter will discuss the three critical control activities from a regulatory perspective. While the focus of this book is one control activity — the validation of computer systems — control cannot be achieved and maintained without careful attention to the related critical activities. The basic goal of validation is to achieve control of the system. This cannot be done if the system is poorly designed. Control cannot be maintained if the system is changed haphazardly.

This discussion will concentrate on the software validation. Hardware qualification is essentially the same process, though there is typically less work to hardware qualification because it is less complex and the work is frequently easier because qualification and validation of physical systems and processes are better understood by the industry. Furthermore, only the validation of applications software will be considered. Applications software is software that solves a specific problem for the pharmaceutical industry. All other software will be considered systems software. The U.S. Food and Drug Administration (FDA) made this distinction in its Compliance Policy Guide [1] where it stated, "applications software consists of programs written to specified user requirements for the purpose of performing a designated task such as process control, laboratory analyses, and acquisition/processing/storage of information required by cGMP regulations." In this same policy guide the FDA stated its intention not to inspect the validation of systems software, a policy that appears to have been adopted by other regulatory bodies covering the pharmaceutical industry.

The FDA policy should not be interpreted to mean system software could be used in an uncontrolled manner. For example, if changes are made to systems software, a company's application software must be evaluated in light of those changes. The application software would need appropriate revalidation to show that the changes to system software do not adversely impact the proper functioning of the applications. A formal process of change control must be applied to systems software, just as it is necessary for applications software. System software is the platform on which the applications that solve a specific problem are built. An effective applications software validation will demonstrate that the underlying platform is performing as intended.

This chapter will not make a distinction between software systems developed by the pharmaceutical industry, those systems developed by contractors to the industry, or COTS (configurable off-the-shelf software). There is no difference in the control activities expected for these software systems by the regulatory authorities if the software is categorized as applications software. The answer to the question of whether an applications software system should be validated does not depend on who developed the system or where the system was obtained. The only important information is exactly how the system is used. It is often true that only the software vendor can successfully execute some of the required tasks. However, regulatory authorities hold the regulated industry responsible for ensuring the quality and performance of all systems used in the manufacture of healthcare products. From a regulatory viewpoint, it is irrelevant who performed the required tasks, as long as that performance was adequately documented.

The following discussion is not intended to cover all the tasks necessary to accomplish the critical control activities effectively. It will focus on the most important tasks as they are normally seen from the viewpoint of a regulatory auditor. Some practical aspects of these tasks will be presented in the other chapters of this book.

DESIGN

The design and documentation of computer hardware essentially follows the same process as the design of other manufacturing equipment. Once it is determined that an automated system will be part of the manufacturing process, a specification should be prepared defining the functions the hardware must perform and providing the criteria to determine if the hardware is performing adequately. Controlled documents, such as engineering drawings, should be prepared and approved showing the actual layout of the system. This should include any computer networks involved in the process. There is little difference in documentation requirements between the design of automated systems, from a hardware perspective, and the engineering of any other physical system, such as a water system or environmental control system.

On the other hand, the software component of automated systems is frequently viewed as not requiring the same rigorous engineering as hardware. One possible reason for this incorrect belief is the fact that software is a logical construct without physical substance, other than the necessary documentation that is an integral part of any software program. Another contributing factor to this mistaken thinking is the relative ease with which a software system can be changed. Since software changes can be made relatively easily compared to the problems of changing physical systems, it is often incorrectly assumed that the engineering of such systems can be more informal, and that any problems can always be just as easily corrected later. This assumption neglects the fact that a computer program is a complex system with many possible interdependencies and internal interfaces. It neglects the critical fact that all changes to a software system are design modifications. This makes it very difficult to make changes without unintended consequence or side effects elsewhere in the program.

Software that impacts the safety, quality, identity, purity, or potency of pharmaceutical products must be developed in accordance with a defined engineering process, commonly called a software life cycle model. The model chosen can be the one that works best for the particular developer or project. Regardless of the model chosen, the activities needed to implement it should be defined in written, approved procedures. Those procedures should define the process in sufficient detail so that it can be executed in a controlled, consistent manner.

A defined software engineering process is required if the pharmaceutical manufacturer develops its own software. The pharmaceutical manufacturer is also required to assure that any software vendors it uses to develop applications software have such a defined process. It can be useful to define a software life cycle model even if the company will use only vendor-supplied software systems. The purpose of doing this is not to force software vendors to follow a process defined by others. Rather, the definition gives that pharmaceutical user a baseline from which to evaluate the engineering processes used by their vendors. By relating what the vendor is doing to the pharmaceutical user's understanding of good engineering practices, the pharmaceutical company will be in a better position to explain to regulatory authorities why it has confidence that its vendors can provide software systems that perform the intended functions accurately and reliably. An assumption that software vendors know good software engineering because they have been developing software for a period of time is incorrect, and unacceptable to regulatory authorities. In addition, such a well-defined software engineering process can provide the basis for the written audit plans required for vendors' user audits.

The chosen life cycle should be defined in written, approved procedures that define the life cycle in sufficient detail, allowing the process to be followed consistently, monitored, and controlled. It is not uncommon to find procedures that provide only a general outline of the intended software engineering process. Such procedures may list some phases for the software project, but fail to define:

- The specific tasks to be accomplished in each phase.
- The inputs to each phase of the model and the deliverables to the next phase.

- Clear criteria that can be used to evaluate the thoroughness and quality of the execution of each phase in the process.

A written procedure is a specification for a process. One critical purpose in writing procedures is to provide the metric by which process execution can be consistently measured and controlled. The more precise the metric, the tighter the control, and the higher the quality of the process output. When procedures are written to allow for unplanned variation in the process without the need for formal change control, a critical purpose of preparing the procedures is defeated. Such procedures indicate to an auditor not only that the process is not well controlled, but also that the company's change control process may be ineffective. That is because two frequent causes of such unspecific procedures are failure to take the time to adequately plan the process or desire to allow for process variations without going through the change control process.

Regulatory agencies do not expect that an engineering process can be repeatedly executed without variation. However, they do expect that unplanned variations will be recognized and appropriate action taken. A clear, precise metric ensures that such variations will be recognized.

The most critical activity in any software engineering project is the analysis and preparation of written requirements for the software. These are the documents that define the intended function of the system, and they are frequently referred to by regulatory bodies as the system specifications. However, they use the term specifications in a broad sense to cover both requirements and design specifications. This is because the regulatory authorities do not prescribe the specific engineering process; they only demand a planned process, sufficient to support the required quality, effectiveness, and reliable maintenance of the system. However, this discussion will separate requirements from design specifications because they are two distinct engineering phases, distinct sets of documents that serve two different purposes. Also, the quality of the second phase and its attendant documents, design specifications, is almost totally dependent on the quality of the first phase requirements.

Requirements are the documents that define the intended system from a user perspective. It is almost irrelevant how the system will accomplish intended functions at this stage. What is important is that the problem that the system is intended to solve is analyzed and thoroughly defined, and that all the requirements for solution are clearly described. The system developers then take these requirements and prepare design specifications that describe precisely how the system will be designed to fulfill the requirements. It is not always possible to keep the *what* totally separate from the *how*, and regulatory authorities do not traditionally worry over this distinction. It is important to keep the distinction in mind during the engineering process because of the close dependence of the design quality on how well the problem was analyzed and on the quality of the requirements.

Unfortunately, the most common cause of poor software design and inadequate software validation is poor requirements. Poor requirements cripple the software project from the beginning, leading to poorly designed software systems that perform unintended functions, do not meet the user's needs, and are difficult and expensive to maintain. The costs of using the system over time increases in direct proportion to the quality of the requirements. Poor requirements mean that the software cannot be validated since the intended function has not been adequately defined. Much validation testing is often done against poor requirements, but that testing does little to raise confidence in the accurate, consistent performance of the software and is, for the most part, wasted effort.

The IEEE Software Engineering Standard 830 [4] for software requirements lists seven characteristics for a good requirement document:

1. Unambiguous.
2. Complete.
3. Verifiable.
4. Consistent.
5. Modifiable.
6. Traceable.
7. Useable during the operation and maintenance phase.

Although all of these characteristics are important, this chapter will discuss four that are key to good software validation — unambiguous, complete, verifiable, and traceable. Failure to ensure that the software requirements possess these characteristics continues to be the most frequent cause for the poor quality of software validation projects and for poor functioning of the software system itself.

A complete software requirements document defines all of the software's intended functions. This is why a thorough analysis of the solution to the problem is so important. The problem is the improvement to the process desired by the addition of a computer system and the other components of the process with which the computer system must interface. When the exact nature of the problem is truly understood, it is much easier to determine precisely what functions will be performed by software and those performed by other processes or personnel. Once the software system functions are determined, it is important to carefully capture the details of all of the intended functionality, including:

- What data the program needs to perform the functions.
- Where that data will come from.
- What validity checking of input and output data should be performed by the software.
- What kinds of error messages are needed by the users so that they may effectively monitor the program.
- What kind of performance characteristics, such as speed, storage capacity, number of simultaneous users, etc. are required.

Determining if a requirements document is complete is quite straightforward for a regulatory auditor. Numerous sources, such as user interviews, operator manuals and procedures, observation of operation, etc., are available to the auditor to determine what functions the software is expected to execute. The auditor then simply requests to see the written definition of selected functionality in the software requirements.

An unambiguous requirement is one that can be interpreted in only one way, the way the author of the requirements intended. Because the exact meaning of normal human language can be notoriously vague, great care must be exercised to define each requirement with sufficient precision to ensure its correct understanding. All too often the requirements documents available define the intended function only at a high level. For example, the requirement may say that the program should automatically perform some calculation, but never define the equation or method that the program should use. It is not uncommon to find a requirement that says the program should typically do some function without ever defining the precise criteria the program will need to determine when it "typically" should, and "typically" should not, execute some action. Such a requirement is absurd since a software system can only perform a function differently over time when it has clear decision criteria for determining when to do it one way and when to do it another. These often lead to the software developer making assumptions about what was intended and those assumptions are all too often incorrect. Such requirements lead to pointless validation testing since many different, and sometimes incompatible, test results could be interpreted as verification of an ambiguous requirement.

A requirement is verifiable if there is some finite process by which a person or machine can demonstrate that the software meets the requirement. The requirements characteristics of unambiguous and verifiable are closely related. A requirement must be written in objective, measurable terms to define a verification process and to recognize when compliance is adequately verified.

A requirements document is traceable if it has been formatted such that each requirement is identified and can be easily and precisely referenced in other documents. Such traceability can make it clear what each item in the design specification is based on and why the item is in the document. This helps assure that the software is designed to perform all of the required functions. Such traceability allows the validation protocols to reference the requirement or requirements that each test case or set of test cases or visual observation is designed to verify. This helps assure that all requirements are verified.

Failure of a requirements document to possess any of the first three critical characteristics — complete, unambiguous, and verifiable — means that the system is not validated. Failure to possess the fourth characteristic — traceable — means it is highly probable that the validation is incomplete since the likelihood of unverified requirements is high. The regulatory auditor supports a conclusion of incomplete validation by finding examples of requirements that were not adequately verified.

One more consideration during the design of software systems is the quality of all the software documentation. The object code, that part of the software system that the computer can understand, is only a small component. The system includes:

- The source code (remember that source code is written to be read by people, not computers).
- The requirement.
- The design specifications.
- The user's manuals.
- All other documents created to record what the system was meant to do, how the system was designed, and how it should be used.

It is never too early to design this complex, interrelated set of documents for ease of use.

Document ease of use means that personnel who need to use the document can accurately and relatively quickly find the required information. Making the software documentation easy to use provides several benefits. The most important is that the documentation becomes more useful during system maintenance. When changes are made to a software system, it is important not only to understand the change made but also to understand the impact of the change on the rest of the system. Clear, useable documentation makes this task easier and more effective. It increases the likelihood that maintenance personnel will use the documents rather than leap to assumptions about the way the system functions. This can lower the costs of the software considerably over its operational lifetime and lead to a safer system. Since the documentation must be created, personnel should take the time to make the documentation as useful as possible. Otherwise, it will be created only to satisfy a regulation and there will truly be little or no return on investment.

Another benefit of easy-to-use documentation is the positive impact on regulatory inspections. When company personnel can produce any requested information efficiently, inspections are completed faster. Such effective use of documentation produces a strong impression of a system under control. That can have a positive impact on how long the regulatory agent takes to inspect the system.

It is tempting to rely on the software developer to write the requirements. As mentioned in the introduction to this chapter, the regulatory authorities do not address who must prepare the required documents, but consider whose problem will be solved by the proposed system and where the process experts reside who can best determine the requirements the system needs to meet in order to solve the problem. Thorough analysis of the problem and development of system requirements establish system control at the proper point — the beginning.

Consider who is in the best position to determine how critical individual requirements are to overall problem solution. Thorough analysis of the problem and development of system requirements allows the company to make decisions about compromises in functionality more effectively, especially when the software is purchased from a vendor. When no available software meets all the requirements, what can be done? There are a number of valid alternatives, but it is critical to system control that the user knows precisely what was done, why it was done, and what constraints might be imposed by the selected alternative.

VALIDATION

The key document that must be developed for a validation project, software or otherwise, is a validation protocol. The U.S. FDA defined a validation protocol this way in 1987 in the document *Guideline on General Principles of Process Validation* [5], "Validation protocol — A written plan stating how validation will be conducted, including test parameters, product characteristics, production equipment, and decision points on what constitutes acceptable test results." The guideline also states, "It is important that the manufacturer prepare a written validation protocol which specifies the procedures (and tests) to be conducted and the data to be collected. The purpose for which data are collected must be clear; the data must reflect facts and be collected carefully and accurately." The FDA reiterated and expanded on this definition in proposed amendments to the cGMPs in 1996 [6]. That document defined a protocol as, "*Validation protocol* means a written plan describing the process to be validated, including production equipment, and how validation will be conducted, including objective test parameters, product and/or process characteristics, predetermined specifications, and factors which will determine acceptable results."

The most common problem with validation protocols is that they are not precise. The validation protocol should clearly indicate what each test case or set of test cases is designed to show, specifically how the verifications should be conducted, and exactly what should occur for each. Validation testing must be carefully planned. It is not up to the test personnel to determine during the test execution what test cases should be used. The protocol should specify this. For example, if an error message is tested to show that the message is displayed when a variable exceeds 25, the test protocol should not instruct personnel to enter some value greater than 25. Such instructions often lead to test personnel selecting some random value that frequently does nothing to verify precise performance by the software of the required function. Rather, it should provide the specific values to use, for example, 25 and 26 if the expected level of precision is integer.

A protocol is a specific procedure for a specific validation study. It must define, in detail, how to carry out the testing. It can be important that the testing follow a specific sequence, since actions taken during a previous test may be necessary to set the machine state for the current test. For a protocol to be useful during revalidation of a system, it is necessary that the test conditions, such as test inputs, or expected outputs, etc. are clearly defined. Note that a good validation protocol, or portions of the protocol, can often be used following software changes to show that the changes have not adversely impacted the software system. This task is commonly known as regression testing.

Another frequent failure of validation protocols is that they do not define adequate test cases designed to find software errors. Since it is not possible to prove that a computer program of any complexity is correct, it is important to raise confidence in the system's ability to perform required tasks accurately and reliably, to look diligently for errors in the programs, i.e., where the program does not behave as required or performs some unintended or unexpected action. The more rigorously the validation protocols are designed to look for such errors, the higher the confidence that the software performs as intended.

The types of test cases that find errors in software include boundary value testing, testing of invalid data inputs, and testing of special values. Boundary value testing means choosing test cases exactly at the maximum and minimum value of the defined valid range, and choosing test cases just outside the valid range for the requirement under test. Invalid values are those that could be input to the system, either intentionally or unintentionally, but which are invalid for the operation. For example, alpha characters might be entered when numeric data are expected from input on a standard computer keyboard. Special values are those with special meaning to the operation undergoing verification and should always be tested. Examples of special values are "0" and "null" entries. Zero can often have special meaning for some computations performed by computers. A "null" entry simply means a return key is hit when the program is expecting some data entry.

This type of testing gives the highest likelihood of finding errors that remain in the system. Simply testing expected values will never prove the system is correct. Such values also are of limited use in finding any remaining errors. These kinds of test values raise confidence in the system by showing that whole classes of values should run properly. Routine, expected values really only eliminate that specific value from consideration when looking for errors in the system.

As with the software requirements documents, the validation protocols must be carefully designed and formatted to facilitate traceability to verify the requirements and specifications. In complex software system validation projects, this traceability is the only way of ensuring that all the requirements have been verified and that the execution of those verification tasks has indeed been adequate to produce a high degree of confidence that the system performs as intended.

A final important validation document is the validation report. While it is not unusual to find a report is generated at the conclusion of each of the planned validation phases, such as IQ (installation qualification), OQ (operational qualification), etc., at least one report must state the conclusions drawn from the validation project and summarize the support for them. It should describe any variations in the planned validation process, the kinds of anomalies or problems with the system found during validation, and what was done about these. The quality unit must approve the report, indicating that the project has been reviewed for compliance with validation plans and procedures, and that the system is approved for use in pharmaceutical manufacturing. If the system is rejected, the report should state what should be done to make it acceptable, if it is decided that the system will be used.

CHANGE CONTROL

Once a system or process has been validated, there are many tasks involved in the on-going evaluation and control of that system or process to keep it in a validated state. One of the most critical tasks is rigorous change control. This is an especially important task for software systems because, unlike hardware and other physical systems, all changes, for any reason, to software systems are design modifications. Design modifications result in a high probability of introduction of new errors to the system as a result of the change. The probability of such new problems increases dramatically as the complexity of the system increases and the quality of the system documentation decreases.

The change control process will be evaluated in almost every regulatory inspection of the computer system. This is not only because of the critical nature of the process, but also because it provides an excellent indicator of the quality of the software system and, thus, can help the regulatory inspector focus the audit on problem systems. A system that has been changed often was probably changed for a reason. This is often the result of poorly designed software, poorly understood requirements, or both. Poor quality is even more strongly indicated when there are patterns in the changes, such as changes to fix errors introduced during past changes.

Failure to recognize that any software change is a design modification also contributes to developing these modifications to a less stringent standard, and not adhering to good software engineering practice during development of the change. As the number of changes developed this way increases, the quality of the software rapidly decreases. The ability to make future changes without introducing new errors decreases until eventually the software system is no longer useable. The widely held belief that software systems improve over time as bugs are found and corrected is only valid for those systems that have had consistent, well-engineered modifications under rigorous change control. An effective change process is the only way to slow the almost inevitable degradation of the software system.

A common failure of change control processes is inconsistent use of change categories. It is almost inevitable that companies will have different categories of changes that demand different levels of change or validation activities based on perceived importance of the change. For example, one common categorization is major, minor, and emergency. There is no regulatory prohibition against such categorization of changes. The failure occurs when the change control procedures do not provide adequate criteria for each category to help ensure consistent categorization of changes. This usually leads to numerous, debatable "minor" changes. Because minor changes usually mean less work, they are popular with personnel who will look for reasons to support the desired conclusion that the change is minor instead of objectively evaluating it. Since the procedure often provides little that would prevent such classification, which in turn means there is small likelihood that later quality review will correct inconsistent classifications, nothing prevents personnel from falling into this trap. Bear in mind that the most basic technique used by any auditor is to look for and question inconsistency in process execution.

As the number of poorly-understood and poorly-designed minor changes grows, the ability to maintain the software system is lessened. Eventually, the system cannot be maintained and its usefulness ends. With great good luck, the end of the software's useful life is all that happens. The change control process should be designed and defined with the goal of preventing this system degradation as much as possible.

Another common problem with change control processes is the failure to track all change requests to closure. Closure means that each change request is evaluated and the change is implemented or rejected. One way to obtain feedback on the quality control of a system or process is through periodic review of the changes that have been requested. This includes rejected changes. For example, if a change has been rejected and later, additional requests are made for the same or similar changes, this is a good indication that a problem exists somewhere and it may not necessarily be with the computer system. It could be in the procedures for using the system, it could be in the training provided to users, or it could be that there is actually a user expectation that the system does not meet, etc. Such useful data will be lost if change requests are not tracked to closure. This loss is in addition to the very real regulatory risk that important changes will disappear in the change control system and not be implemented in a timely manner.

The software system must be appropriately revalidated following any changes. Appropriate revalidation means validating that the change performs according to its requirement, and that the software system as a whole still performs according to its requirements. This includes any modifications in the system requirements necessitated by the change. The amount of work involved in this revalidation depends on the complexity of the change, the software system as a whole, the quality of the software design and documentation, and the quality of the baseline system validation. That more work would be required to validate more complex changes is obvious. But it is also likely to be more difficult to revalidate after changes, as the software system becomes more complex. This is because of the increased interdependence of different parts of complex software systems — a change in one place is more likely to cause effects elsewhere in the system. The software documentation impacts the ability of maintenance personnel to understand the possible effects of their changes on the remainder of the software system. The baseline validation, or initial complete system validation, provides increased knowledge about specifically how the system functions, once again, making it easier for change developers to design effective modifications without undesired side-effects. The only appropriate revalidation if one cannot demonstrate this level of understanding of the software system, is completely validating the system after each modification. One important return on investment from a good, well documented validation project is the reduction in revalidation effort.

Regardless of the level of revalidation executed following changes, it is important to record the justification for the amount of revalidation chosen. Every step of revalidation is always subject to question by regulatory authorities. It is usually difficult to remember complex details and reasoning months or years afterwards. Good documentation of the rationale for such decisions leaves any personnel who must face regulatory authorities in a more comfortable position.

CLOSING REMARKS

Two popular myths about the validation of computer systems seem to have persisted over the 20 or more years since regulatory authorities began inspecting computer systems. The first is that a system is validated because it is widely used or has been used for many years, i.e., validation through use. The second myth is that the system can be considered compliant if the regulatory authorities do not have objections during inspections. Belief in either of these myths will lead a company into a false sense of security.

Validation of a system or process is a scientific study. It should be designed to find flaws in the theory that the system or process performs its intended function accurately and reliably. The more closely the computer system complies with its requirements in the face of such a concerted effort to reveal the flaws, the higher the confidence that the system or process can be controlled. A critical characteristic of any scientific study is that it can be independently verified, i.e., it is reproducible. Simply using the system for a long time, or the knowledge that many people have used the system, does not lead to clearly documented, reproducible evidence. There are simply too many variations in exactly how a computer system is used by different users, and in what it is used for, to draw justifiable conclusions from, normally poorly documented, system use. In addition, normal system use does not intentionally seek to find system flaws. If it did, many of the most popular software programs used by business today would be validated and thus performing their intended functions accurately and reliably. Anyone who has used a computer system running the more popular operating systems software and business applications can refute that conclusion.

The second myth, that failure of the regulatory authorities to object to a system equates to regulatory acceptance, tacitly assumes that all systems and processes are reviewed by the regulatory agents, in detail, during each inspection. It also assumes that the system or process will continue to be used in exactly the same way over its useful life or, at least, that it has not changed since the last inspection. Modern manufacturing processes are too complex for either of these assumptions to hold true. A regulatory inspection is a sample taken at a point in time. It is limited by any number of variables, including the inspector's specific knowledge of the systems and processes covered during the inspection. A different inspector will approach the same system from a different viewpoint, with different background knowledge, will sample the documents in different ways, and find different problems. Belief in this myth often leads to failure to devote the time and effort to continuous improvement of the system under the assumption that it is acceptable as is to the regulatory bodies. This frequently leads to relaxing control of the system so that the resources can be used elsewhere. Any company that has undergone severe regulatory sanctions can testify that reestablishing that control once lost is an expensive, resource-intensive job.

The following chapters will provide some practical considerations for individual tasks involved in the validation of computer systems. This chapter has tried to provide an overview of minimum regulatory expectations. All healthcare companies are encouraged to far exceed these minimum expectations. The benefits of continuous improvement in the quality of computer system development and validation are many, and include:

- Software systems of higher quality that perform as the user intended and expects, and that do surprise the user with unintended actions.
- Lower development costs by catching problems early in the development cycle, when they are easier and less expensive to correct.
- Systems that are better understood and, thus, better controlled.
- More effective, less expensive software maintenance.
- Software systems with longer useful lives.

The more complex the system, the more difficult it is to establish and maintain control. But failure to establish and maintain control of the system is simply not acceptable when the ultimate product of the manufacturing processes impacts human lives in so critical a fashion as do healthcare products.

REFERENCES

1. Title 21 Code of Federal Regulations, Part 210 and 211, Current Good Manufacturing Practices (cGMP) in Manufacturing, Processing, Packing, or Holding of Drugs and Finished Pharmaceuticals.
2. Title 21 Code of Federal Regulations, Part 11, Electronic Records; Electronic Signatures.
3. U.S. Food & Drug Administration Compliance Policy Guide, Section 425.100.
4. ANSI-IEEE Std 830-1984, IEEE Guide to Software Requirements Specifications, The Institute of Electrical & Electronic Engineers, 345 East 47th Street, New York, NY 10017.
5. Guideline on General Principles of Process Validation, Center for Drugs and

Biologics, & Center For Devices and Radiological Health, Food and Drug Administration, May 1987.

6. Federal Register, Vol. 61, No. 87, Friday, May 3, 1996. Proposed Rules; Current Good Manufacturing Practice; Proposed Amendment of Certain Requirements for Finished Pharmaceuticals.

Chapter 3

State-of-the-Art Risk Assessment and Management

John Andrews

CONTENTS

INTRODUCTION

To understand risk assessment one must first understand the meaning of taking risks. “Combination of the probability of occurrence of harm and the severity of that harm.” Taking risks means that you deliberately undertake an action that is, in essence, not safe, understanding the consequences if you get it wrong. Safe means nothing adverse will happen to you if you do nothing. In other words you compare the odds to doing something against the odds of not doing something, and because they are in your favor to a large degree, which will be discussed later, to move forward, hoping you are right.

This may sound a bit risky when put it like that, but do not be too concerned. We do this all the time and a vast majority of people make it through life without too many hitches. In fact “man” has only evolved out of the caves because of his ability to take risks and win. The secret to getting this right is to be careful which bets to make. Take the civil aviation industry; it employs a maintenance management approach, which is shared across the globe that enables it to keep a whole fleet of aircraft in the air safely without large amounts of downtime. But remember when it goes wrong we all get to hear about it, because the results are so catastrophic.

How does it do this? It all comes down to risk assessment and management of component failure. This requires tremendous discipline and you must stand by your decisions, even if it means letting down a whole planeload of angry passengers who want to board a plane home when returning from their holiday in the Canaries at 2:00 A.M. because the public address system does not work.

In this chapter we review a selection of different formal techniques, look at their strengths and weaknesses, and discuss the potential application to the healthcare industry when applied to the validation of computerized systems.

Whatever the process selected it is essential to document both the approach and the conclusions. When asked, possibly years later, about how a decision was reached not to challenge test something, then it must be clear how the decision was reached.

RISK ASSESSMENT TECHNIQUES

Failure Mode Effect Analysis (FMEA)

Introduction

Failure mode effect analysis (FMEA) is a structured method to study a "product" design or "process" to anticipate and minimize unwanted performance or unexpected failures, or what could go wrong even if the process or product meets the specifications.

Key component activities include:

- Determine possible defects.
- Determine undesired events that can occur.
- Quantify "risk."
- Identify corrective action in product and process design to mitigate the "risk."

FMEA was first developed originally by the defense and the aviation industries in the early 1940s. Later the automotive industries started to use it in the 1970s followed by the semiconductor and the consumer health industries in the 1980 and 1990s. ISO has even referenced it in ISO–14971 Application of Risk Management to Medical Devices.

Method

The first steps involve drawing and defining your process, e.g., developing a process flow diagram defining the inputs and outputs and the interfaces to other systems. Then define some performance characteristics, such as throughput of a machine, number of transactions per minute, etc. Finally, you must differentiate between process and subprocess operations. They should be written in terms of functions or items listed.

You are now ready to start to complete the evaluation chart (Figure 3.1). This chart will ask a number of questions relating to the listed functions or items you previously documented. The first question asks you to list the potential failure modes for each listed function or item. For each failure mode you must then ask what would be the effect of each failure in the operation condition. The process continues until you have identified a risk and defined a priority to resolving it. This often results in a redesign for the higher priority issues or extra testing for the medium defined issues and maybe a reduction in testing or validation effort for the lower priority issues.

The chart is completed by asking the following questions and populating the chart (shown in Figure 3.1) with the responses to each question.

Item/ Function	Potential failure mode	Potential effect of failure	Severity	Potential cause of failure	Occurrence	Current controls	Detection	RPN

Figure 3.1 Evaluation chart.

- Function or item:
  - Description of process or operation performed.
  - Differentiate between process and subprocess operations.
- Potential failure modes:
  - Elements in which process could potentially fail to meet process requirements or design intent.
  - Description of nonconformances related to the specific operations.
- Potential effects of failure:
  - Effects of a failure mode on the end-user of process operation or the product.
  - Defined in terms of product and system performance.
- Severity:
  - Assessment of the seriousness of the effect of the potential failure mode to the product.
  - Severity applies only to the "effect" number or scaled value 1–10 ranking correlating to "no issue" up to "hazardous," or low to high.
- Potential cause of failure:
  - "Mechanism" as to how the failure could occur.
  - Describe relative to the element that can be controlled or mitigated.
- Occurrence:
  - Frequency that the specific failure "cause" is "projected" to occur.
  - Only occurrence resulting in a failure mode should be considered.
  - Failure detection measures are not captured here.
  - Number or scaled value 1–10 ranking correlating to "remote" up to "very high likelihood" or low to high.
  - Correlate from process capability or possible failure rates.
- Current process controls:
  - Controls or measures that either prevent the failure mode from occurring or mechanism to detect the failure mode occurrence.

- Detection:
  - Assessment of the probability that the proposed process controls will detect the potential failure mode.
  - Number or scaled value 1–10 ranking correlating to "almost certain" up to "almost impossible."
- Risk priority number (RPN):
  - The RPN is the product of severity, occurrence, detection (RPN = severity multiplied by the occurrence multiplied by the likelihood of detection).

Once the process has been completed and actions and responsibilities for reducing risks have been employed, the whole process must be completed to ensure that the resultant actions have reduced the actual original perceived risks.

Strengths

The benefits of FMEA applied to the development and validation computerized system are as follows.

- Identifies key critical and significant characteristics of a design.
- Identifies potential deficiencies of design parameters for the integrated system.
- Identifies potential design related failure modes within a system, subsystem, or component level which adversely affect product achieving specification requirements.
- Provides reference to aid in analyzing "issues" in future designs.
- Provides objective evaluation of design requirements and alternatives.
- Aids in determining, evaluating, and improving design verification tests.
- Provides organized, structured, systematic approach to identify potential affects on subsystem assembly and failure modes.
- Identifies potential systemic failure modes caused by system interaction with other systems or subsystems.
- Aids in determining if redundancy is required in order to meet the reliability requirements.

Weaknesses

The FMEA process is very methodical and can tie up resources for some time, very heavy-going for a novice, so the process must be facilitated by an expert. All practitioners must be trained to understand the process and the objectives. There must be a clear business benefit or objective established before the process starts to ensure the process is focused.

The process can take on a life of its own, i.e., it can grow to include subcomponent or functional elements, so be clear at what level you apply this tool, i.e., it is best applied to the requirements level as opposed to the module code level of a computerized system. Be clear regarding the boundaries and scope of the review. Because this tool is very methodical it will ask questions relating to interfaces to other systems, so ensure you close out these links with either an action to review these systems later or with an individual assessment relating to the likely impact of not evaluating that interface.

Failure Mode Effect Cause Analysis (FMECA)

Introduction

Failure mode effect *cause* analysis (FMECA) is exactly what its name indicates: it is FMCA but looks for the reasons for the failure to enable focused resolution. The process itself follows the same rules as FMCA, then introduces a step looking at the components failure and the effect in a production environment or within software, the inputs to a function that result in that function not performing as intended.

Strengths and Weaknesses

FMECA benefits include those for FMCA but add on the ability to focus resolution on the causes. The process is very powerful with this step included: it allows for design corrections and focused testing to ensure correct performance etc.

Hazard Analysis Critical Control Points (HACCP)

Introduction

Hazard analysis critical control points (HACCP) is a management tool used for a systematic approach to the identification, evaluation, and control of hazards. It is designed to be a preventive tool, not reactive methodology. In other words, it must be utilized to identify hazards in advance. HACCP is not a zero-risk method; it is primarily designed to minimize the risks of hazards. Its focus is on the strength of "controls" for the risk hazards. Its application should be on cross-functional system design via audits utilizing preplanned corrective actions.

HACCP was originally developed by the chemical industry in the 1940s and 1950s, then pioneered in the 1960s in the U.S. space program food development. Adopted by many food processing companies and even the U.S. government, HACCP-like systems are now used by many other industries. The FDA Medical Device Quality System Regulation recommends that the HACCP approach be adopted by all regulatory agencies and should be mandatory for all food processors, e.g., the FDA enforcement in seafood and juice industries (ASQ CQA-HACCP).

In order to perform a HACCP analysis it is important to understand some key terms.

Term	Description
Hazard	Condition that results in an adverse consequence detrimental user and safety, either actual or potential.
Hazard analysis	Identification of hazards and their initiating causes.
Control point	Any point, step, or procedure at which a variable, parameter, or quality factor can be controlled within established specifications.
Critical control point	A point, step, or procedure at which control can be applied and is essential to prevent, eliminate or reduce a hazard to an acceptable level.
Critical limits	A maximum or minimum value to which a product, process or quality parameter must be controlled at a critical control point (CCP) to prevent, eliminate, or reduce to an acceptable level the occurrence of the hazard.

Method

The first action is as previously discussed for FMEA and FMECA methodologies, to define your process by developing an overview of each process step. Then a team of experts conducts a hazard analysis on each of these process steps in an attempt to determine the CCPs. Once the CCPs have been determined then you must:

- Establish critical limits.
- Monitor each CCP.
- Establish corrective actions.
- Establish verification procedures.
- Establish record-keeping and documentation procedures.

There is also an evaluation form to assist in the process (Figure 3.2). This asks all the relevant questions to enable the team to fully exploit the risk areas and a suitable mitigation strategy:

- Identify processing steps and identify materials and components.
- Identify potential product hazards. These may be:
  - Process introduced product hazards.
  - Process controlled product hazards.

Material/ components processing steps	Identify potential hazards introduced, controlled, or enhanced at this step	Are any potential safety hazards significant? (Yes/No?)	Justify your decision for column 3	What preventative measures can be applied to prevent the significant hazard?	Is this step a CCP? (Yes/No?)

Figure 3.2 Hazards from the hazard analysis worksheet.

  - Process enhanced product hazards.
- Determine significance of potential safety hazards. Information is transferred from severity column on the hazard table.
  - "Yes" for potential significant hazard.
  - "No" for nonsignificant hazard.
- Provide rationale and justify your decision for column 3.
  - Response required if column 3 is "no."
  - Response desirable but not required if column 3 is "yes."
- Identify "preventative measures" to prevent significant hazards.
  - Identify controls that are in place.
  - Identify quality systems that are in place.
- Determine if this step is a CCP?
  - The team may choose to use a CCP decision tree process (Figure 3.3), discussed next.

Each critical control point is then transferred to the corrective action form to evaluate the required actions and confirm activities necessary to verify that the risk has been reduced (Figure 3.4).

- Transfer the CCPs and significant hazards from the hazard analysis worksheet to the HACCP plan form.
- Identify and insert the "critical limits" for each CCP.
- Identify those "controls" that are in place for "monitoring" the CCP.
- Identify those corrective actions that are in place in the event that the monitoring elements "fail."
- Identify preplanned corrective action for each CCP:
  - Assess the adequacy of the controls that are in place to mitigate the hazard upon occurrence.

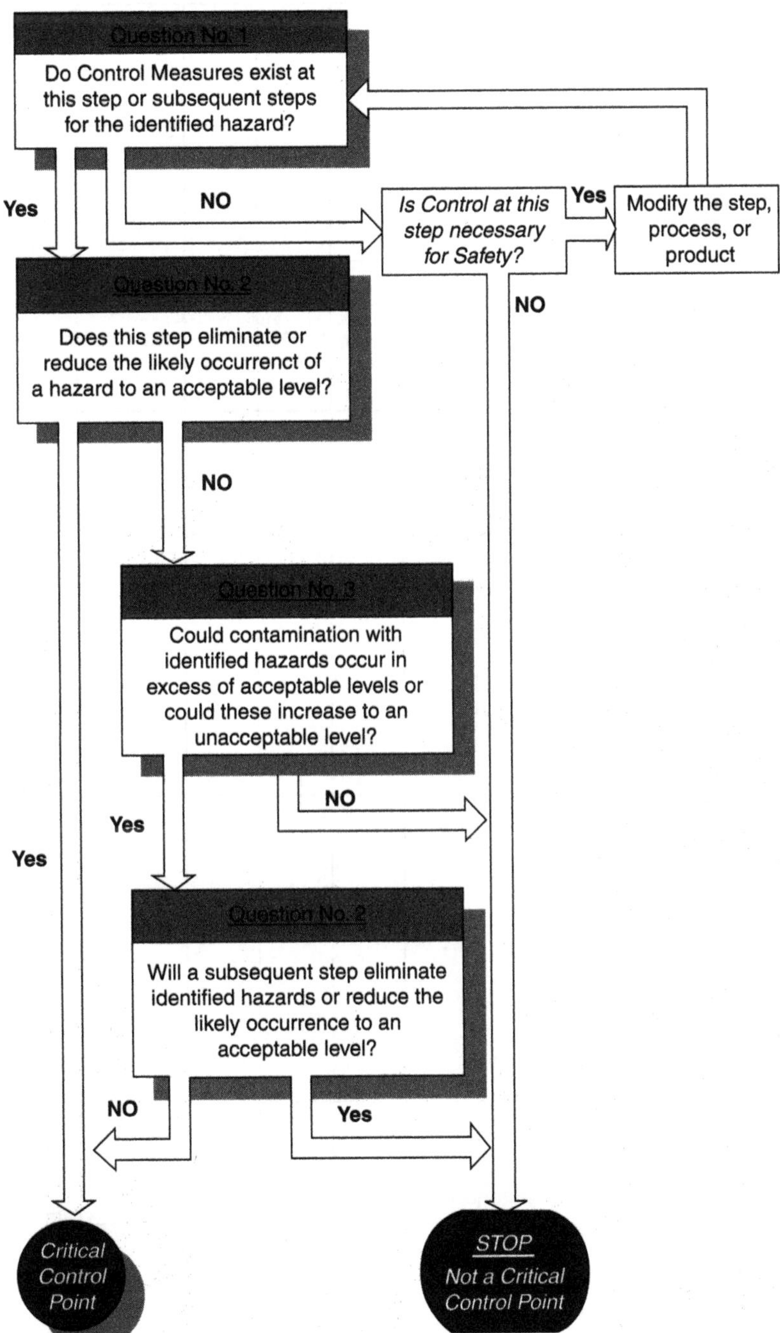

Figure 3.3 CCP decison tree process.

1 Critical control point (CCP)	2 Significant hazard	3 Critical limits for each preventive measure	4 Monitoring	5	6	7	8 Corrective action(s)	9 Verification	10 Records
			What	How	Frequency	Who			

Figure 3.4 HACCP plan form.

  - Determine the strength of controls.
  - Determine whether other controls may be needed.
  - Determine remediation activities that may be required.
- Specify the verification "procedures" or mechanism for each CCP.
- Specify the record-keeping procedures, outputs, documents for each CCP.

Remaining activities include:

- Review.
- Approval.
- Document control.
- Periodic reevaluation.

Strengths

The strength of this process lies in the simplicity of application and documentation. The process allows for cross-functional system interface and assessment, with the focus on the risks and the actions needed to control or mitigate them. The process relies on what you have now in terms of the system or process current design or performance to identify the relevant resolution actions.

Weaknesses

This approach was developed to control food manufacture, therefore, during analysis, you could find that parts of the methodology may not be appropriate to computerized systems in the pharmaceutical industry. Training in the techniques is required to ensure correct application. The process requires auditing to manage resolution of identified issues, so resources are needed to perform these actions.

Fault Tree Analysis (FTA)

Introduction

Fault tree analysis (FTA) is used to identify and analyze conditions and factors that cause or contribute to the occurrence of a defined undesirable event. The methodology uses graphical depiction of pathways in a system or process which lead to an undesirable event or failure. It is a top-down assessment of interconnecting events and conditions using logic symbols. Analysis is via numerical probabilities or reliability factors to evaluate events or failures.

Sy	Description
	Top-level event
	Event — Event or fault that results from combination of more basic faults and that can be further developed
	"AND" Gate — Provides an output event only if all the input events occur
	"OR" Gate — Provides an output event if one or more of the input events are present or occur
	"INHIBIT" Gate — Conditional event where input produces output directly only when the conditional input is satisfied
	Undeveloped event — Event that is not developed further either because further development is of insufficient consequence or because the necessary info is unavailable
	Initiating event — Event that does not need further development. Type of event is independent of other events and indicated termination at that point

Figure 3.5 FTA Overview: commonly used components.

Again the principles were developed in the 1960s by Boeing and NASA via the Minuteman launch and control system. The principles were adopted by nuclear power industry in the 1970s to investigate the Three Mile Island accident. Also adopted by the chemical industry in the 1980s, and recently adopted in the PC and robotics industries (Figure 3.5).

The FTA process uses a graphic display of chains of events or conditions leading to a loss event. Identification of those potential contributors to failure, which are "critical" leads to improved understanding of system characteristics. The process uses qualitative and quantitative insight into probability of a loss event.

This process also helps the identification of resources committed to preventing failure and guidance for redeploying resources to optimize control of risk. The methodology allows for full documentation of analytical results (Figures 3.6 and 3.7).

Key steps

- Identify top level event.
- Identify "gates."
- Identify "next" level events.
- Repeat until identify "initiating event."

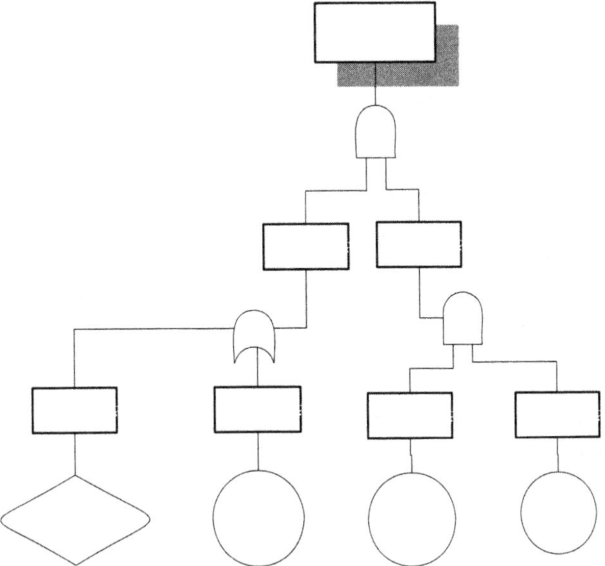

Figure 3.6 FTA overview: what it looks like...

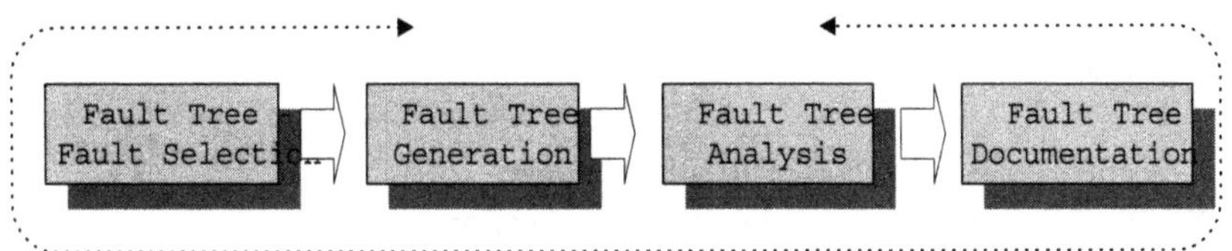

Figure 3.7 FTA process.

- Precursory steps.
  - Develop and verify process flow chart.
  - Identify process and product "characteristics."
  - Extract input information from design "risk assessment" data.
- Fault tree selection.
  - Identify product steps.
  - Identify process steps.
  - Identify process attributes.

- Fault tree generation.
  - Identify undesired outcomes, via brainstorming in groups, confirm via known events.
  - Refine undesired outcomes into groups, prioritize against known data.
  - Construct FTA.
- Fault tree analysis.
  - Conduct FTA using quantitative and qualitative analysis. Identify unique sets of events that together cause the top level event to occur. Confirm one of many root causes and the events that cause the top level event.
  - Qualitative and quantitative analysis asks logical questions relating to probability and reliability.
- Fault tree documentation.
  - Identify corrective actions.
  - Map critical events into process control diagrams.
  - Summarize findings.

Strengths

- Multiple potential contributors to a mishap or situation.
- Complex multielement systems or processes.
- Large perceived threats of loss (high risk).
- Already identified undesirable events.
- Lessons learned — "crisis autopsy."

Weaknesses

- Requires an understanding of Boolean algebra.
- Requires training and discipline in its application.

The GAMP Model

The GAMP version 4 risk assessment model is one of the best-known in the pharmaceutical industry, but it owes most of its content and method to FMCA and as such could be accused of being a little unwieldy for general use. This is because the review team needs to be fully trained in the methodology to successfully take part in a review, be clear about its objectives and ensure that objectives and boundaries are clearly defined. See the FMCA section for the benefits and weakness of the method.

GAMP 4 also recommends evaluation of systems construction using the GAMP software categories to identify the level of likely risk with the system development, e.g., for a system operating system (software category 1), then the risks of this performing incorrectly are relatively low because of the stable nature of such software products. Bespoke-developed code (software category 5) however, is more likely to contain errors. A more methodical approach to design and testing is therefore necessary. There are five software and two hardware categories within the GAMP Guide that provide guidance on their application to system development and the validation of such systems.

Other factors to be considered within the GAMP 4 guidance include the results of the impact the system will have on product quality. The supplier audit, the structure of the design documentation and the traceability of requirements can all be used to manage the risk inherent within the design of a computerized system.

APPLICATION TO THE VALIDATION OF COMPUTERIZED SYSTEMS

The application to risk assessment to the validation of computerized systems is becoming essential to ensure that valuable resourses are appropriately directed. Gone are the days when GMP meant "great mounds of paper" with the emphasis on documenting everything, just in case. Validation activities are increasingly regarded as a method to manage a project, rather than a bolt-on after the development activities are complete.

In the past there has been much debate and many misconceptions about validation. Some have maintained that a lot of the unnecessary costs associated with an automation project are attributable to validation effort required and, therefore, the validation effort should be reduced. Conversely, others have argued that more should be spent, because the costs of getting it wrong are potentially huge, with figures of 20–30% of the overheads cited. This has resulted in a seesaw approach to managing validation within projects, normally in response to regulatory interest, observations, and warning letters.

What seems to have been overlooked is that the amount spent on validation is not what counts — it is the quality of the workmanship of those individuals involved in system development, operation, and maintenance, and how that quality is recorded as documentary evidence.

A blend of risk assessment techniques should be used to ensure that relevant questions are asked at appropriate points in a system development to ensure that the risks are reduced and the design is captured in documentation at the appropriate level. These assumptions can then be fed into the validation or project planning cycle to ensure all activities are appropriate to the identified risks.

Figure 3.8 shows an example of the application of a risk-based approach to system testing during acceptance testing.

Risk grades should have been established for each design intention from the risk assessment of the user requirements and system design specifications. This will show what requirements are perceived to be high, medium, and low risk. This risk assessment should be reviewed to ensure that it is still appropriate for the built

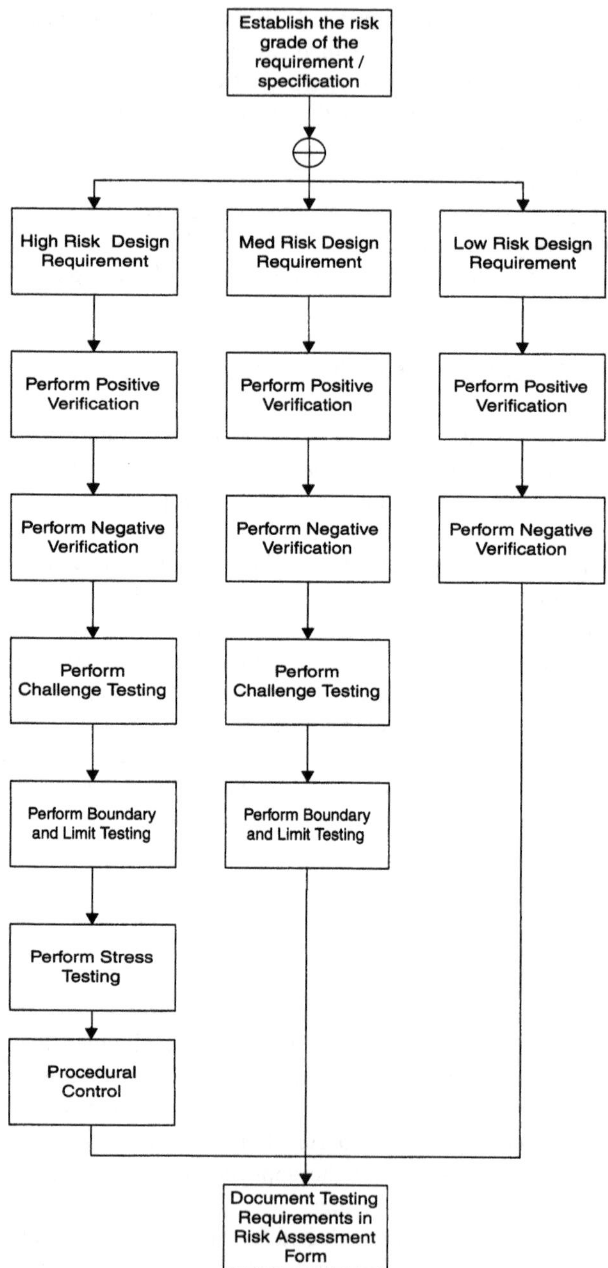

Figure 3.8 Risk-based approach to system testing.

system; if this assessment was incomplete, then risk grade should be established for the design. This can now be used to analyze the level of detail required within the testing phase of the life cycle.

Depending on the risk grade that has been established for the system design, mere verification testing may only assure that the system meets the specified design, but it might not ensure that the system is capable of consistently meeting those design intentions. Therefore extra procedural controls may need to be established to mitigate further risk within the organization.

RISK MANAGEMENT

The proposed method outlined below employs the use of risk assessments. These risk assessments are conducted at different levels of a system to determine the area in which to focus the validation effort. This suggested approach considers the likely impact on GxP. GxP is an industry term to cover the requirements of GMP, GLP, GDP, etc.

- High level to determine which of a company's systems impact on GxP.
- Lower level to determine the GxP impact of a subsystem.
- Assigning priorities.

This will help determine which functions require either redesigning or detailed confirmation and challenging, as opposed to just high-level confirmation and verification.

High-Level GxP Determination

The first step is to determine whether a system or subsystem represents a risk to GxP when assessed against a series of GxP questions. First, does a system impact on GxP?

System Impact Assessment

- Is the system used to monitor, control, or supervise a GxP drug manufacturing or packaging process?
- Is the system used for GxP analytical quality control?
- Is the system used to monitor, control, or supervise warehousing or distribution with a GxP implication?
- Does the system support the maintenance of GxP systems?
- Does the system manipulate data, or produce reports, to be used by GxP quality-related decision authorization or approval processes?

- Is the system used for GxP batch sentencing or batch records?

If the assessment of a system concludes that it does not impact on GxP then this decision should be documented on the assessment sheet.

This is followed up by a series of subsystem questions (if it is a business system application, replace "subsystem" with "functions"). These questions help determine how the subsystems or functions for any given system, deemed to have an impact on GxP, actually impact individually on GxP.

Subsystem Impact Assessment

- Is the subsystem used to demonstrate compliance with the registered process?
- Does normal operation or control of the subsystem have a direct effect on product quality?
- Will failure or alarm of the subsystem have a direct effect on product quality or efficacy?
- Is information from this subsystem recorded as part of the batch record, lot release data, or other GMP documentation?
- Does the subsystem interact with elements that come into contact with product or product components?
- Does the subsystem control critical process elements in such a way to affect product quality?

If the assessment of a particular subsystem or function determines that there is no risk to GxP, the justification for making this judgment should also be documented on the assessment sheet.

This process will provide a list of subsystems that can be assessed for their individual functional impact on GxP by using a risk assessment method.

Functional Risk Assessment

The methodology below uses FMECA and starts by asking eight very simple questions. These have been slightly modified to fit the healthcare industry's GxP requirements.

- *What are the major GxP functions and associated performance requirements of the subsystem?* List all the subsystems functions and any performance criteria. This information can be derived from the user requirement specification and functional specification for the given system.
- *From the major functions, what are the subfunctions and their associated performance requirements?* This information can be derived from the system's design documents.

- *What are the failure events?* From the list of subfunctions look at the different types of failures that may exist in the operating environment.
- *What is the effect of each failure event?* From the list of failures events look at all the likely effects of each type of failure in the production environment.
- *Is there a GxP consequence for each failure effect?* Assess if there is an impact GxP for each failure effect, yes or no.
- *What is the probability of detecting each failure effect?* Categorize into low, medium, or high probability of detection in a normal production environment.
- *Assess the probability of each failure effect.* Categorize into low, medium, or high probability of it happening.
- *What modifications to the design can be made to reduce GxP risks?* Review findings and modify design to eliminate the high risk, high probability of it happening functions.

For the purpose of illustration, the example form in Table 3.1 is of a barcode reading system, which is a subsystem of a labeling machine deemed to have a GxP impact. Its function is to detect a wrong, misplaced, or missing bar-coded label, and stops the machine. This example illustrates the methodology by taking the example through six of the eight questions listed above, looking at the main function, the subfunctions, and how these can fail. In addition, a review of the GxP effect of any failure and the probability of detection in a normal production environment is considered. The probability of a failure happening is explored further in Table 3.2 where risk prioritization is assigned. The purpose of Table 3.2 is to understand if any high GxP risks exist that necessitate a redesign of the system, or demonstrate how error checking or system intervention methodologies can be employed to reduce any GxP risk that may exist if the redesign is not possible.

The resulting review of the system example in Table 3.1 and after applying Table 3.2 would determine that a review of the "medium probability of its detection" functions (highlighted with an asterisk in Table 3.1) versus a high risk of it happening is a "high priority" and would require either a change to the design or the introduction of an intervention SOP to challenge the integrity of the barcode reading systems. This is where the eighth question comes in — "What modifications to the design can be made to reduce GxP risks"? As with the example for the barcode reader, sometimes there is no possible modification, therefore alternative methods will need to be employed, e.g., an intervention SOP. The intervention SOP will need to be designed to interact at suitable frequencies to increase the likelihood of detection and therefore decrease the probability of it happening, along with a suitable follow-up process if an error is detected.

During the system development life cycle risk assessments should be conducted at several stages because risk priorities are likely to change. The following should be considered as a guide to the minimum requirements for risk assessment reviews during a development life cycle.

Table 3.1 Example risk assessment form

Major functions	Subfunctions	Failure events	Possible effects in production environment	Impact on GxP		Probability of detection		
				Y	N	L	M	H
Reading barcode and stopping machine if incorrect	Detects when to read barcode by detecting leading black stripe	Fails to see barcode leading black stripe	Machine will stop		✓			✓
			Machine does not stop and puts labels in wrong place on cartons	✓				✓
		Looks for barcode at wrong position	Labels read as incorrect and machine stops		✓			✓
			*Labels are not seen and machine continues to run	✓			✓	
	Reads barcode	Fails to read correct barcode	Machine will stop		✓			✓
			*Machine continues to run	✓			✓	
		Fails to read incorrect barcode	Machine will stop		✓			✓
			*Machine continues to run	✓			✓	
	Makes decision pass or fail	Makes no decision	*Machine does not stop	✓			✓	
		Makes incorrect decision	*Machine does not stop	✓			✓	

Note: Above example for illustration purposes only.

Table 3.2 Risk prioritization

Probability of it happening		Probability of detection: High	Probability of detection: Medium	Probability of detection: Low
	High	Medium priority	High priority	High priority
	Medium	Low priority	Medium priority	High priority
	Low	Low priority	Low priority	Medium priority

Note: Above example for illustration purposes only.

- The generation of the user requirements specification.
- The supplier assessment and audit.
- The development of the functional specification.
- The completion of the design review prior to validation testing.
- Change management — whenever any major changes are applied to the system or there is a major change to regulations. This is intended to be a maintenance tool to ensure continued GxP compliance.

From the assessment process a suitable validation strategy can be devised.

- For high priority risks — avoidance, system redesign or a suitable challenging program must be employed along with increased verification and testing.
- For medium priority risks — process redesign should be considered, risks managed through procedures and testing.
- For low priority risks — decrease testing as appropriate.

APPLICATION TO PART 11

This section looks at applying the approach discussed above to the assessment of legacy systems applications for impact on the regulation 21 CFR Part 11 Electronic Records Electronic Signatures. Following the three steps, the records deemed high or medium risk from the results of the risk assessment should then be further assessed against audit trails and record retention requirements of relevant predicate rules. Using this assessment tool appears easy, but it will highlight the gaps in normal operational expectations to comply with the narrowed interpretation of Part 11.

Step 1 — Does the System Impact Part 11?

Does the system manage, store, or use GxP electronic records? Y/N

Consider: Are the records required by predicate rules and maintained in electronic format? Also, are the records required by predicate rules maintained in electronic format and paper format where the electronic format is relied on to perform regulated activity?

Note: Review business practices to ensure the electronic format of a record is or is not performing a regulated activity. Is this document in a SOP?

Does the system impact predicate rule requirements? Y/N

Consider: Was the system in place before August 20, 1997? If the answer to the question is yes, Part 11 may not apply. Review current use against predicate rule requirements.

If the answer to the above question is yes, have there been any major upgrades made to the system since August 20, 1997? If yes, Part 11 may apply.

Note: Are records in electronic format in place of paper format. If yes, Part 11 would apply. *Or*: Is the system used to generate paper printouts of electronic records, and do those records meet the requirements of the predicate rules? Do persons rely on the paper to perform regulated activities? If yes, Part 11 would not apply. Is this document in an SOP? Also, what happens to the electronic record?

Is the system used to approve or authorize GxP operations, or to authenticate GxP electronic records by means of an electronic signature or other electronic mechanism? Y/N

Note: Paper and e-records and signature components can coexist as long as predicate rule requirements are met and the content and meaning of the records is preserved. If the answer to the above three questions is no, then Part 11 does not apply.

Step 2 — Risk Management

Produce a process flow diagram identifying all major functions and interdependencies, i.e., network connections, other computer systems, and peripherals like printers, interfaces with people including the SOPs.

- What are the major GxP functions and associated performance requirements of the system? List all the major systems functions and any performance criteria. This information can be derived from the flow diagram and the user requirement specification or functional specification for the given system.
- From the major functions, what GxP data is produced and how does it impact predicate rule requirements? This information can be derived from the system design documents.
- If the system fails to perform a function that impacts on predicate rule requirements correctly, what are the failure events? From the list of major

Table 3.3 Part II Checklist

Major functions	What GxP data is produced	Failure events – identify the risks	What is the effect on GxP of each failure event?	Impact on GxP		Probability of detection		
				Y	N	L	M	H
Patient history file	Baseline data recording patient first visit and history information	Incorrect baseline data recorded	Incorrect dose	✓		✓		
			Incorrect study results	✓		✓		
		Baseline data lost	Study delayed		✓			✓
			Patient removed from study	✓				✓
	Study data results of all subsequent visits and test results	Incorrect study data recorded	Study results wrong	✓		✓		
			Study abandoned		✓	✓		
	Visit data lists the number and dates of all visits and tests	Incorrect visits scheduled	Study results wrong	✓			✓	
		Visit history missing	Patient removed from study	✓			✓	

Note: Above example for illustration only.

functions, look at the different types of failures that may exist in the operating environment.

- What is the effect on GxP of each failure event? Assess if there is an impact GxP for each failure event.
- What is the probability of detecting each failure effect? Categorize into low, medium, or high probability of detection in a normal production environment.
- Assess the probability of each failure effect happening. Categorize into low, medium, or high probability.
- What modifications to the design or enhancements to SOPs can be made to reduce GxP risks. Review findings and modify design to eliminate the high risk or high probability of it happening functions. Enhance SOPs to cover lower priorities. Use a Part 11 checklist to assess system compliance and likely resolution requirements (Table 3.3).

In Table 3.4, the baseline study data are considered to be high priority if there is a medium to high probability of it happening, and a medium to high priority if there is a low probability of it happening. Therefore it is important to assess the full compliance status of this system and address any compliance deficiencies in relation to handling baseline study data.

Having established the priorities, work can commence on designing the necessary corrective measures. When this is done, the risk assessment can then be reexecuted to determine the residual risk. This is an iterative process where secondary risks may be identified along the way. When the risk assessment team is satisfied that it can achieve a "minimum risk" solution, the risk assessment report can be compiled.

Step 3 — Part 11 Assessment

Conduct a 21 CFR Part 11 assessment of the system using a standard checklist, e.g.,

Table 3.4 Baseline Study Data

		Probability of detection		
		High	**Medium**	**Low**
Probability of it happening	**High**	Medium priority	High priority	High priority
	Medium	Low priority	Medium priority	High priority
	Low	Low priority	Low priority	Medium priority

Note: Above example for illustration purposes only.

Table 3.5 Risk Assessment Report

Section	Preamble Ref.	Question to consider	Part 11 guideline comment
11.10(b)	69,70	11.10 (b) The ability to generate accurate and complete copies of records in both human readable and electronic form suitable for inspection, review, and copying by the agency. Persons should contact the agency if there are any questions regarding the ability of the agency to perform such review and copying of the electronic records. • Can a copy of a single record (in electronic format) be supplied to an inspector? In paper format? • Can a copy of the entire database (in electronic format) be supplied to an inspector? • Are procedures in place to describe *how* to accomplish these inspection tasks? • Are procedures in place to define what format the electronic records will be provided?	You should provide the inspector with reasonable and useful access to records during an inspection. Provide copies in common format where records are kept in these formats, or, using established automated conversion methods make copies into a more common format. If you sort, trend, etc., copies to the agency should also have the same capability. Consider procedures and techniques to access records.

Note: Above example for illustration purposes only

using the ISPE GAMP Guide, to assess the likely remediation requirements to meet full compliance. The structure of the risk assessment report should clearly document the process you followed and it helps if you include the Part 11 requirements together with the questions you need to consider, as shown in Table 3.5.

PROCESS ANALYTICAL TECHNOLOGY (PAT)

Implementation of Process Analytical Technology (PAT) for pharmaceutical manufacturing has continued to advance and enable operations that monitor, control, and analyze critical quality attributes of processes and products while manufacturing is in progress, i.e., continuous quality verification. Pharmaceutical industry and regulatory agencies such as the FDA have emphasized the benefits of using PAT in support of a risk-based approach to cGMPs that recognizes the extent of scientific knowledge supporting process validation and process control. Implementation of PAT challenges the current validation paradigm to change towards supporting quality by design so that a balance is maintained between compliance and innovation. Therefore, it is necessary to define PAT system validation that is appropriate, commensurate with intended use of data, and practical for a risk-based approach to cGMPs. In this chapter the risk management validation methods and example approach is equal with the FDA's stated objectives for validation of PAT systems.

CONCLUSION

Pharmaceutical manufacturers must validate, otherwise their license to market a drug is revoked or not issued in the first place. The cost of validation should be related to the potential impact on GxP (and subsequently the business). If there is a potential impact on GxP then the whole system should be validated, with particular attention on the GxP aspects of the system's functionality. There is increasing pressure from other "regulators," such as financial auditors, data protection authorities, the U.S. Drug Enforcement Agency, or the U.K. Home Office (for the control of certain classes of active ingredient). It is also good business practice to validate systems because of the added payback from systems working more efficiently from day one, and the benefits must be clearly understood. The risk-based approach to validation ensures that resources are appropriately focused to ensure that a system is designed, built, and tested to ensure it correctly performs as intended.

FURTHER READING

ISO 61508 applies to *safety-related systems* when one or more of such systems incorporate electrical or electronic or programable electronic (*E/E/PE*) devices. It covers possible hazards caused by failure of the safety functions to be performed by the E/E/PE safety-related systems, as distinct from hazards arising from the E/E/PE equipment itself (for example, electric shock, etc.). It is generically based and applicable to all E/E/PE safety-related systems irrespective of the application.

It is recognized that the consequences of failure could also have serious economic implications and in such cases the standard could be used to specify any E/E/PE safety-related system used for the protection of equipment or product.

REFERENCES

1. The underlying requirements set forth in The Federal Food, Drug, and Cosmetic Act (the Act) Public Health Service Act (the PHS Act) and FDA regulations are referred to as the predicate rules.

2. Andrews, J. "Effective Cost Control for Automated Systems Validation Projects and Procedures." Published by ISPE, in *Pharmaceutical Engineering*.
3. Andrews, J., Phoenix, K. "Adopting a Risk-Based Approach to 21 CFR Part 11 Assessments." Published by ISPE in *Pharmaceutical Engineering*.
4. Schadt, R. PhD. *Process Analytical Technology — Changing the Validation Paradigm*. Pfizer Global Manufacturing, Pfizer Inc.
5. KMI PAREXEL LLC — training methodology on risk management techniques.
6. U.S. FDA. *Regulation: 21 CFR Part 11; Electronic Records; Electronic Signatures, Electronic Copies of Electronic Records*.
7. U.S. FDA. *Pharmaceutical Current Good Manufacturing Practices (cGMPs) for the 21st Century: A Risk Based Approach*.
8. U.S. FDA. *Guidance for Industry Part 11, Electronic Records; Electronic Signatures — Scope and Application*. August 2003.
9. *GAMP 4, GAMP Guide for Validation of Automated Systems*. ISPE, 2001.

Chapter 4

Validation Planning and Reporting

Chris Clark

CONTENTS

INTRODUCTION

The purpose of this chapter is to provide an overview of the key initiation and ending phases for the validation of GxP-critical computerized systems, namely the use of formal validation plans and the associated close out documentation related to validation reporting. It will also cover how to go about managing and creating such documents. At the same time it attempts to clarify the roles and responsibilities in both validation planning and reporting, and draws attention to the benefits that good planning and reporting activities bring to the implementation of a successful project. Finally, the chapter provides checklists to aid the user in developing validation plans and reports that are suitable for any specific application to which they may be applied.

We discuss the principles (both regulatory and business related) behind the need to create validation plans and reports and go on to identify where they fit within the typical project life cycle. These principles should be applied whenever there is a requirement to validate either a specific computerized system or a group of related computerized systems in an area or site. In particular these requirements should be formally applied when the system under consideration has been identified as being GxP-critical.* It is worth noting that the methodology may also be applied to other business-critical systems if deemed necessary following an assessment of business risk.

This chapter is divided into two subsections. The first covers validation planning, and the second covers the closely related activity of validation reporting.

Both of these documents are internal user-generated documents, the content of which must provide an accurate summary of the proposed validation strategy or activities (validation plan) and the actual history and events surrounding the whole validation effort (validation report). They must be of a suitable standard to allow them to be presented to outside regulatory agencies such as the U.S. Food and Drug Administration (FDA) and the Medicines and Healthcare Products Regulatory Agency (MHRA) in the U.K.

VALIDATION PLANNING

Overview of Planning in the Validation Life Cycle

There are as many differing depictions of the project life cycle that can be applied to the validation of computerized systems as there are books written on the subject, but in general they all can be illustrated as shown in Figure 4.1.

The key observation to note from Figure 4.1 is that the creation and approval of the validation plan is one of the earliest, if not one of the very first, activities undertaken in a project. In reality, and due to the tight time-scales often imposed upon modern day implementations, the development of the validation plan generally occurs as a parallel activity with that of requirements definition (creation of the URS, etc.).

Before looking at the activities, inputs, roles, and other elements surrounding the creation and management of this document, it is necessary to define exactly what is meant by the expressions "validation plans" and "validation master plans." Are these documents one and the same or do they represent different things to different people?

The difference is really determined by their scope. Generally the term "validation master plan" (VMP) will refer to the more generic validation activities associated with a corporation, single facility or a large site-wide (or multisite) system or group

---

* Where the term cGxP or GxP is utilized throughout this chapter, this can be equally applied to GMP, GLP, and GCP related systems.

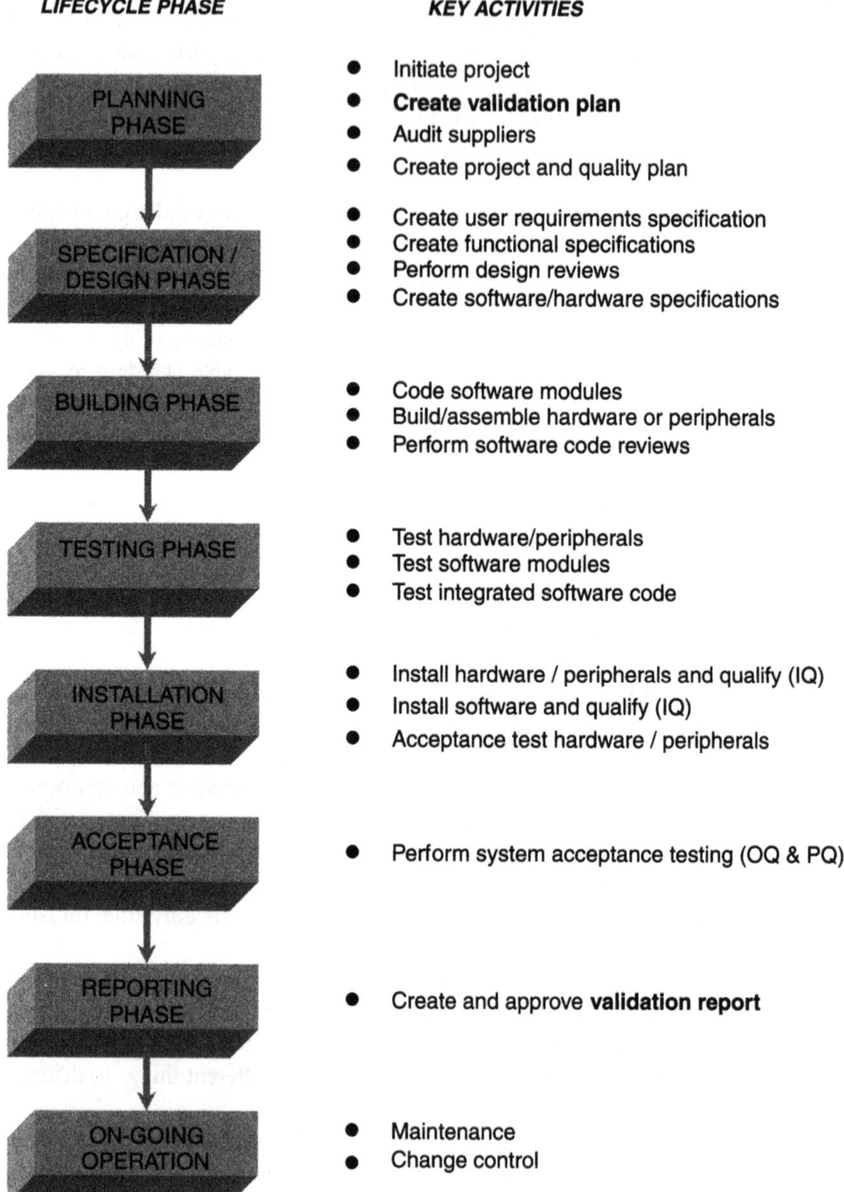

Figure 4.1 Generic life cycle model.

of systems. The term “validation plan” (VP), on the other hand, is generally used to refer to the document defining the specific validation activities associated with an individual given system or a piece of equipment within an area or department. Due to the fact that the VMP is more generic in nature and does not provide a high level of detail regarding specifics, this guideline will concentrate on the VP. The guide will indicate, where necessary, any additions or omissions that would be relevant when creating a VMP.

Purpose of the Validation Plan

The VP is the key document in the overall validation process. Its importance is not only relevant for internal project control but is also of specific interest to external regulatory bodies, for example, the U.S. FDA and the U.K. MHRA. It is by examination of this document that these authorities can see how organizations intend to control the implementation of a new computerized system from the initial requirements definition, via the build process, installation, acceptance testing and through to ongoing operation and maintenance. Furthermore, the authorities can understand the controls employed to ensure that the system not only meets its user requirements (and will continue to do so in the future), but that the company can formally demonstrate how the implementation has complied with the requirements laid down in the relevant cGMPs. A VP will therefore define certain critical aspects of the project. These include, but are not limited to:

- Project background and system definition.
- Organizational structure of the project team — both internal and external (if applicable).
- Life cycle definition.
- Overview and justification of validation approach and testing strategy.
- Standard operating procedures to be followed.
- Project team roles and responsibilities.
- Key milestones and deliverable items required at each stage.
- Clearly-defined set of acceptance criteria by which to measure the success of the implementation.

Once developed, the VP can be utilized as part of the selection process for both the system components and suppliers (including third party implementation services if applicable). It is generally accepted that during the selection process the prospective suppliers will be forwarded a copy of the user requirements specification (URS) (usually as part of a request for proposal (RFP)). However, the suppliers should also receive a copy of the VP for the proposed system as this will define what additional services and roles they may be required to supply within the project. For example, the plan will most likely identify the requirement for a functional specification which has been developed either for a specific bespoke system or is readily available for "configurable off-the-shelf" software. The readiness of the supplier to be involved in the creation of such a document or its availability will have a critical bearing on the decision making process during selection, and possibly a bearing on the success of the final implementation.

Relationships with Other Life Cycle Phases and Documents

Figure 4.1 depicted a simplified generic view of the validation process and some of the main activities that usually take place at the different phases within the life cycle. In trying to understand the relationship of VPs with other life cycle phases and documents, it is useful to consider a more complex view of the life cycle. An extension of the "V-model," found in the GAMP 4 Guide [1] and illustrated in Figure 4.2, provides one such view. The illustration shows that there is a *direct relationship* between the VP and the validation report. In practice this means that the requirements and activities for validation proposed within the validation plan need to be adequately documented by the resultant project output generated and discussed or summarized in the validation report. Further information on the purpose and content of the validation report will be found elsewhere. At this point it is sufficient to state that all the deliverables, activities, or milestones identified as required within the VP must have some form of evidence documented in the report that either confirms successful completion or justifies an acceptable status when not fully meeting the original requirements.

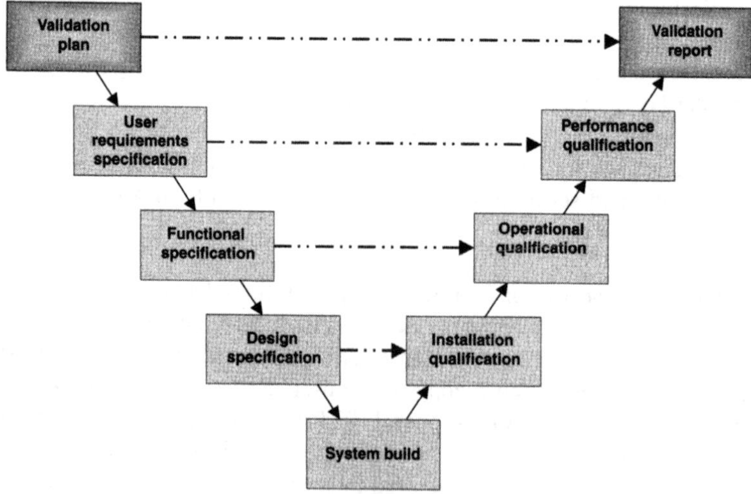

Figure 4.2 Extended "V- model."

When one considers the overall purpose of a VP it can be said that it is a formal statement of those activities, that when combined, have the ultimate intent to ensure:

- The computer system delivered is that which was originally required by the users.
- The delivered system performs as required under the operating conditions specified.
- The delivered system will continue to perform as required in the future.

Deeper interpretation of these statements shows there is a stronger relationship between the VP and the URS than at first meets the eye. Consider that the URS is the formal documentation of what the proposed system should do and the business processes it may replace. Therefore, not only is it a statement of intent, but it is also a means to measure the success of an implementation. The URS, like the VP, should be developed prior to system selection or build. Some would even argue that a comprehensive system VP could not be created and approved without the determination of system requirements (and an assessment of possible risks). Hence the relationship between these two documents is closer and more parallel in nature than that suggested by the V-model in Figure 4.2.

Further reflection on the purpose of the VPs shows that it must have either a direct or indirect relationship with *all* other phases in the life cycle. The plan is designed to cover the requirements and activities for design, build, testing, acceptance and long term operation and control of the computer system. A further consequence of this project term relationship is that the VP must also be maintained as a "live" document. At the initiation of the project the team may have created a high level VP. This plan may have contained many vague statements regarding the validation approach and strategy because at this stage the system details were only conceptual and not finalized. The process of system and supplier selection will have added further detail to the final concept of the proposed solution and consequently led to a greater understanding of the validation requirements. These requirements must be documented and maintained as a history of the project and therefore the VP will require an update. This means that the plan is not fixed at one point in time and it should be allowed to develop as the project develops.

KEY PLANNING ACTIVITIES

Formation of Project Team

The initiation phase of a project includes the nomination of a project leader or manager, who will organize the project team around them. One of the first activities of the project team is to discuss and agree upon the validation approach and strategy to be used. To ensure these discussions are as complete and successful as possible, the constituent team membership should consist of personnel with appropriate qualifications, skills, and experience. It is usual for some, if not all, of the following attributes to be represented by the team (although not all necessarily together in a single individual):

- Adequate level of authority within the company to make and implement critical project and business decisions.
- Suitable knowledge of the business areas affected by the project scope.
- Extensive knowledge of international regulatory requirements covering cGMP and computer systems validation.
- Computer literacy and reasonable knowledge of current IT trends.

The composition of the team may change depending upon the size of the project, the length of time it has run, or the current stage. However, each team must contain at least one member of the quality assurance department (and the validation department if separate), one member of the IT department, and one user.

Tables 4.1 through 4.4 show examples of the possible constituent membership for the different projects listed.

Table 4.1 Manufacturing resource planning (MRPII) project

Member	Roles
Warehouse and distribution	User/process ownership
Customer services	User/process ownership
Purchasing	User/process ownership, supplier/system selection process
Finance	User/process ownership, project budget control
Planning	User/process ownership
Production	User/process ownership
Senior management/directors	Facilitators/project management
Quality assurance/quality control	User/process ownership, regulatory compliance, supplier assessment, validation management
Engineering	User/process ownership, hardware, peripherals, and cabling installation
Information technology	User, IT systems development, implementation, and management
Third party implementation specialist (optional)	Systems integration, interface and software development, project management, validation consultant and support services

Table 4.2 Capsule filling machine with integrated check-weighing device

Member	Roles
Production operations	Users
Production management	Process ownership
Production director	Facilitator
Quality assurance	Regulatory compliance, supplier assessment, validation management
Engineering	User, supplier liaison, equipment (hardware and software) installation, utilities installation
Information technology	IT consultant, review of software development (process and code)

Table 4.3 Laboratory information management system (LIMS)

Member	Roles
Laboratory staff	Users
Laboratory management	Process ownership
Senior management/directors	Facilitators
Quality control	User, technical, analytical and regulatory support
Quality assurance	Regulatory compliance, supplier assessment, validation management
Information technology	IT systems development, implementation and management
Third party implementation specialist (optional)	Systems integration, interface and software development, project management, validation consultant and support services

Table 4.4 Clinical trials management system

Member	Roles
Data handlers, coordinators	Users/process owners
Senior medical research management	Facilitators/project management
Quality assurance	User, regulatory compliance, supplier assessment, validation management
Information technology	User, IT systems development, implementation and management
Third party implementation specialist (optional)	Systems integration, interface and software development, project management, validation consultant and support services

The project team membership will vary depending upon the size of the organization involved (due to availability of resources) and the scope of the project. However, it is generally possible to summarize the team membership in the following terms:

- Project manager.
- Process owner.
- Facilitator.
- Users.
- Quality assurance.
- Information technology.

Analyze the GMP Implications

At the start of any computer systems implementation project, the most commonly asked question is: “How much validation is necessary?”

This is not such an unreasonable question given that since the early 1990s the regulatory bodies have focused an immense amount of attention upon computer systems validation. The result of this attention has been a number of well-documented citations against some of the industry's major global companies. These citations have covered a large variety of noncompliance issues ranging from inadequate retrospective validation documentation, poor project management and control, insufficient evidence of validation activity, poor specification and testing of error messages and the lack of controls surrounding system security. The result of this attention has been that the industry has reacted, or possibly overreacted, to ensure that the gaps are closed. It has done this mainly by producing mountains of paperwork documenting and specifying the smallest detail of a system, all backed up with an immense and complex series of test protocols. The situation toward the end of the 1990s was that more often than not the practice of validation resulted in a major spend item on the project budget and was seen to add considerably to the project timescales and for very little perceived benefit.

All of this can be avoided by spending a little time planning the validation carefully and adequately for the particular project to which it is being applied. To aid this process ask the question: "What are GxP implications of this project?"

Whether the regulatory inspector is from the U.S. or the EU, the prime motivator in questions regarding validation is to ensure that the computer system will not adversely affect the product quality and, ultimately, patient safety. Hence, they will focus very clearly on the statutory regulations and guidelines as their source of reference. This leads to the conclusion that one of the initial activities of the project team must be to fully disseminate the *direct* GMP relationships that many of the system components (software *and* hardware) may have. More recently, the regulators have expressed their wish to see a more "risk-based" approach to meeting GxP compliance, and this provides the team with a key tool to aid the development of a suitable validation approach. There are many different ways in which risk can be assessed, and a good introduction can be found by reference to the ISO14971 — "Medical devices — Application of risk management to medical devices." There are many other reference documents, one of which can be found in Appendix M3 of the GAMP 4 Guide. Further guidance can be found in the "Develop Validation Approach and Strategy" section of this chapter.

Once this information has been distilled, the team can better visualize the extent of the problem in front of them. This puts them in a position to develop a testing strategy of the appropriate level of detail and depth according to the GMP implications revealed by the analysis.

One problem area is that most systems implementers see computer systems as business tools and do not fully appreciate the direct GxP relationship that many of the system modules have. This is the reason for ensuring a wide knowledge base in the project team. This should therefore include people with experience in regulatory compliance who can help negotiate the complex web of rules and regulations that may be applied to the project. Furthermore, they can, with the support of other suitably qualified team members, assimilate this information, together with the knowledge of the business process under review.

As an example of such an analysis is one of the more complex and convoluted of business systems, namely a MRPII system.

Most modern-day MRPII systems are modular. Each module generally deals with a different aspect of the business, with some element of crossover between the modules. Some of these modules include inventory control, quality control, lot control and traceability and storage and distribution. These modules can handle some very GMP specific data, some examples of which are listed in Tables 4.5 through 4.11.

Table 4.5

Information associated with a lot	Lot number Lot status Dates associated with a lot (e.g., expiry date, traceability) Quantity/potency Conversion factors Lot notes Quality

Table 4.6

Information associated with a shop order	Shop order number Quantities Receipt date Transactions (e.g., material allocations, issues) Shelf days/retest day

Table 4.7

Information associated with a purchase order Dates	Purchase order number Vendor lot number Transactions

Table 4.8

Information associated with an item	Item number Item notes Bill of material (e.g., units of measure, conversion factors, yield factors, quantity per, approval) Location (including storage conditions and cycle counting) Type Quality

Table 4.9

Information associated with a customer order	Customer order number

Table 4.10

Information associated with a supplier	Quality approval/status (e.g., fully approved, provisional approval)

Table 4.11

Information associated with a user	People (e.g., user ID, password, names, job title, security access levels, authority)

The validation of any system functionality surrounding the transaction and collection of the above data is of critical interest to the regulatory bodies. They will require adequate documentary evidence of the tasks performed in obtaining that validation. This can be achieved by following a life cycle approach similar to that defined in Figures 4.1 and 4.2, an approach that will be further refined in the validation plan.

Develop Validation Approach and Strategy

The analysis of the GxP aspects of a system helps define the approach to validation, but before finalizing the strategy it is also worth considering those elements of the system that could be classified as **business-critical** functions. After all, an organization's objective is to achieve, upon implementation of the new system, one that functions successfully to meet as fully as possible *all* the business needs originally defined. For example, it is necessary to take into account the requirements of the company financial auditors, customs and excise, and other government agencies (e.g., the U.K. Home Office — in relation to controlled drugs). All must be considered and included in plans for validation.

A useful tool for carrying out this task is to perform a **risk assessment** of the processes within the scope of the project. Risk assessment is a process that allows the project team to focus on the likelihood and the potential impact of all forms of possible failure and disruption so that appropriate measures can be taken to reduce or even eliminate them. When applied to computer systems validation the risk assessment process must address the ways in which differing types of activity could be disrupted, stopped, or have their performance degraded to unacceptable levels. Some examples are:

- Readiness and operation of business processes required as obligations under GMP regulations or under statute (e.g., health and safety).
- Readiness and operation of normal business processes that directly affect product quality and therefore patient safety.
- Readiness and operation of business processes that support business reputation or cost of operations.

There are many different ways in which risk assessment can be carried out and it is outside the scope of this chapter to describe them. However, all forms of risk assessment follow a similar route, as summarized in Figure 4.3, which indicates the main steps to be applied in the risk assessment process.

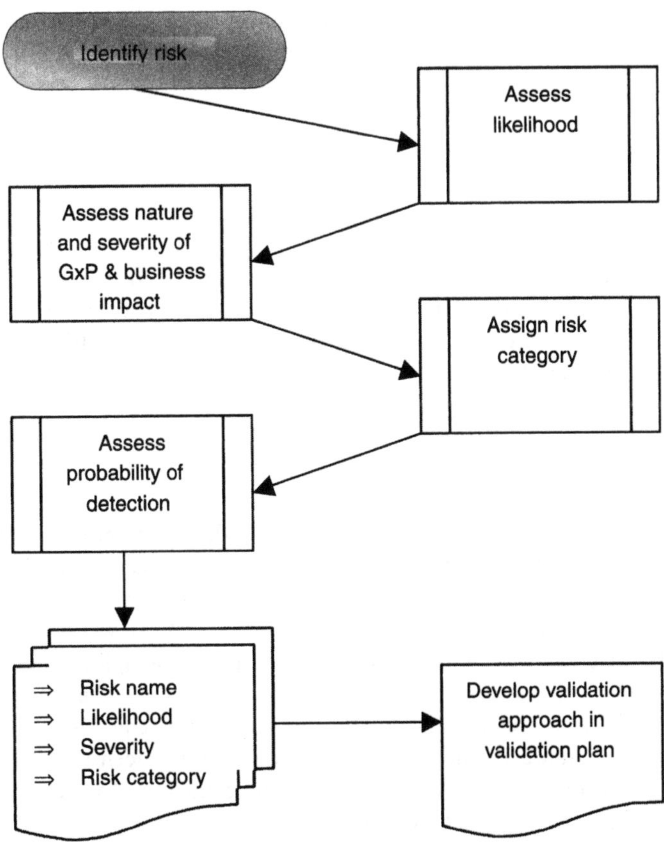

Figure 4.3 Overview of a risk assessment process.

The key to performing successful risk assessment for a validation project is to follow a formal procedure and ensure that all conclusions are fully documented. It should be noted that risk assessment should occur more than once throughout the life cycle of the project. The primary activities are as follows.

Identify Risk

In assessing the types of risk to which the project may be subject, it is important to ensure that the assessment is well informed and based on verifiable evidence. Where possible and appropriate, the views of acknowledged experts should be called upon to ensure that the assessment of the nature and likelihood of a particular risk is as realistic as possible.

At this stage it is only necessary to record summary details for each risk. These details should include a name, which should convey something of the nature of the risk, and a one- or two-sentence description of the nature of the risk.

Assess Likelihood

The most straightforward way to define the likelihood of a risk occurring is to use some simple criteria.

Low: probability of the risk occurring perceived as less than 10%.
Medium: probability of the risk occurring perceived as between 10% and 50%.
High: probability of the risk occurring perceived as between 50% and 80%.
Very high: probability of the risk occurring perceived as over 80%.

Assess Nature and Severity of Business Impact

The risk assessment process should result in the identification of the immediate effects of the risk happening and also the impact on the business of those effects. For example, the immediate effect of a hard disk problem may be the corruption of some inventory and distribution data stored on that disk. However, the longterm effect will impact upon the ability of the business to have a high level of assurance that GMP- and business-critical data relating to product distribution is accurate. This is a significant noncompliance with the regulatory requirements that could lead to the withdrawal of the company's manufacturing license and hence will adversely affect the company's ability to continue trading. As a minimum, risk assessment should consider the impact on:

- Product quality and safety.
- Regulatory compliance.

- Health and safety (employees and public).
- Financial performance.
- Company reputation with customers, suppliers, staff, and investors.

A simple grading system can be used, ensuring that the assessment is well informed and based upon verifiable evidence.

Low: a minor negative impact, having no long-term detrimental effects.

Medium: a moderate negative impact, with short- to medium-term detrimental effects.

High: a significant negative impact, having significant medium- to long-term effects.

Very high: an immediate and very significant negative impact, having significant long-term effects and potentially catastrophic short-term effects.

Assign Risk Category

An example of risk categorization is provided in Figure 4.4.

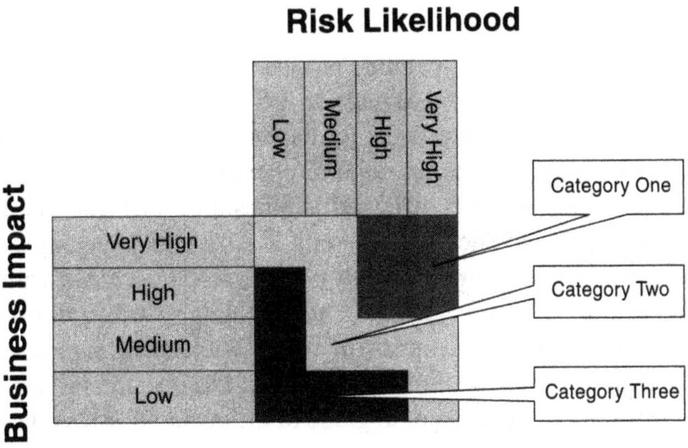

Figure 4.4 Risk category matrix.

Assess Probability of Detection

The probability of risk detection can be graded using a simple scheme as follows:

Low: probability of risk detection perceived as less than 10%.
Medium: probability of risk detection perceived as between 10% and 50%.
High: probability of risk detection perceived as between 50% and 80%.

Very high: probability of risk detection perceived as over 80%.

Another factor to be considered when defining the validation strategy is the construction of the software in the system itself. One approach is to categorize the system components (software and hardware) to segregate those that are common and have a low risk of failure from those that are less common and have a higher risk of failure.

Does the implemented solution consist of software based on standard or bespoke code?

One such approach is defined in the GAMP 4 Guide, [1] which classifies software commonly found in manufacturing systems into five types. These categories may then be used, along with the GMP and business criticality factors previously discussed, as a basis for determining an appropriate validation approach. At the lower end of the scale the validation effort will be restricted to simple recording of the name and version number in the hardware acceptance tests or equipment IQ. However, at the higher end of the scale the requirement is more likely to be for following a full life cycle for all parts of the system.

The five categories defined within the GAMP 4 Guide are as follows.

Category 1 — Operating Systems

Where the application software is operating on an established, commercially available operating system (e.g., Windows98, Windows NT), the operating system may be validated as part of the validation process for the application software. Currently the U.S. and EU regulatory bodies do not require operating systems to be specifically validated other than as part of particular applications that run on them. The recommended validation approach is to use only well-known operating systems and record the name and version number as part of the installation qualification. Before implementation and use of a new version of an operating system, a thorough review must be undertaken to consider the impact of any new, amended, or removed features upon the application running on it. Such a review could lead to formal retesting of the application, particularly where a major upgrade of the operating system has occurred.

Category 2 — Firmware

This group of systems includes equipment like weigh scales, bar code scanners, label printers. Because of their standard nature hard coded programs or "firmware" drives them. These programs, while non user-programmable, are configurable and the approach during validation of such items is to formally record the configuration in the equipment installation qualification. As with Category 1, the unplanned and informal introduction of new versions of firmware during maintenance must be prevented by the application of rigorous change control. Again it is important to assess the impact of new versions on the validity of the IQ documentation and the necessary corrective action planned, initiated, and confirmed.

Category 3 — Standard Software Packages

Typical examples include Lotus 1-2-3, Microsoft Excel and other spreadsheet packages, Microsoft Access and other database packages (SAS). They are sometimes also referred to as canned or COTS (commercial off-the-shelf) configurable packages. There is no requirement to validate the software package, however new versions should be treated with caution. Validation effort should concentrate on the application, which includes:

- System requirements and functionality.
- The high level language or macros used to build the application.
- Critical algorithms and parameters.
- Data integrity, security, accuracy, and reliability.
- Operational procedures.

As for other categories, change control should be applied stringently, since changing these applications is often very easy, and with limited security. User training should emphasize the importance of change control and the validated integrity of these systems.

Category 4 — Configurable Software Packages

Such systems include MRP packages, LIMS, manufacturing execution systems (MES), distributed control systems (DCS), and supervisory control and data acquisition packages (SCADA).

A typical feature of these systems is that they permit users to develop their own applications by configuring or amending predefined software modules and also developing new application software modules. Each application (of the standard product) is therefore specific to the user process, and maintenance becomes a key issue, particularly when new versions of the standard product are produced.

The full life cycle approach should be used to specify, design, test, and maintain the application. Particular attention should be paid to any additional or amended code and to the configuration of the standard modules. A software review of the modified code (including any algorithms in the configuration) should be undertaken.

In addition, an audit of the supplier is required to determine the level of quality and structural testing built into the standard product. The audit needs to consider the development of the standard product that may have followed a prototyping methodology without user involvement. In such cases it is recommended that suppliers use a formally documented quality management structure and documentation during the development of the standard product. If the system and platform are not well known and mature, it may be more prudent to consider them in Category 5 rather than in Category 4.

Category 5 — Custom (Bespoke) Software

The full life cycle should be followed for all parts of such systems. An audit of the supplier is required to examine their existing quality systems. The VP should only be finally prepared after this audit to document precisely what activities are necessary, based on the results of the audit and on the complexity of the proposed bespoke system.

Use of the above categorization regime provides invaluable aid toward defining a suitable and appropriate validation approach in the VP. Nevertheless, care should be exercised as complex systems will most often have many layers of software, each with its own degree of categorization, and therefore one system could exhibit several or even all of the above categories. One such example is that of the MRPII system that could be constructed as follows:

- Application layer regarded as a configurable software package (Category 4).
- Running on a commercially available operating system (Category 1).
- Utilizing bespoke interfaces to other corporate systems (Category 5).
- User interfaces via standard desktop PCs, label printers, weigh scales, and barcode readers (Category 2).
- Based upon a corporate network built from standard software and hardware (Category 3).

Write the Validation Plan

The first section of this chapter indicated that there are two types of plans we could consider creating — the VMP and the VP. This section will concentrate upon the creation of the VP, but first it is wise to briefly consider some features of the VMP. The VMP is an *internal* user company document, written at a high level, the purpose of which is to document the areas, systems, and projects to be managed. Because it is a high-level document it should only indicate:

- The level to which these systems require validation.
  - *Primarily based on the GxP impact.*
- Whether they are "old" or "new" systems.
  - *Consideration of handling legacy systems, for example.*
- Who has responsibility for owning the system.

  - *Specifying the person or department that will retain responsibility for the implementation and management of the implemented system.*
- Who is managing the validation and change control.
  - *Enable clearer definition of roles and responsibilities.*
- The timescales anticipated for completion of the stated tasks.
  - *Providing for improved management of resources.*
- Who is responsible for approval of the validation.
  - Designate specific responsibility for project completion and sign off.

The style of this document is often no more than an expanded Gantt Chart or project plan, with the additional feature of formal maintenance in a quality assurance system and approved by senior management. However, other styles are more formal, with structured paragraphs, diagrams and tables, and follow the strict rules applied for the control of compliance critical documentation. Whatever the style, the prime concern is the availability of a plan. This plan should provide an overview of the company's approach to validation, show that they know the extent of the challenge (an inventory of the systems under consideration for validation, and even those not considered for validation) and have a planned way for resolving it.

The individual systems identified in the VMP inventory will have their own VPs. As with the VMP, the VP is an *internal* user company document and should be provided by the customer organization to the supplier or implementor of the system. This type of plan will indicate, in detail:

- What validation must be done.
- How this validation will be achieved.
- When it is anticipated the validation (and phases within) will be completed.
- Who is responsible.

These validation requirements must be communicated to the supplier or implementor at the start of the project because it will help determine the mix of activities required, assignment of resources and project timescales. To achieve this, the user organization will supply the approved VP to the supplier or implementor, together with the URS. These combined documents will provide the supplier or implementor with all the basic information required to understand both the technical requirements (URS) and the regulatory constraints (VP) to be imposed on the project.

Who should actually write the VP? Conventional wisdom indicates this is best driven by and assigned to the QA department, or, if applicable, the compliance and validation department. Members of these departments will have the specific knowledge enabling them to interpret the regulatory requirements, together with the analysis of GMP impact to produce a suitable plan. However, these groups cannot perform this task in isolation and it will be necessary for them to consult with other key team members such as the users and the information systems and technology department. This process will eventually produce the first issue of the VP, and it will be this version of the document that will be used in early discussions with the supplier or implementor. Commonly this revision undergoes further refinement following these discussions, as the technical design becomes clearer and the implications for the original validation approach become obvious. For more complex systems (i.e., MRPII) it is not unusual at this stage to define parallel life cycles of activity for different aspects of the system (standard application software, bespoke software, hardware, peripherals). Each cycle will have its activity emphasized at different parts of the V-model depending upon the GxP criticality assessment identified during the earlier planning of the project.

What about the scope that the VP will cover and what should the content look like? These issues will be discussed more fully in Section 3, but it is sufficient to state that the document should cover the following aspects.

- Project team and validation team organization.
- Life cycle to be followed.
- Standard operating procedures to be followed.
- Roles and responsibilities of different parties.
- Activities and phases.
- Deliverable items.
- Overall project acceptance criteria.

Review the Validation Plan

One of the important factors for consideration when creating and managing validation plans is to make certain that the validation approach, related activities, and deliverables called for by the plan are agreed upon by as wide an audience as possible. This ensures that those responsible for overseeing (or even performing) the stated tasks and providing the deliverables are committed to their successful completion. Clearly the best way to achieve this is to carry out a thorough review of the VP with these parties involved. In most cases this may not prove too difficult because it is usual to find that many of the reviewers may have already participated in the writing of the plan.

It is also imperative that this audience has the appropriate levels of authority and responsibility within their relevant organizations to make approval decisions about the VP.

Table 4.12 lists the minimum number of participants it is advisable to involve in the review process. Where possible, the table also provides an indication of some potential reviewers' roles and responsibilities.

Table 4.12

Reviewer	Role/responsibility
Project manager	Ensures that the defined approach fits with the overall project objectives and does not conflict with budgetary limits. Responsible to the senior management for the successful implementation of the project.
Users	Understand and agree user roles in validation approach (could involve participation in acceptance testing for example) and that the validation approach and strategy fits with their requirements and the overall project objectives. Users could be from a number of differing functions and each may have a separate perspective on the project.
Quality assurance	Ensure the plans meet the company standards for project control and compliance critical documentation. Responsible for all GMP regulatory aspects, both in terms of system design and implementation.
Validation	Ensure plans comply with current accepted practices for validation of computer systems and meet company standards for validation. Act as general validation consultants internally and, if required, liaison with external validation services or implementor.
Research and development	Where the system involves a new process ensure definition of specifications, limits, and other technical assistance.
Information technology	Technical expertise regarding hardware, software, and systems suitability and compatibility. Ensure compliance with company IT strategy. Management of day-to-day IT systems operations and controls.
Engineering	Surveys for suitability for siting of hardware, cabling, and peripherals. Definition of capacity and maintenance requirements. Supply of suitable utilities and organization of installation or liaison with supplier or implementor.
Supplier or implementor	Agree and understand validation approach and what is required for compliance.

Approve the Validation Plan

When a company is subject to regulatory inspections of computer systems validation, it is usual for the inspectors to begin the review by understanding what validation activities were planned initially. In order to find the clearest demonstration of this, they will request to see a VP and they will expect it to be adequately approved and controlled. The approval of the plan should be clear and unambiguous, and should have been performed by suitably expert and experienced persons. Each individual should sign the VP as appropriate, with the approval signature indicating their name, job or function and the date the approval was given.

As for who should be involved in this approval process, the list is similar to the list for reviewing the plan given in the "Review the Validation Plan" section of this chapter. The approval process followed should be exactly the same as that for any other compliance critical document managed by the company's QA documentation control system.

Document Management and Control

It is not unusual for the approach defined in the VP to change as the project progresses and more is understood about the issues surrounding the system's implementation. Also the length of time it takes for some projects to reach completion means that invariably there will be personnel changes or even job or organization restructuring. Once approved, the VP must be formally controlled by a documentation control system to ensure such changes happen in an organized manner. While documentation systems can vary from company to company, the features to be aware of are generally encapsulated in the following basic principles.

- Documents to be assigned a unique reference code.
- Version control from one edition to the next to identify when a document has been superseded.
- Laid out in an orderly format so as to ensure unambiguous and clear content.
- Ability to conduct formal review process and update document as required.
- Change control process to track change requests — who, why, when.
- Clear document approval, involving only those with suitable authority to approve.
- Approvals to be dated.
- Control of document issue and return or destruction of old versions.
- Documents should be subjected to regular documented review and amended as necessary in order to stay current.

Within the U.K. (and the EU) the requirements for documentation control are contained within the rules and guidance governing GMP and are as applicable to validation documents as they are to any other compliance critical document.

The responsibility for managing and controlling documents is generally given to the quality assurance function and this applies equally to VPs. However it is important that the project or validation team is conscious of the need for document control and the team should be given the necessary training to build and improve this awareness.

FORMAT AND CONTENT OF THE VALIDATION PLAN

This section defines the typical contents of the VP. While all the sections listed here should not be regarded as mandatory, careful consideration must be given to the scope of the project when deciding which ones to omit. If any sections are excluded from the final plan it is recommended that some form of justification be provided.

The primary sections for inclusion in a VP are:

- Introduction and project overview.

- System description.
- Validation approach.
- Validation documentation.
- Validation documentation procedures.
- Training requirements.
- Validation organization.
- Validation activity schedule and timeline.
- Maintenance of validation status.
- Constraints and assumptions.
- Appendices.

Introduction and Project Overview

The author of the VP should use this section to set the scene for the content of the remainder of the document and provide the correct context for the reader to understand the approach taken. It is therefore important that this section contain information relating to some, if not all of the following topics.

- Background to, and reasons for, the project.
- Who produced, reviewed, and approved the document, under what authority and for what purpose.
- The scope of validation for the system.
- The objectives of the validation.
- The period within which the plan will next be reviewed.

An example of such text is as follows:

> Currently the Novocastrian Pharmaceutical Company Limited (NPCL) uses a wide range of computer systems for the day to day running of the business. These range from manufacturing inventory and planning systems to finance systems, collectively known as the "MYOPE" system. In addition the company operates office automation packages (MS Office, e-mail, etc.). The "MYOPE" system is now old and is not easy to upgrade. In addition, the system contains large amounts of important data that could be of use to management to improve the business. However, the constituent parts of the system are based on different operating systems and databases, and hence it is very difficult to access this data in a simple way. It has also been recognized that there is an issue regarding the regulatory compliance of this older system to current MCA/FDA computer systems validation guidelines.
>
> To resolve the above problems, and to gain business improvement through the use of new electronic computer systems, NPCL have decided to introduce a series of new computer systems that will all form part of an integrated strategy. This VP defines the strategy to validate these new computer systems for the production and financial management processes. These processes are defined in the URS (reference URS-NPCL-001) and include, but are not limited to:

- Production planning.
- Manufacturing and filling and packaging.
- Quality department (QC, QA).
- Engineering.
- Warehousing.
- Purchasing.
- Production costing, nominal ledger, sales ledger, purchase ledger, fixed assets.

This document was produced under the authority of the production director at NPCL and has been reviewed and approved by the head of information systems and the head of quality assurance. It follows the standard company procedure for the preparation of a VMP (reference QUA-VAL-002) and complies with the company validation policy (reference QUA-POL-001).

This VP is to be regarded as an active document. It controls the generation of all validation related documents, and this documentation will be produced in stages during the phased implementation of the chosen software packages, therefore it may be necessary to review this VP at regular intervals or as and when major changes to the documentation occurs. Such updates will be reviewed and issued as a new version of the VP under standard company change control procedures.

System Description

The URS will have already described in some detail the process that the computer system will automate, support or replace. This needs to be reinforced by a high-level description of what the proposed system will be like. In earlier versions of the VP this may only be a sketchy overview of some conceptual designs, but as the project progresses through the tendering process, a more tangible proposal will emerge. It is useful to include such a description in the VP in order to allow the reader to comprehend the structure of the approach defined in the remainder of the document.

The usual form of a system description is a text description of the system as in the example below.

The computer systems to be installed will cover the following functional areas:

- Manufacturing and inventory.
- Purchasing.
- Sales.
- Finance.

Over the last 2 years NPCL has been creating documents outlining the way in which the current manufacturing and financial functions operate on a day-to-day basis, both computer and noncomputer related. This was then followed by documenting, in a comprehensive user requirement document, the functionality ideally desired in a new series of computer systems (refer to document URS-NPCL-001, Edition B, dated February 1997).

As part of the initial stages of application software selection, many varying packages were reviewed. It was decided that no single package met all the requirements, and an integrated approach was needed to provide the overall functionality required.

Reliability and ease of integration is gained by use of the Hewlett Packard (HP) computer systems as the hardware standard, and the HP Unix operating system is the basis on which all the packages will operate. The Oracle database is the base relational database package on which the application software will run. Microsoft Windows NT is the preferred client operating system, the overall company IT strategy based on client/server architecture.

The final application packages selected are:

Oracle GEMMS – Manufacturing requirements planning.
Oracle Financials – Financial management.
Base10 FS – Dispensary system.
Documentum – Enterprise document management system.

However, this can be simplified by using a flowchart, showing the main systems and the links and interfaces between them, the hardware, the users, and peripherals. An example is given in Figure 4.5.

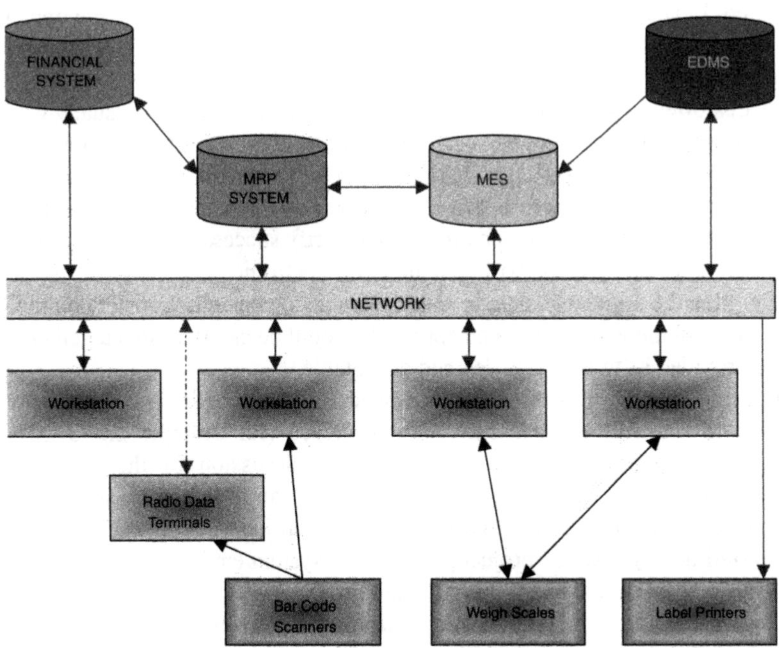

Figure 4.5 Example system diagram.

The key to creating these descriptions is to keep them as simple as possible. They should be easy to understand by a reader with little or very limited knowledge of computer systems, but they should also be sufficiently detailed for the more expert eye to be able to comprehend the objective of the project.

Validation Approach

The purpose of this section is to document the life cycle model that has been decided upon following the analysis of the system GxP criticality. In addition, it should note any special validation requirements accounting for any compliance issues that may have been identified following further investigations into software suitability and the adequacy of the development processes.

The opening paragraphs of this section ought to cover the overall definition of the approach taken. For example, the text must indicate whether the validation is performed prospectively, concurrently, or retrospectively.

The discussion in subsequent paragraphs must be designed to consider whether the software applications purchased will be implemented as modified or unmodified packages. Emphasis should be placed upon the use of any bespoke software, and the development process behind it, together with how compliance will be assured. Indication should be given as to the exact nature of these developments, what they are being used for and what impact they have from a GxP or business critical viewpoint.

One area often overlooked in writing VPs is that of data transfer. Usually when a modern system updates or replaces an older or obsolete system, there is a great deal of critical business and GxP data that may need to be transferred. The same is true if a new computerized system is brought in to replace a manual one. In such cases the VP must describe the approach proposed to verify successful data transition, and indicate whether this process will be manual or electronic.

Quite often the approach taken in many plans is to concentrate solely on the GxP critical areas of the system. Such an approach should be clearly stated together with reasons provided as to why it is deemed acceptable.

It is often valuable to define the life cycle and support this with diagrams or examples to illustrate the particular model chosen (for example the GAMP V-model). This should be further developed by discussion of the use of any categorization of hardware system, peripherals and software, showing the categories assigned by the team to each item in the project. It is also valuable at this stage to outline any planned project phasing and system environment management to support system development, testing, and go-live.

As a final point, this section must identify any special requirements to be undertaken due to issues raised during vendor assessments. For example, the software development process of a standard COTS software package may be found to have some compliance issues with it during the vendor assessment process. The project team may still decide to purchase the software for many other valid reasons. Consequently the validation team may decide to perform some additional testing to close out any potential shortfalls that may be perceived to exist within the package.

Validation Documentation

The purpose of this section is to list documents that the team feels will be required to provide sufficient evidence of compliance and control over the entire validation process. Clearly this means that the eventual listing presented in the VP is entirely dependent upon the particular life cycle model chosen for the specific project under discussion. Therefore, for the purposes of this chapter consideration is given to the documents that could be generated if following a generic life cycle similar to that described in Figure 4.1. It should be noted that no discussion regarding these documents is considered at this point as they will be encompassed elsewhere.

- Planning phase:
  - URS.
  - Invitation to tender, response to proposal.
  - Company searches, vendor questionnaires, audit reports.
  - VPs.
  - Quality and project plan.
- Specification and design phase:
  - Functional specification.
  - Hardware design specifications.
  - Mechanical and electrical diagrams.
  - Software design specifications.
  - Software module design specifications.
  - Network design specifications.
  - Minutes of design review meetings.
  - Change notices.
- Building phase:
  - Hardware manufacture and assembly records.
  - Peripherals and equipment manufacture and assembly records.
  - Software code reviews.
  - Network manufacture and assembly records.
  - Change notices.
- Testing phase:
  - Hardware testing protocols and records.
  - Software module testing protocols and records.
  - Software integration testing protocols and records.
  - Peripherals and equipment testing protocols and records.
  - Change notices.

- Installation phase:
  - Hardware installation qualification protocols and records.
  - Software installation qualification protocols and records.
  - Peripherals and equipment installation qualification protocols and records.
  - Network installation qualification protocols and records.
  - Hardware acceptance testing protocols and records (OQ).
  - Network acceptance testing protocols and records (OQ).
  - Change notices.
  - Acceptance reports and certification.
- Acceptance phase:
  - Factory acceptance testing (FAT) protocols and records (OQ/PQ).
  - System acceptance testing protocols and records (OQ/PQ).
  - Go-live testing protocols and records (OQ/PQ).
  - Change notices.
  - Acceptance reports and certification.
- Reporting phase:
  - Final validation reports and sign off.
- Ongoing operation:
  - Standard operating procedure — user manuals and data center operations.
  - Change control procedures.
  - Configuration management procedures.

Validation Documentation Procedures

Why does the VP need to have a section covering the procedures applicable to the validation documentation? There are several reasons for this.

The most obvious reason can be seen from the listing in the above section. It shows that the range of validation documentation can be very wide. Some of these documents are very technical and complex in nature.

Second, these documents will not all be produced by the same person or group of people. Some of them are likely to be generated internally by the project team (e.g., URS, acceptance protocols) while others may be produced externally depending upon the complexity of the project (e.g., functional specification, design specifications, assembly records).

The third reason for defining rules and guidelines around validation documentation is to ensure consistency in both document format, content, and management procedures. All documentation must have some form of unique coding and version or date control. They must undergo a formal documented review and approval process, resulting in the unambiguous signature of approval by suitably qualified and authorized personnel, either internal or external to the company. The definition of controls around document content reduces the risk of information being erroneously omitted.

The most successful way to deal with such issues is to ensure that at the outset of a validation project it is clearly stated **why** these documents exist, **what** they are expected to contain, **how** they are to be controlled, and to **whom** this responsibility will fall. For smaller projects it is usual to handle these via the normal internal company standard operating procedures, but what about a more complex project where many documents may be generated externally by a third party implementor or have already been created by the software or hardware vendor? In such circumstances the validation team should reach agreement, both internally and externally, on the basic documentation formats and control requirements and state them in the VP. Note that they should bear in mind that they must comply with company policy and GxP requirements.

Training Requirements

A critical area often overlooked when planning validation projects is that connected with training, and it is an area that tends to need attention at different times during the project. Some training needs are more obvious than others. It may be necessary to embark upon some form of training for the groups that are to produce the various different documents during the project. After all, special rules may have been generated and personnel need to be made aware of them. Another aspect of training is more obvious — the training of the users in the operation of the new system. But what does "training" mean? Quite often it can take many different forms and the VP can be used to consider this and to identify key requirements. Some members of the company may only require a high level of information about the project, as they are not direct users. This is classed as "**communication**" and it takes the form of briefings or some other form of project overview — for example the use of video presentations. Other personnel will be directly affected and must be brought up to speed in a more controlled fashion. To achieve this they could undergo a number of project awareness sessions to prepare them for the next phase. These sessions form the basis of "**education.**" Finally, they can undergo the more formal and directly applicable "**training**" process for their day-to-day interaction with the system.

The VP must be used to provide details of all the above requirements and indicate the standard operating procedures that will control and formally record the process in adequate training records.

Validation Organization

This is a key section of the VP and must give an overview of the internal (and when applicable, external organization) requirements for its the successful execution. The first important item for inclusion is a full definition of the critical roles and responsibilities for the project. These will comprise critical roles such as:

- Phase or task ownership.
- Documentation ownership.
- Technical support.
- Quality assurance.

The section should go on to identify these key persons, including an indication of job titles to aid determination of the individual qualification and authority for the role.

Validation Activity Schedule and Timeline

The purpose of this section of the VP is to allow a high-level description of the tasks and activities associated with the project, and to link them with the overall expected schedule for the successful validation of the proposed system.

It should indicate the key phases of the project together with proposed planned end dates for the validation milestones in the project. It is usual to present this information in the form of a Gantt chart or some other widely recognized project-planning chart or tool.

The author of the VP should be aware that when writing this section timescales provided ought to be regarded for the purposes of indication only. The main purpose of this section is to show the time-related relationships between the phases and activities in the overall plan. It is usual for a detailed analysis of resource allocation activities and timing to be provided in another document, the quality and project plan.

Maintenance of Validation Status

The aim in this section of the VP is to indicate required procedures once the system has been validated and is "live." The purpose of these procedures is to ensure the maintenance of the validation status gained through compliance with the activities listed in the VP. Such procedures will include some, if not all, of the following.

- Change control.
- Access and security.
- Configuration management.
- Business continuity planning.
- Backup and recovery process.
- System start-up and shutdown.
- Help desk operation.
- Routine system audit.
- Upgrade strategy and plans.

- Revalidation policy.
- Ongoing training.

Appendices

This section should contain the following information.

- Definition of technical terms and abbreviations used in the document or reference to a glossary.
- References to other relevant documentation (internal company policies and procedures, regulatory guides, international standards, etc.).

CHECKLIST FOR COMPLETION OF A VALIDATION PLAN

This section provides a checklist of typical questions that the document author may ask in order to obtain the information required to populate the relevant sections of the VP.

Question	Y/N	Details (if applicable)
Has a project team been formed with the relevant: • Authority? • Business process knowledge? • Regulatory knowledge and experience? • Computer literacy?		List team membership and job titles.
Has the team performed an analysis of the GxP implications of the project?		Quote any references to formal documentation or meeting minutes.
Has the team defined a validation approach or strategy based upon: • GxP/business criticality? • Risk assessment? • Software and hardware categorization?		Quote any references to formal documentation or meeting minutes.
Does the document meet the company requirements for layout and format, including: • Approvals page • Titles page		

Question	Y/N	Details (if applicable)
• Unique project specific code		Record code number.
• Text format and numbering		
• Clear identification of author or owner		Record name and job title
Does the creation, review, approval, and control of the VP comply with the formal company document management procedures?		Record relevant company SOPs and any change control references.
Is there a contents page or list?		
Does the plan contain a detailed project overview that details the following:		
• Background and justification for the project? • Who produced the plan, under what authority and for what purpose? • Scope of the system validation? • Objectives of the validation? • Review periods?		
Does the system description include: • A process or system flow diagram? • A detailed description of components? • List of manufacturer or suppliers? • Data and information flows? • System and user interfaces? • Constraints?		
Does the plan contain a definition of the validation approach, including:		Record any reference documents used to arrive at decisions.
• Strategy for package modification? • Handling of bespoke software? • Issues surrounding data transfer? • Potential for phased implementation? • Follow up from vendor assessments?		
Is there a list of each possible document type that could be required to satisfy validation?		Record any documentation standards that may apply.
• URS? • Vendor assessment reports? • Quality and project plan? • Functional specifications? • Design specifications?		

Question	Y/N	Details (if applicable)
• Design meeting minutes? • Change control system or notices? • Hardware and equipment assembly records? • Software code reviews? • Hardware testing protocols and records? • Software testing protocols and records? • Hardware IQ protocols and records? • Software IQ protocols and records? • Hardware OQ protocols and records? • Factory acceptance protocols and records? • System acceptance protocols and records? • Go-live protocols and records? • Acceptance reports and certification? • User manuals and SOPs? • Ongoing operational procedures? • Configuration management and control? • Final validation report and sign-off?		
Does the plan clearly state the requirements for validation documentation management?		Quote relevant SOP reference.
Is there a section covering the potential requirements for training, including communication and education?		
Does the plan contain a detailed description of the team organization with respect to validation?		
Are details provided of the overall expected timescales and activities associated with validation of the system?		
Is there a section within the plan that provides an indication of the ongoing requirements for validation maintenance?		
Are the relevant appendices incorporated within the plan?		
Have the following reviewers commented upon the plan content (list only those relevant for the project): • Project manager? • Users?		

Question	Y/N	Details (if applicable)
• Quality assurance?		
• Validation?		
• Research and development?		
• Information technology?		
• Engineering?		
• Supplier or implementor?		
• Others?		
Have the following approvers provided signed acceptance of the plan content (list only those relevant for the project):		
• Project manager?		
• Users?		
• Quality assurance?		
• Validation?		
• Research and development?		
• Information technology?		
• Engineering?		
• Supplier or implementor?		
• Others?		

VALIDATION REPORTING

Overview of Validation Life Cycle

It is necessary to re-examine the simplified depiction of the generic validation life cycle for computerized systems as shown in Figure 4.1.

Initial examination of this figure seems to indicate that the validation report is one of the final activities of the life cycle and as such has the apparent function of summarizing all the activities that have gone on before. It also shows that it has a particularly close link to the project **VP**. Closer examination and discussion of the report and its role in the validation life cycle show that this relationship is not always as simple as depicted.

Purpose of the Validation Report

While the simplified view in Figure 4.1 indicates the need for a validation report at the end of the project, in reality this final report is more than likely to be one in a series of reports produced throughout the life of the project. This will particularly be the case when involved in lengthy complex implementations across several departments, with multiple applications linked together (for example, an MRPII system). In such cases it is usual for other types of reports to be produced at regular intervals throughout the project, primarily dealing with recording the progress made, issues raised, and acceptance of different phases of the project. Generally these "phase" reports are used as the formal documentation indicating completion of one phase and approval to commence the next. Hence they form a vital part of the control process surrounding the project's management. In analyzing the subject of writing the validation report, it is necessary to consider at what stage the report is written and any relationship between the various reports produced. It is important to note that there is always a need to have a final validation report, whatever the project, which summarizes the entire project and measures its ultimate success and acceptance by the user.

An often-quoted phrase regarding validation is that: "If it isn't written down then it's a rumor" (attributed to Sam Clark, a former FDA investigator). This provides a major clue as to the necessity for the creation of a validation report. When attempting to determine if pharmaceutical companies are complying with the GxPs, regulators such as the U.S. FDA and the U.K. MHRA want to see written evidence of task completion and controlled written evidence in particular. It is not acceptable to state verbally that some activity has occurred without the backup of some form of written evidence. The validation report has come to be seen to be of specific interest to these external regulatory bodies, so much so that inspectors from these bodies are more than likely to request such documents during regular inspection or surveillance visits. It is through examination of this document that regulatory authorities can see how organizations conducted and controlled the implementation of a new computerized system from the initial requirements definition, via the build process, installation, acceptance testing, and through to ongoing operation and maintenance. Furthermore, the regulatory authorities can understand, via a suitably constructed report, the degree of demonstrable compliance with the requirements laid down in the relevant GxPs.

Due to the highly crucial role that it can play in providing regulatory assurance, a validation report must record certain critical items, including, but not limited to:

- Introduction and brief project background.
- Overview and definition of phase or testing.
- Organizational or procedural arrangements for phase execution.
- Prerequisites considered.
- Environment.
- Planned deviations from VP (including justifications).
- Summary of phase output.
- Detailed description of phase output.
- Problem reporting and resolution or actions.
- Clear statement of status at end of phase.

Relationships with Other Life Cycle Phases and Documents

The term "validation report" can be applied to a series of reports rather than to a single entity. But what might these other reports be? By viewing an extension of the "V-model", found in the GAMP 4 Guide and illustrated in Figure 4.6, it is possible to see that there is a direct relationship between the VP and the validation report. However, it is also possible to gain an insight into the other reports that could be created during the project life cycle.

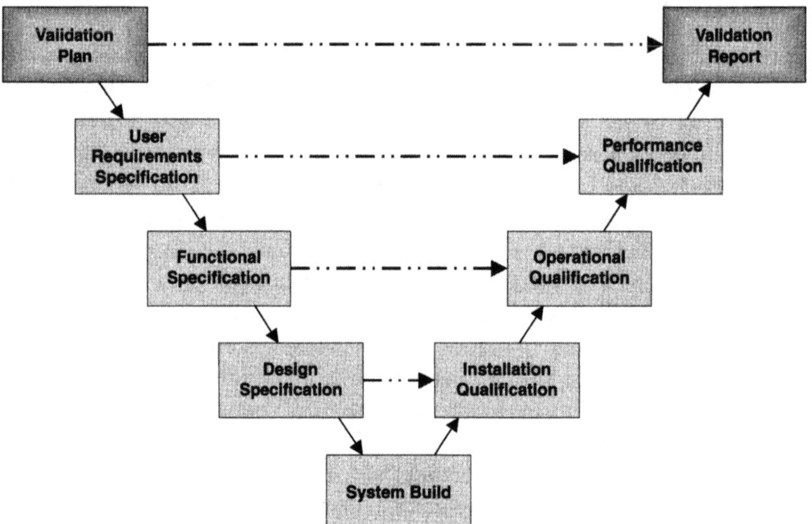

Figure 4.6 Extended V-model.

Figure 4.6 illustrates that for each stage or phase of the project there is a natural progression to the next phase. However, what is not clear from this illustration is that each of these phases will, of necessity, generate some form of output or deliverables. Take the example of the process of creating, reviewing, and approving the functional and design specifications, a vital step in the life cycle. Any errors or omissions at this stage of the project can lead to costly amendments or delays at a later stage. It is usual to document this review process formally to ensure that the initial requirements are adequately catered for by the proposed design, and any problems, variations, decisions, and exceptions raised during this time are recorded, acted upon, or carried forward. This exercise is collectively known as design qualification (DQ). The most advantageous method of summarizing these various activities is via a design qualification report. The DQ report is therefore the key deliverable from this project

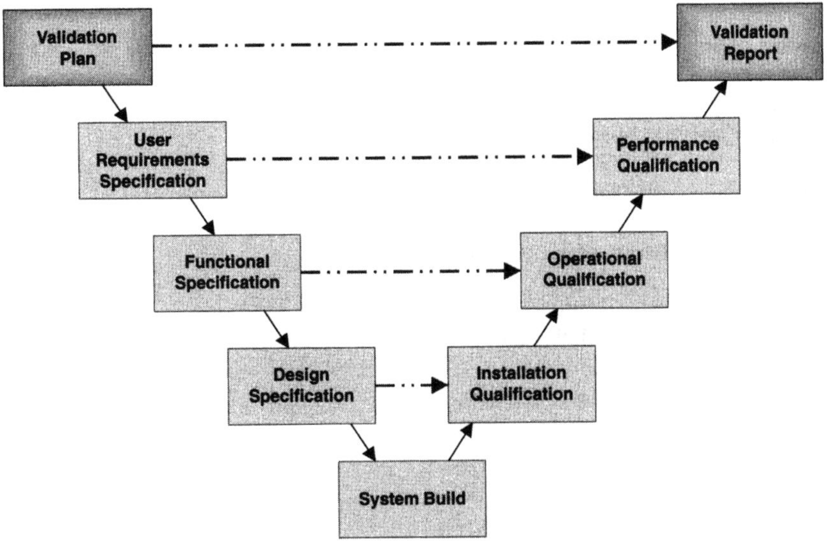

Figure 4.7 V-model reports relationships.

phase, and this is illustrated in Figure 4.7 which also shows that similar interactions exist between the other phases of the life cycle and also with the "final" report. It is possible to see that these phase reports form a subset of supporting information for the "final" validation report. As such they represent a depiction of the critical pathway from the beginning to the end of the project.

KEY REPORTING ACTIVITIES

Review Phase Requirements

The process of transferring from one phase of the life cycle to the next is a significant milestone in the project. During the project lifetime there will be several of these phase transfers, all of which lead to the final transfer of the system into the "live" state. Such points in the life cycle provide a focal point when the project team is required to provide confirmation that one phase has been completed to a satisfactory standard, while simultaneously granting approval for the next phase to commence. These points in time are also an opportunity for the project team to review progress against the overall project plan and to manage resources accordingly. The key output from this process should be the creation and approval of a "phase report." The phase requirements review process should take the form of

Table 4.13 Items that may require review.

Planning phase:
- URS.
- Invitation to tender, response to proposal.
- Company searches, vendor questionnaires, audit reports.
- VPs.
- Quality and project plan.

Specification and design phase (design qualification):
- Functional specification.
- Hardware design specifications.
- Mechanical and electrical diagrams.
- Software design specifications.
- Software module design specifications.
- Network design specifications.
- Minutes of design review meetings.
- Change notices.

Building phase:
- Hardware manufacture and assembly records.
- Peripherals and equipment manufacture and assembly records.
- Software code reviews.
- Network manufacture and assembly records.
- Change notices.

Testing phase:
- Hardware testing protocols and records.
- Software module testing protocols and records.
- Software integration testing protocols and records.
- Peripherals and equipment testing protocols and records.
- Change notices.

Installation phase (IQ/OQ):
- Hardware installation qualification protocols and records.
- Software installation qualification protocols and records.
- Peripherals and equipment installation qualification protocols and records.
- Network installation qualification protocols and records.
- Hardware acceptance testing protocols and records (OQ).
- Network acceptance testing protocols and records (OQ).
- Change notices.
- Acceptance reports and certification.

Acceptance phase (OQ/PQ):
- FAT protocols and records (OQ/PQ).
- System acceptance testing protocols and records (OQ/PQ).
- Go-live testing protocols and records (OQ/PQ).

- Change notices.
- Acceptance reports and certification.

Final reporting phase:
- Ongoing operation.
- Standard operating procedure — user manuals, data center operations.
- Change control procedures.
- Configuration management procedures.
- Final validation reports and sign off.

---

verifying that all the planned activities are complete and the planned deliverables for the phase are present and correct. This is not a detailed review at this stage, more a preparation for the subsequent collation and analysis of test results and issues. If this process reveals any unusual occurrences, deviations, or variations from the planned activities and project deliverables, they can be noted and further discussed within the main body of the phase report. Table 4.13 indicates some examples of the items that could require review as part of each of the indicated phases.

Collate and Analyze the Results Obtained

The project team should nominate an individual or, in the case of large projects, a subteam to perform this task. Generally these people should have the appropriate experience and qualifications to understand the GxP and business impact of the results and be able to present their conclusions to the remainder of the project team in a clear and concise manner.

A useful approach is for this group to tabulate the outcomes and results to make review easier, highlighting any deviations from the planned activities or outcomes at the same time. They should then prepare to summarize the outcome and conclusions to the rest of the team, using the deviations noted to stimulate discussions on possible resolution.

Collate and Analyze the Issues Raised

All deviations must be addressed to the satisfaction of the project team and within the project's scope and objectives. Each one must be assessed for any potential GxP impact. The nature and severity of the deviation could well determine the approach to its resolution. If the deviation is the result of an incomplete activity or deliverable then the reasons for noncompletion must be determined and the project team must decide if it needs to be completed before the phase can be accepted. If some critical documentation is not available, an action plan must be formulated either to obtain it or to justify its noninclusion. However, if the deviation is the result of a test failure it may be necessary to make a controlled change to the system and repeat the relevant tests.

The project team must decide which, if any, of these issues must be completed in order to accept the phase, and conversely, if any may be carried forward to the next phase. All such decisions must be formally documented and approved. The phase report provides the ideal mechanism for achieving this.

Write the Validation Report

The task of writing the validation report (or phase report) is the responsibility of the project team. It is more efficient and usual for the team to nominate an individual to perform this task rather than attempt to create a report by committee. If the project has already created a number of report formats or templates, the task of creating the report will be relatively simple, with the author required only to enter the relevant information or data into predefined sections.

It is advisable to begin the process of drafting the report at almost the same time as the phase begins, creating it in parallel with the activities of the phase. This will not only save time at the end of the phase when the report is undergoing the review and approval process, but it can also act as a focal point for the collation of the information required by the review team as discussed in the "Review Phase Requirements" section.

Review the Validation Report

The draft report should be presented to the project team for a review process. The entire team may not need to perform this process; an appointed subteam may well suffice. However this subteam must be made up of members who have the relevant technical expertise and qualifications, including detailed knowledge of any issues raised and the implications that they may have on the project as a whole (in particular GxP and business impact).

Table 4.14 lists the recommended minimum number of participants needed in the review process, together with an indication of reviewers' roles and responsibilities.

It may be necessary for the report to undergo two or three cycles of the review process in order to reach agreement with the whole team (including QA). This fact should not be overlooked and it is important that time is allowed in the project planning process for this. All to often a project plan will assign one day for approval of the report, with no time allowance built in for an adequate review and modification process. If the report is used to signal the end of one phase and the start of another it is entirely possible that the next phase will be delayed while the report is undergoing this process.

Table 4.14 Participants in the report review process

Users	Ensure the reports meet the requirements of the planned activities.
Project manager	Ensure the conclusions detailed in the report adequately reflect the status of the phase or project. Ensure issues or deviations have been resolved, justified, or corrective actions agreed and carried forward if necessary.
Validation	Ensure the conclusions detailed in the report adequately reflect the status of the phase or project and comply with current accepted industry or company standards for validation of computer systems.
Information technology	Technical expertise regarding hardware, software, and systems acceptability and compatibility. Ensure compliance with company IT strategy. Management of day-to-day IT systems operations and controls.
Engineering	Acceptance of hardware siting, cabling and peripherals, and compliance with capacity and maintenance requirements.
Supplier or implementer	Ensure the conclusions detailed in the report adequately reflect the status of the phase/project.
Quality assurance	Ensure the report complies with predefined format and structure requirements. Review all deviations and issues and ensure GxP or business impact has been assessed. Ensure issues and deviations have been resolved, justified, or corrective actions agreed and carried forward if necessary. Ensure compliance with any relevant regulatory requirements.

Approve the Validation Report

Regulatory inspectors often seek to assess the approach to and levels of compliance with the approved validation requirements by asking to review the validation activities that were initially planned. Hence they will request to see a VP, which should be adequately approved and controlled. The next logical question following this review will be to request evidence that the planned activities were satisfactorily completed. In addition they will attempt to determine that throughout the duration of the project adequate controls were in place. By providing the phase reports the company is able to demonstrate that it can meet these requirements, but these reports need to carry the suitable level of authority that can only be granted full approval. The approval of the reports should be clear and unambiguous, and should be performed by suitably competent and experienced persons. Each individual should sign each report as appropriate, with the approval signature indicating name, job or function and the approval date.

As for who should be involved in this approval process, the list is similar to that given in the preceding section for phase reports review. The approval process followed should be exactly the same as that for any other compliance critical document managed by the company's QA documentation control system.

Document Management and Control

Validation reports are usually classed as critical documents in the same way as one would regard a standard operating procedure or a master batch record. However, in the context of their importance in the validation life cycle as illustrated in this chapter, the author considers that such documents should be treated similarly to other "compliance critical" documents and should, once approved, be formally controlled by a documentation control system. This will ensure they are adequately issued and stored so as to be available for subsequent inhouse review (maybe as part of a system modification or upgrade project) or by regulatory agencies, without fear of any adulteration having taken place.

While documentation systems can vary from company to company, reports should include the following basic principles.

- Documents should be assigned a unique reference code, linked to the original VP.
- Version control must be in operation from one edition to the next to identify when a document has been superseded.
- Documents should be laid out in an orderly format so as to ensure unambiguous and clear content.
- The ability to conduct formal review processes and update documents as required must exist.
- There must be a clear change control process to track change requests — who, why, when?
- There must be clear document approval involving only those with appropriate qualifications and with suitable authority to approve.
- Approvals must be dated.
- Control of document issue and distribution should be in operation, including return or destruction of old versions.

The responsibility for managing and controlling documents is generally given to the quality assurance function and this applies equally to validation reports. However, it is important that the project team are conscious of the need for document control and they should be given the necessary training to build and improve this awareness.

FORMAT AND CONTENT OF A VALIDATION REPORT

This section defines the typical contents of a validation report. While none of the sections listed here should be regarded as mandatory, careful consideration must be given to the scope, criticality, and phase of the project when deciding which to omit. If any sections are excluded it is recommended that some form of justification is provided.

The primary sections for placing within a validation report, irrespective of project phase, are:

- Introduction.
- Summary of phase results.
- Phase execution.
- Problem reporting and resolution.
- Validation phase status.
- Glossary.
- Appendices.

Introduction

The introduction to any formal document is vital to setting the scene for the reader and should place the main content and conclusions into their correct context. Therefore the author of a validation report should spend a reasonably significant amount of time in constructing this section and structuring it to meet these needs adequately. Examples of the typical themes to be covered by the introduction include:

- Purpose of the report.
- Who created it.
- Under what authority (with cross references to key documents).
- Definition of the phase requirements.
- Summary of the approach adopted.
- Scope of phase.

Although many of the items listed seem to require a high level of detail, it is possible to encompass them in a few well-chosen sentences. An example of some suitable text is as shown in Table 4.15.

Table 4.15 Example text.

INTRODUCTION

The purpose of this report is to review and summarize those activities connected with the system acceptance testing (SAT) phase of the Novocastrian Pharmaceutical Company

Limited (NPCL) ERP project. These activities are defined in the System Acceptance Test Specification (document ref. OQ-123/002, Issue 1.00, dated 5 November 1998).

In addition this report presents a summary of the issues raised during SAT with indications of their satisfactory resolution or, if unresolved, details of the action plans to allow successful resolution.

This report supplements the information contained within the SAT certificate (document reference OQ-123-003) signifying acceptance of the system by NPCL and approval to move into full system implementation and go-live.

[*NPCL Validation Manager*], in accordance with the system acceptance test specification (document ref. OQ-123/002), has prepared this report.

Definition of System Acceptance Testing

The definition of "system acceptance testing" is the culmination of all major system testing work, and is the second and final phase of formal OQ acceptance testing by the client. SAT consists of those tests that show that the system operates correctly in its final operating environment and interfaces correctly with other systems and equipment.

SAT, together with the results of FAT, provides sufficient evidence to validate the system in accordance with the approach defined within the NPCL Validation Plan VP-123, the requirements of the pharmaceutical industry regulatory authorities and in compliance with the standards defined by GAMP.

Summary of System Acceptance Testing Approach

System acceptance testing was executed between November 6, 2000 and December 22, 2000. It was hosted on the Mercedes/Jaguar servers using the standard NPCL Desktop environment.

In totality SAT included:

- IQ (hardware acceptance testing) of hardware configuration to be used for SAT.
- IQ of software configuration and software setup on Mercedes/Jaguar servers and on the PC clients used for SAT.
- IQ of peripheral devices used during SAT.
- OQ — run of agreed, specified acceptance tests on Mercedes/Jaguar servers using the total solution.
- PQ–SAT was executed in the final target environment using production peripheral equipment in their Go-Live environment, and utilized test databases {GFSAT, FSSAT} with a high proportion of the static data to be used for go-live.

Scope of Testing

- The functional testing of all the four core applications — Oracle GEMMS, Oracle Financials, FlowStream, and Documentum.
- The functional testing of all interfaces between the core application systems, interfaces to legacy systems and peripheral interfaces (balances, radio data terminals, barcode scanners, label printers).
- The execution of SAT included, where possible, the use of the draft SOP.

Summary of Phase Results

It is normal, and aids the readability of the report, if a short section is included early on to provide a brief summary of the test results. This could take the form of a short text description of the overall outcome of the testing and activities performed, giving an indication of the levels of success or failure. More simply, the results could be tabulated to indicate the total numbers passed, the numbers failed, those tests not performed, and any with inconclusive outcomes.

Finally, the summary should briefly indicate any unusual occurrences, deviations and variations from the expected outcome, and raise key issues for further discussion within the main body of the report.

Phase Execution

This section of the report will probably be the longest and most detailed. It provides a comprehensive breakdown of the outcome of all the activities required for completion of the phase, including test results, test certificates, documentation, etc.

A suggested list of themes to be covered within this section is as follows:

- Prerequisites.
- Project environment.
- Exclusions.
- Details of phase execution.
- Comprehensive results breakdown.

Each of the above is briefly discussed in the subsequent paragraphs. However this list is not exhaustive and consideration should be given to any other relevant information which can be used to provide a historical record of the events that occurred to support the implementation and validation of the system.

Prerequisites

The objective of this subsection is to present a detailed itemization of the tasks, conditions, and actions deemed to be satisfactorily completed before beginning any phase specific activities such as testing. There is no idealized list of the items that can be created as they will very much depend upon the individual requirements of each and every project, but an example list is given in Table 4.16. In practice not all of these items may have reached such a suitable conclusion and it may be necessary to indicate where some of these cannot be satisfied and to justify the reasons for continuing the implementation uninterrupted. In constructing the report and using a table to list prerequisite status, it is useful to indicate these actions and responsibilities at the same time, and this routine is also illustrated in Table 4.16. This table is constructed on the basis of the pre-requisites that may be considered necessary when moving from the FAT to the system acceptance testing (SAT) phase. The example project is a fictional ERP implementation for the Novocastrian Pharmaceutical Company Limited (NPCL), which is supported by a third-party systems implementor (SI).

Project Environment

Within the context of this chapter the phrase "project environment" is used to refer to the different combinations of hardware and software at various stages of the project. Hence the combination may develop from that housed on a development server and simple client to the more complex client/server combination of the live system. The project environment used for the various phases should be described in sufficient detail so as to give an overview of the software configuration, master databases, hardware, and peripherals involved. The origin of this environment should be indicated, for example, where was it initially created, and when was it copied over. The text should go on to describe how and when it was finally migrated to the live server and the clients, and if any special configuration requirements were implemented. Indication must also be provided of the change control procedures applied to the software configuration and master databases.

Exclusions

Quite often it is necessary to modify the original approach taken to reach a satisfactory conclusion to the different phases of a project as a result of changing circumstances throughout the lifetime of that project. For example, because of the need to satisfy certain SAT prerequisites before executing some SAT tests, and the need to continue specific business processes in some areas, it could be found that a number of planned tests could not be executed in the manner expected, or at all. It is vital that when this happens the validation report must not only highlight these exclusions, but also justify them in terms of the overall risk to the successful completion of the project and the satisfactory validation of the system.

Some example situations are:

- Tests involving equipment that could not be tested outside its normal environment (e.g., floor-mounted balances in a dispensing area).
- Activities associated with an area undergoing a parallel refurbishment program, that was not completed on time.
- Activities including full operational testing of legacy system interfaces where a test legacy system could not be implemented.

Table 4.16 Possible prerequisites for SAT

Description	Resp.	Status/Action	Reference
FAT test results for each module	SI	Complete	FAT test report ref. TR/VP123/001
Approved FAT reports	NPCL	Complete	N/A
Migration of application and bespoke software from "test server" to "live server"	NPCL/SI	Complete	IT operations report ref. PE/VP123/050
"Live server" system environment complete	NPCL/SI	Complete	IT operations report ref. PE/VP123/061
System installation qualification	NPCL/SI	Complete	IQ system – ref. TR/VP123/210
Complete test script amendments resulting from execution of FAT	NPCL/SI	Complete	Document change request ref. 10099
Updated FDS and application setup documents	SI	Held pending completion and approval of SAT	NA
Technical document changes	NPCL	Complete	PE/VP123/063
Final draft and reviewed SOPs	NPCL	Still in progress – for completion before "go-live"	Document change request ref. 10100
Input static and dynamic data for SAT	NPCL	Detailed as per each test prerequisite	See SAT specification
Collate and record data, hardware and software changes to database plus bespoke and core applications as a result of execution of FAT	NPCL/SI	Complete	FAT test report ref. TR/VP123/001
Install and qualify hardware, peripherals and interfaces required for SAT	NPCL/SI	Complete	IQ project environment – ref. TR/VP123/213 IQ peripherals – Ref. TR/VP123/280
Bespoke software modifications excluding label formatting and additional core label are installed	SI	Incomplete at start of SAT – to be completed during SAT and tested before completion of phase	N/A
Required security in place	NPCL	Complete	TR/VP123/133
Required system support capability in place	NPCL	Complete	PE/VP123/038

Details of Phase Execution

It is good practice to include in the report a short description of the underlying details of the phase execution. At the outset it is customary to refer to the controlling specification for the phase (the acceptance test specification, for example). The text should then proceed to confirm that all completed tests were executed and witnessed by suitably qualified and authorized personnel, indicating any support resources that were available and specifying the names, job titles, and qualifications of those involved. As far as reasonably possible the testing and witnessing personnel should be selected on the basis of their knowledge of that area of the business under test, and past experience of the proposed solution.

The description should then continue with a discussion regarding the location of the testing. This is particularly important, as it is necessary to explain the level of control exercised during the development of a system, demonstrating the reduction of any risk to existing live systems during the implementation and before acceptance.

Another detail that should be considered for inclusion in this part of the report, particularly in relation to tracing the project history, is confirmation of the dates over which the phase occurred, together with explanations of reasons for delays and actions taken to resolve them.

Finally it is recommended that the text include confirmation that all tests and activities are subjected to a regular project team review process, indicating the evidence to support this statement.

Comprehensive Results Breakdown

This section forms the main body of the report and it is important to ensure that it is both comprehensive and concise. The recommended way to achieve this is to record the summarized results in a tabular form. In designing the table format it is necessary to consider what information is conveyed to the reader. The validation report is a summary of the activities that took place during the phase. Hard copy original test records or documents containing detailed information of the activity, reference to any other documents (e.g., URS, FDS) and the outcome of those activities will back it up. Therefore the summary table only needs to indicate the test reference, what it applies to, the title of the test or activity, the outcome and a reference to the incident log for follow-up if required. Table 4.17 provides some examples of the type of issues to be recorded and a possible format for use in other reports.

Problem Reporting and Resolution

As can be observed from the discussion in the previous section of this chapter, it will be most unusual for the activities or tests performed during a phase to complete

Table 4.17 Example test result summary

Test	Module	Description	Result	Incident #
T130/009	Purchasing	Long receipt: lot controlled items	**Fail** Did not save records – software bug	530
T131/015	Sales	Sales order acknowledgement	**Pass**	–
T131/016	Sales	Perform stock checks during order processing through to despatch	**Pass**	–
T132/005	Finance	Capital/revenue mix – revenue is recorded	**Pass**	–
T132/006	Finance	Run standard reports	**Fail** Printer set-up problem	531
T132/007	Finance	Accounts inquiry on budgets	**Pass**	–
T135/010	Legacy	U.K. sales data extract	**Fail** Extract files contained sales data and raw materials data	532
T138/001	Quality	Sampling raw material, intermediate product or packaging component	**Fail** Label L_MAI_001 not produced due to system error	533
T138/002	Quality	Sample raw material or packaging component (inventory adjusted, interface test)	**Pass**	–
T138/003	Quality	Sampling water	**Pass**	–
T138/004	Quality	Extract data for inclusion in external template	**Pass**	–
T138/005	Quality	Recall finished goods	**Pass**	–
T142/064	Dispensing	Stock check (no inventory adjustment required)	**Fail** Report not available at time of test	534
T142/065	Dispensing	Stock check (inventory adjustment required)	**Pass**	–

without any problems or deviation from the expected outcome. In such circumstances it is vital that the validation report accurately reflects these issues and discusses them in sufficient detail to clarify the required actions and timescales for resolution and justification for the chosen courses of action. A full assessment of system readiness before proceeding from one phase to the next requires a review of not only the test results (see previous section), but also the solutions to the issues and problems raised during the total testing period.

The documentation of these issues is very much a matter of individual taste, but again the use of a tabular format provides a disciplined approach that will ensure all the required issues are highlighted for each adverse event or deviation. Table 4.18 provides an example of one such format that provides details of what the variance is, when and where it occurred, what the effect has been, an indication of a resolution route, and a statement of its status at the time of writing the validation report.

The use of such a simple format for recording these problems means that the author and readers of the report can quickly observe the main issues and trace the resolution during future stages of the project.

Table 4.18 Example problem reporting summary

Incident #	Test	Problem description	Cause/Solution	Action
530	T130/009	Test failure — software does not save updated records in the purchasing module	• Identified as software error — confirmed by vendor • Install patch fix ref. 1223444, confirm IQ and retest function	Change notice 1642
531	T132/006	Test failure — standard reports would not print when requested	• Printer setup error • Update printer configuration and retest	Change notice 1643
532	T135/010	Test failure — erroneous data contained within U.K. sales data extract into legacy forecast system	• Design of extract routine code specifying incorrect database database tables • Modify code and retest	Change notice 1644

Validation Status

The opening to this section of the chapter indicated that an important feature of any formal document is the need to set the document into its correct context. It is also equally important that the status at the conclusion of the activities covered by the validation report is clearly defined.

The structure of the report proposed in this chapter naturally guides the reader to this statement of the validation phase status. Such statements need not be excessively complex, but should attempt to covey the following basic messages.

- Who has reviewed the report and under what authority?
- What does their signature on the report represent?
- Is the status acceptable or unacceptable?
- Can the project proceed to the next phase?

In cases where the report is the final validation report, the last bullet point would be more akin to a statement that the system is validated in accordance with the planned activities originally defined in the VP.

Glossary

The inclusion of a glossary is a useful aid for the reader who is unfamiliar with specific terminology employed within the project or the technology adopted for the final implemented system. The glossary should limit itself to brief but meaningful definitions of technical terms and abbreviations used within the report and any other reference documentation.

Appendices

This section should contain the following information.

- For validation reports that cover a wide number of events it may be useful to provide listings of cross-reference documentation.
- References to other relevant documentation (internal company policies and procedures, regulatory guides, international standards, etc.).

CHECKLIST FOR COMPLETION OF A VALIDATION REPORT

This section provides a checklist of typical questions that the document author may ask in order to obtain the information required to populate the relevant sections of the validation report.

Question	Y/N	Details (if applicable)
Does the report meet the company requirements for layout and format, including:		
• Approvals page?		
• Titles page?		
• Unique project specific code?		Record code number
• Text format and numbering?		
• Clear identification of author or owner?		Record name and job title
Does the creation, review, approval, and control of the validation report comply with the formal company document management procedures?		Record relevant company SOPs and any change control references
Is there a contents page or list?		
Does the report contain an introduction which details the following:		
• Purpose of the report?		
• Who produced the report and under what authority?		
• Definition of the phase requirements?		
• Summary of the approach adopted?		
• Scope of the phase and report?		
Does the report provide an easily readable summary of the results?		
Does the report contain the following details of the execution of the phase:		Record any reference documents used to arrive at decisions
• Prerequisites?		
• Project environment?		
• Exclusions?		
• Details of the phase execution?		
• Comprehensive results breakdown?		
Does the report highlight any deviations or variations from the expected results and actions for resolution or closure?		
Does the report indicate that any deviations or variations from the expected results have been assessed for:		

Question	Y/N	Details (if applicable)
• GxP and business criticality?		
• Risk analysis?		
Are the relevant appendices incorporated within the report?		
Is there a clear statement of the validation status of the project or system following approval of the report?		
Have the following reviewers commented upon the report content (list only those relevant for the project):		
• Project manager?		
• Users?		
• Quality assurance?		
• Validation?		
• Information technology?		
• Engineering?		
• Supplier or implementer?		
• Others?		
Have the following approvers provided signed acceptance of the report content (list only those relevant for the project):		
• Project manager?		
• Users?		
• Quality assurance?		
• Validation?		
• Information technology?		
• Engineering?		
• Supplier or implementer?		
• Others?		

GLOSSARY

Computerized system. Consists of hardware, software, and network components, together with the controlled functions and associated documentation. Sometimes referred to as an automated system.

Configuration. The documented physical and functional characteristics of an item or system.

Environment. This term, when unqualified, usually refers to the combination of hardware and software in a computerized system.

ERP. Enterprise resource planning is an industry term for the broad set of activities supported by multimodule application software that helps a manufacturer or other business manage the important parts of its business. Such activities include product planning, purchasing, maintaining inventories, interacting with suppliers, providing customer service, tracking orders, finance, and human resources.

Factory acceptance test (FAT). The factory acceptance tests are those tests of the functions and facilities that can be tested outside the system's operating environment with the aid of test hardware and software.

Functional specification. A functional specification defines a system to meet the customer's needs, which should be set out in a URS. It defines what the system should do, and what functions and facilities are to be provided. It provides a list of design objectives for the system.

GAMP. Good automated manufacturing practice.

Installation qualification. Documented verification that all key aspects of software and hardware installation adhere to appropriate codes and approved design intentions.

MRPII system. Similar to an ERP but usually without such activities as human resources or finance.

Operational qualification. Documented verification that the equipment-related system or sub-system performs as intended throughout representative or anticipated operating ranges.

Performance qualification. Documented verification that the process and the total process related system performs as intended throughout all anticipated operating ranges.

System acceptance test (SAT). The system acceptance tests are those tests that show the system operates correctly in its final operating environment and interfaces correctly with other systems and equipment.

REFERENCES

1. International Society for Pharmaceutical Engineering. *The Good Automated Manufacturing Practice (GAMP) Guide for the Validation of Automated Systems in Pharmaceutical Manufacture*, Version 4, December 2001.
2. Medicines and Healthcare Products Regulatory Agency. "Rules and Guidance for Pharmaceutical Manufacturers and Distributors 2002."

Chapter 5

Supplier Audits: Questions and Answers

Guy Wingate

CONTENTS

INTRODUCTION: TWENTY FREQUENTLY ASKED QUESTIONS

This chapter is intended for users and suppliers involved in the auditing of computer systems, software, and associated services to the pharmaceutical and healthcare industries.

This chapter will help users and suppliers prepare for audit, complete their audits efficiently, and present themselves professionally to the regulatory sector. This is especially important where a potential manufacturer or customer conducts an audit as part of a supplier selection exercise.

Suppliers can help themselves and their customers so much more if they are prepared for such audits. It is vital to the manufacturer that a true reflection of the supplier's quality and compliance be established. It is not in the interests of the supplier or user that the supplier's capability is either under- or overestimated.

This chapter aims to help suppliers understand the audit process adopted in the pharmaceutical and healthcare industries, and how best to prepare and manage user audits.

It has been structured to pose and then answer a series of 20 questions about what, why, and how a supplier should prepare and manage an audit by a manufacturer or customer.

Based on work conducted by the author with the Supplier Forum, it should be read in conjunction with the pharmaceutical and healthcare manufacturer's own auditing procedure, and general industry guidance given to pharmaceutical and healthcare industry auditors in the GAMP Guide (Version 4, December 2001).

Q1 WHAT IS COMPUTER VALIDATION?

It is vital that computer systems are suitable for their intended use, especially when used to support the development, manufacture, and distribution of healthcare and drug products. The healthcare and pharmaceutical industries use the term "computer systems validation" (CSV), to describe those activities deemed appropriate to ensure computer systems are fit for purpose.

Computer systems validation is largely based on adopting the basic principles and good practices of quality assurance. It necessitates: "Establishing documented evidence which provides a high degree of assurance that a specific process will consistently produce a product meeting its pre-determined specifications and quality attributes." (U.S. Food and Drug Administration, 1995)

The key phrases are "meeting pre-determined specifications," "documentary evidence," and "high degree of assurance."

1. The requirements and specification of a system should be defined before testing is conducted.
2. Testing should confirm that requirements are met.
3. Requirements, specifications, and testing should all be carefully documented.

If activities are not documented, they cannot be reviewed afterwards to confirm they were conducted in an appropriate manner. The overall aim is to *build a level of confidence* in a system, rather than simply to *prove* it. There are practical limitations on testing, but it is important to demonstrate to the regulators that a reasonable level of testing has been successfully concluded.

A life cycle approach — preferred for validation activities — covers planning, specification, design, build, testing, authorization for use, operation and maintenance, archive, and decommissioning.

Q2 HOW AND BY WHOM ARE COMPUTER SYSTEMS VALIDATION ACTIVITIES REGULATED?

Regulatory authorities such as the U.S. Food and Drug Administration (FDA) and U.K. Medicines Control Agency (MHRA) monitor the compliance of validation to various regulations and standards set out for their respective domestic markets.

The regulations governing validation are generically known as "GxP" or "good practice regulations" and cover good clinical practice (GCP), good laboratory practice (GLP), good manufacturing practice (GMP), and good distribution practice (GDP). "Good automated manufacturing practice" (GAMP) is a term developed from GMP and is documented in the GAMP Guide Version 4 (GAMP Forum, 2001).

If a pharmaceutical and healthcare manufacturer's computer system fails to satisfy a regulatory authority's requirements, that regulatory authority can revoke the manufacturer's license to sell any drug products supported by the system in question.

This can of course have serious adverse consequences for supplier and manufacturer and is best avoided by early correct actions and procedures, to ensure compliance.

Q3 WHO IS RESPONSIBLE FOR VALIDATING COMPUTER SYSTEMS?

Pharmaceutical and healthcare manufacturers are accountable to regulatory authorities for the validation of computer systems used to support the manufacture of drug products.

Pharmaceutical and healthcare manufacturers expect suppliers to provide solutions to satisfy their needs and to demonstrate control of the work assigned to them.

Any shortfalls in the supplier's capability uncovered in the audit will have to be made up by the pharmaceutical and healthcare manufacturers, either directly or through third-party support.

Suppliers must remember, however, that they have an inherent legal responsibility to all their users that their products and services are fit for purpose.

Q4 WHY DO CUSTOMERS CONDUCT AUDITS?

Pharmaceutical and healthcare manufacturers will often conduct an audit of a supplier to assess the supplier's quality systems and management. The audit may be part of a supplier selection exercise; or alternatively audits may be used to confirm the present compliance status of a preselected preferred supplier.

Regulators expect supplier audits to be conducted to a defined procedure and be properly documented to demonstrate compliance. They expect the results of such audits to be acted upon and any necessary corrective actions to be taken in a timely fashion.

If an audit determines any persistent deficiencies with the supplier, the pharmaceutical and healthcare manufacturer will be expected to review whether a suitable alternative supplier is more appropriate.

Q5 IS THERE A STANDARD AUDIT PROCESS?

A typical audit process (illustrated in Figure 5.1) is initiated by determining if an audit is required. Once the need for an audit has been defined, the supplier concerned should be contacted, and an audit request made explaining its context.

The supplier may require a briefing in the proposed audit process.

The audit is then conducted and a report prepared by the pharmaceutical and healthcare manufacturer. The supplier should be given a chance to review and comment on the report so that any necessary clarifications can be made at an early stage.

Any corrective actions undertaken by the supplier should be followed up, and so the audit process loops back to arranging another audit.

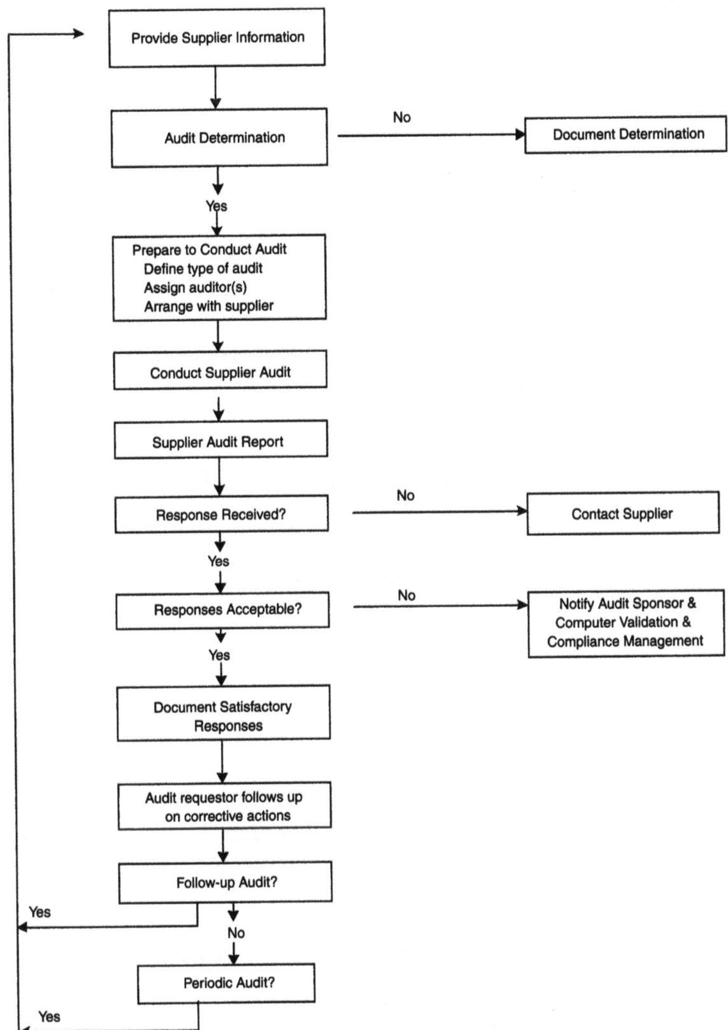

Figure 5.1 The audit process table.

Q6 WHEN IS AN AUDIT REQUIRED?

The latest edition of the GAMP Guide suggests that pharmaceutical and healthcare manufacturers should conduct audits of suppliers for:

- Standard software used in all critical applications.

- Configurable commercial software used in complex or critical applications.
- Bespoke or custom software.
- Bespoke or custom hardware.

This scope includes laboratory instrumentation, process control systems, IT systems, spreadsheets, databases, and networks.

Audits are not normally expected for widely distributed standard software or configurable commercial software packages. The basis for this decision is that the software or system has been satisfactorily market tested.

There is a general expectation that software must have been released for over six months, and have been successfully deployed by more than 100 active users to satisfy market testing criteria. Software under beta testing is not considered as formally released to market.

Q7 WHAT IS THE SCOPE OF AN AUDIT?

The scope of an audit can be summarized as indicated below. Topics have been grouped as suggested in the GAMP Guide, though not all topics will be relevant to all suppliers.

Company Overview

Supplier viability:

- Evidence must exist to assure users that the supplier will be able to provide continuing support of the computer system, based on factors such as company history, growth, business plans, legal commitments, and financial success.

Systems viability:

- The history and customer base of the supplier's systems and development process do not reflect negatively on system viability.
- The system's viability is not at risk from associations with third party or contracted products or services.
- The source code is available for any required regulatory review or use, in the event the supplier can no longer support the product.
- New releases of the system will enable the user to access or convert data created by previous releases.
- The supplier demonstrates control over systems via an inventory of their systems and versions.
- The supplier has ensured that the system is fully operational.

Organization and Quality Management

- The supplier has a current organization chart and structure to address the key aspects of the supplier's responsibilities concerning the computer system.
- The supplier has written qualification requirements or job descriptions for persons in the positions that impact the computer system.
- The supplier has evidence that the personnel currently in place meet the requirements for their positions.
- The supplier has evidence that key personnel maintain the education, experience, and training required for their positions.

Planning and Product or Project Management

Project management:

- The supplier uses project management tools and methods to ensure that development or implementation activities are properly organized, documented, and controlled.

Quality management:

- The supplier has a quality function in place, to ensure documentation of both the initial and ongoing quality of the system.
- The supplier's quality function is independent of the software development group.
- The supplier can demonstrate how the quality function is assigned to members of the supplier's organization.

Specifications

- The supplier maintains a current requirements specification to document the required content of functions for the computer system.
- The supplier maintains a current design specification to document how the requirements for the system will be met.
- For bespoke hardware, the supplier has applicable hardware layout diagrams for the system.

Implementation

- The supplier constructs source code in accordance with predefined programing standards.
- The supplier's programing standards address programing conventions to be used, including annotations and dead code handling.

- The supplier reviews code for conformance with programing standards.
- The supplier has (available for inspection) written documentation detailing the instructions for installation, configuration, operation, and any applicable calibration and maintenance for the system.
- The written documentation includes plans for installation activities, and a verification test plan for the installation system.
- If the supplier participates in the installation of hardware or software for the customer's system, it produces installation reports and has procedures for documenting and resolving installation problems.
- The supplier has written procedures to verify that proper controls, calibrations and standards were used to implement modules interfaced to instruments or other devices.
- Source code will be made available when requested by a regulator.

Testing

- The supplier performs documented testing to demonstrate that the structure and functionality of the computer system meet the predetermined requirements.
- The testing complies with written system development procedures.
- The testing is based on the predetermined and predefined approved requirements and specifications, and is traceable to these documents.
- The supplier has a procedure in place to resolve test failures and errors discovered during testing.
- The supplier's testing includes written test plans with defined expected results, documented test results, and documented release of the system.

Completion and Release

- The supplier maintains a secure environment for system development, to ensure that physical and electronic access to the computer system is limited to authorized personnel.
- The supplier has procedures for contingency planning, virus handling and backup and restoration of software, to ensure security from natural disasters and malfunctions.
- The supplier periodically backs up its software.
- The supplier has documented testing of their contingency plan available.
- Service level agreements (SLA) and/or warrantees are in place.

Support and Maintenance

Customer training:

- The supplier has a customer-training program, with regularly scheduled instruction courses or with optional customer-training facilities at the client site.
- This customer-training program provides complete training materials to the client, and includes information required to install, administer, and operate the system.

Technical support:

- The supplier maintains a technical support program to support the customer's use of the computer system.
- The supplier maintains a process to adequately record, track, analyze, and correct defects reported or discovered in the computer system.

Supporting Procedures and Activities

Procedures:

- Ensure supplier has current written procedures in place to control the development, testing, and maintenance of the computer system.
- Ensure that development, modification, approval, and use of these procedures is controlled.

Change control:

- The supplier controls, implements, and tracks changes to the system.
- The system is controled to ensure traceability and security through the use of a configuration management system or procedures.
- The supplier can recreate past and present software versions.
- The supplier maintains a link between their fault-reporting mechanism and the change control program.

Document control:

- The supplier uses documented practices to control the preparation, approval, issuing, and modification of documents related to the computer system.

Q8 WHAT ABOUT ELECTRONIC RECORDS AND ELECTRONIC SIGNATURES?

Currently the main driver for particular attention towards electronic records and electronic signatures (ERES) comes from the U.S. and Europe. Pharmaceutical and healthcare manufacturers supplying drug products to these markets must ensure their computer systems satisfy electronic record and electronic signature requirements.

Steps they must take are related to:

- Electronic records

The supplier has procedures and processes in place to comply with the electronic records requirements in 21 CFR Part 11 and EU GMP Annex 11, for systems supporting drugs manufactured for the U.S. and EU markets, respectively.

- Electronic Signatures:

The supplier has procedures and processes in place to comply with the electronic signature requirements in 21 CFR Part 11 and EU Directive 1999/93/EU for systems supporting drugs manufactured for the U.S. and EU markets respectively.

Even if a supplier is not directly asked about electronic records and electronic signature compliance, it is recommended that this topic be raised and discussed. Regulatory requirements are emerging around the world, perhaps the most well-known is the U.S. 21 Code of Federal Regulation Part 11. This is sometimes referred to as 21 CFR Part 11, or just 21 CFR 11.

The precise need for compliance with these regulations is not always entirely clear: much industry debate continues. Indeed, the U.S. FDA is currently preparing draft guidance documents to help define their regulatory expectations on what can be an extremely complex topic.

Suppliers should be wary of not *over stating* their compliance with such regulatory requirements, particularly as the baseline requirements themselves are open to differing interpretations. Just because a supplier satisfies one pharmaceutical and healthcare manufacturer, does not necessarily mean all pharmaceutical and healthcare manufacturers will deem the same supplier compliant.

Q9 WHO CONDUCTS THE AUDIT?

Pharmaceutical and healthcare manufacturers will nominate an internal or third party auditor to conduct their supplier audits. This is normally specified in the pharmaceutical and healthcare manufacturer's validation plan.

Suppliers should consider asking who the auditors will be and what audit experience they have; the supplier is best advised to avoid audit by any one person who is either currently or previously associated with the supplier.

If the customer puts forward a strong objection to individual auditors, then an alternative auditor should be requested, with an explanation supporting the request.

Q10 HOW WILL THE AUDIT BE CONDUCTED?

The audit itself usually takes one of three courses. It is important to formally agree on the scope and method of a proposed audit.

Quality Review

A quality review involves using available information, both formal (product or service literature, previous audit reports) and informal (hearsay, telephone conversations with supplier, taking up references from other users, etc.) to determine the general quality of a suppliers' product or service. Quality reviews may, in turn, recommend a postal audit or full supplier audit.

Postal Audit

A postal audit assesses a supplier's response to a postal checklist or questionnaire examining its quality management system in relation to a product or service. Postal audits may in turn recommend a full supplier audit.

Full Supplier Audit

The full supplier audit assesses a supplier's quality management system at first hand at the supplier's premises with detailed examination of procedures and documentation relating to a product or service.

Q11 WHEN AND HOW WILL SUPPLIERS BE CONTACTED IN REGARD TO AN AUDIT?

A supplier may be contacted informally to discuss the most appropriate audit route prior to any formal invitation to audit. Any proposal or bid made by a supplier should contain all the correct contact details of quality managers and personnel, so that the auditor can easily contact the appropriate person in the supplier organization with whom to discuss such options.

When the auditor contacts the supplier to organize an audit, he should supply full details (full name, postal address, telephone, fax, e-mail, and even video conference details where appropriate) for future communication.

It is important — even at this early stage — that formal confidentiality agreements be signed for nondisclosure of proprietary information to unauthorized third parties.

Suppliers should consider preparing a standard proforma agreement, which can be completed and faxed or posted to the auditor. The agreement must state the full name and precise role of signatories.

Where a pharmaceutical and healthcare manufacturer uses a third party auditor, then the supplier must ensure that the agreement covers both the pharmaceutical and healthcare manufacturers *and* the third party.

It must be made abundantly clear that written permission must be received from the supplier to authorize *any* disclosure of the audit findings, regardless of whether the audit is favorable or otherwise towards the supplier.

Q12 WHAT HAPPENS IN A QUALITY REVIEW?

The quality review — the benchmark for a supplier's adherence to ISO 9000 standards – ensures that, regardless of whether a supplier is accredited to ISO 9000, suppliers show *complete awareness* of how they line up against this standard/code of practice.

Suppliers should consider preparing a short report mapping their current working practices to the clauses of ISO 9000. This report could then be supplied quickly and easily, if requested, to existing and prospective users. In addition, suppliers should collect reference site material (possibly as sales literature), and user contacts which can be supplied to potential new users.

Suppliers may wish to consider collecting testimonials at the end of projects rather than try to locate users at a later date, as such personnel may have moved on by that time.

Q13 WHAT HAPPENS IN A POSTAL AUDIT?

Postal audits are usually only used where a supplier's product, or at least the version to be used by the pharmaceutical and healthcare manufacturer, is established and stable. If this is not the case then an audit of the supplier premises is usually deemed appropriate.

The supplier should retain a copy of the auditor's postal questionnaire and his own responses, together with any communication with the auditor clarifying the scope of method of the questionnaire.

If a postal questionnaire is requested, then the supplier's response time should be agreed. A busy contract period, illness, holiday, and staff turnover may all affect the timing of a response. Before agreeing to a response time, the supplier should ask to see a copy of the questionnaire so that the amount of work in reply to the questionnaire can be gauged.

If the supplier has already prepared an internal ISO 9000 mapping, or an internal audit report on how they align to GAMP, this can be offered as an alternative to the auditor's postal questionnaire, or at least a reduced postal questionnaire may be agreed.

A postal audit checklist providing a framework is presented in Appendix B; it is suggested that an internal GAMP audit report be prepared against this checklist. Wherever possible, photocopies of actual example documents and test records should be included in the report.

Remember that the pharmaceutical and healthcare manufacturers are themselves inspected for documentary evidence of validation.

Q14 WHAT HAPPENS IN A FULL SUPPLIER AUDIT?

At this stage the supplier should agree to the audit schedule in advance of the audit. The supplier can take the initiative and suggest a schedule that can be adapted to meet the auditor's needs. A typical audit schedule might consist of:

- A general introduction by the supplier giving details of:
  - The audit plan.
  - An overview of the supplier's business operations.
  - Quality department organization.
- A presentation by the supplier of its own quality management system, perhaps reviewing the supplier's internal ISO 9000 mapping report and internal GAMP audit report.
- A presentation by the suppler of the quality process adopted for the particular product or service under scrutiny, possibly even including a review of other user quality expectations — with emphasis on pharmaceutical and healthcare industry users.
- An opportunity for the auditor to view actual quality documents and records.
- A summary by the auditor of his preliminary findings, with an opportunity for the supplier to discuss and clarify.

With this auditing process, it is useful if the supplier has a nominated person to receive the audit, a person trained in auditing who can understand and anticipate the auditor's perspective. ISO 10011 gives an industry standard for auditing.

Audits normally take one to two days to conduct. There may a number of user auditors, and of course a number of supplier representatives will be needed.

There are no hard and fast rules on the composition of audit teams. Suppliers should take time to discuss who is, and who is not, appropriate. As a general rule, try to minimize the size of the audit team while ensuring the team has sufficient breadth and depth of experience to satisfy the scope of the audit.

The timing of the audit in relation to the personnel involved should also be considered here.

- Are some potential members of the team unavailable due to holidays?
- Are there qualified deputies in place to deal with any unforeseen unavailability?
- The logistics of the audit should not be underestimated.

Items to consider when audit planning

- Who is the auditor by name and function?
- Is the auditor assisted by anybody (name and function)?
- Who is the auditee by name and function?

- Who is assisting the auditee (name and function)?
- Where will the audit be conducted, have maps and times been sent out to participants?
- Has hotel accommodation been organized where needed?
- Have presentation slides and materials been prepared?
- Are copies of same available for the auditor?
- Will relevant information be brought to audit by auditees?
- Has a tour of the supplier premises been organized?

It is useful to assign a base camp room for the duration of the audit, dedicated to the audit team, even if they are not permanently located in the room. This room provides a focus for the audit team; a place for them to leave personal baggage, and collect files of information pending review, or leave information that has completed review.

Visits to supplier premises are expensive, not only to the supplier, but also to the pharmaceutical and healthcare manufacturer. It is important to both parties that such visits be conducted quickly and efficiently.

Reimbursement to suppliers to cover the costs associated with audits are not normally offered or requested. Some suppliers have tried to levy fees, but this has not been well accepted. Suppliers who have adopted this approach are generally felt to have tarnished their public relations in the marketplace.

After all, a quality culture should already be established in the supplier firm, and the audit should be seen not as an opportunity to defend a quality stance, but to sell quality as a distinguishing feature of the product or service on offer.

Some suppliers have offered pharmaceutical and healthcare manufacturers the chance to audit collectively in managed groups, perhaps through a user group structure. Suppliers offering this facility, and limiting the number of audits to two or three per year, have reduced their annual audit costs by up to 80%.

Q15 WHAT HAPPENS AFTER AN AUDIT?

It is very important that the auditor does not disappear into a black hole after an audit. Suppliers should agree at the outset their right to review and correct a draft of the audit report before it is issued. There should also be some agreement as to the timescales expected for the issue of a draft report.

It is not appropriate that a supplier ask to approve the audit report, the content of which is the auditor's opinions and should not be influenced except where based on misconceptions, which should be clarified by the supplier.

The supplier should retain a copy of the draft audit report, together with a note of any review comment, and should also request a final copy of the approved and issued report.

The audit report will normally contain a number of observations and recommendations — or some other system of gauging the significance or importance of findings — together with an indication of the priorities for remedial action. It is then the supplier's job to agree upon follow-up actions and timescales. The supplier should try never to be defensive at this point, but recognize issues and problem areas.

An opportunity exists to build audit findings into an ongoing program of continuous improvement, and an ability to demonstrate such an attitude to improvement will nearly always impress the user. Consider using the auditor's expertise to debate options for quality improvement, usually a free resource.

Finally, agree upon how to communicate completion of agreed follow-up actions with the auditor.

Not all recommendations have to be accepted by the supplier but try to accommodate the auditor's findings. This will enhance the relationships between suppliers, their auditors, and manufacturing customers.

Q16 ARE AUDIT REPORTS CONFIDENTIAL?

Audit reports and associated documents are confidential to the supplier and the customer: neither party should share them without written permission.

A pharmaceutical or healthcare manufacturer may be unhappy if through a favorable audit report to promote a supplier's capabilities its name is used without prior knowledge.

Equally a supplier is unlikely to be happy if an audit report is circulated to other potential customers if it highlights supplier deficiencies.

Confidentiality agreements should be reached and signed as soon as possible in the audit process (see Q11).

Q17 CAN A REGULATOR SUCH AS FDA OR MHRA INSPECT A SUPPLIER?

It is highly unlikely at the present time that a supplier could be directly inspected at its own premises by a regulator. Remember that in the perspective of regulators like FDA and MHRA, pharmaceutical and healthcare *manufacturers* (not their suppliers) are fully accountable for validation. However, this may change and should not excuse suppliers from showing an equally responsible approach to the quality and compliance of the systems they produce for crucial applications such as drug manufacturing. A supplier will be infinitely more successful if it demonstrates a total awareness of, or willingness to adapt to, regulatory requirements.

The site of a supplier's computer system is expected to have available all the necessary validation to demonstrate regulatory compliance.

Some suppliers may be requested by their customers to help support a regulatory inspection, either by providing technical information during an inspection, or by providing additional documentation only available at the supplier's premises.

Supplier personnel should avoid interfacing with a regulator directly in an inspection without appropriate inspection training.

Q18 CAN SUPPLIERS BE APPROVED BY REGULATORS?

Regulators to the pharmaceutical and healthcare industry do not (as yet) approve suppliers. Regulatory inspections are based on an audit process, and only take a sample approach to regulatory compliance. Even when a computer system is selected for detailed review, just a fraction of the validation will be examined.

Inspectors are looking for a high degree of assurance that a computer system is fit for purpose — once they have this assurance, they will typically quickly move onto another inspection topic. If deficiencies are discovered, then the inspector will dig deeper to determine the extent of any problems.

The lack of any identified deficiencies does not imply there are none to be found. A successful inspection by a regulator at one customer site could easily be followed by an unsuccessful inspection by a different regulator with a different customer.

Suppliers whose products have been reviewed by a regulator during an inspection at a customer site are definitely wiser *not* to claim their products as, for instance, "*FDA approved*."

Q19 WHAT IS AN ESCROW ACCOUNT?

Some suppliers may be asked to establish an escrow account by their customers. A common request is for a computer source code to be deposited in an escrow account, together with any required design documentation to maintain its application.

Escrow accounts are agreements with third party organizations to hold proprietary information about a supplier's product, in the event that the supplier becomes insolvent, or for other unforeseen circumstance can no longer support their customer.

Such an eventuality would be very serious to a customer from business and regulatory standpoints, should they no longer be able to maintain their computer systems, or demonstrate their compliance during regulatory inspections. Escrow accounts can be very expensive. Suppliers should not inadvertently agree to establish escrow accounts with the manufacturer unless both parties fully appreciate the costs involved.

Q20 WHERE CAN I GET MORE GUIDANCE AND ADVICE?

Further guidance on supplier audits can be found in the GAMP 4 Guide (GAMP

Forum 2002), Howard Garston-Smith's *Software Quality Assurance: A Guide for Developers and Auditors*, and *Computer System Validation: Quality Assurance, Risk Management and Regulatory Compliance*. All three are very practical and easy to read.

Additionally, the Sue Horwood Desktop Guides series, *Computer Systems Validation Life Cycle Activities*, contains guidance on a range of issues appertaining to topics such as electronic records and signatures, 21 CFR Part 11 compliance, change control, function and user design specification, and validation master planning and reporting, design documentation and testing (see bibliography).

For advice and discussion participation in the GAMP Forum is recommended.* The GAMP Forum is a computer validation group of pharmaceutical and healthcare manufacturers and their suppliers, who meet with the regulators to discuss topical issues and produce industry guidance. The GAMP Forum has a special interest group for suppliers known as the Supplier Forum, which meets regularly to discuss topical issues and learn about regulatory updates. These forums are held several times each year, and are very affordable to suppliers, manufacturers, and all concerned with the safe manufacture of drug compounds.

SUMMARY

The guidance provided to suppliers in this chapter is summarized in the checklist given in Appendix D and can be used to monitor progress during audits.

It is suggested that suppliers consider photocopying the checklist or create a similar one, to annotate with user details (proposal number or contract number), together with comments as appropriate to the audit, and to retain the checklist with their user files.

By planning audit schedules and conducting preparatory work, much of the stress associated with audits can be avoided, and unwanted audit outcomes avoided.

ABBREVIATIONS

EMEA	European Medicines Evaluation Agency, London, U.K.
EPS	European Parenteral Society, Swindon, U.K.
EU	European Union.
FDA	Food and Drug Administration, Department of Health & Human Services, Bethesda, MD, U.S.A.
IEE	Institute of Electrical Engineers, U.S.A.
ISO	International Standards Organization.
IQA	Institute of Quality Assurance, U.K.

*Contact details can be found at www.ispe.org.

IVT	Institute of Validation Technology, Duluth, MN, U.S.A.
IPSE	International Society of Pharmaceutical Engineers, U.S.A.
MHRA	Medicines and Healthcare Products Regulatory Agency, U.K.
PDA	Parenteral Drug Association, Bethesda, MD, U.S.A.

TERMINOLOGY IN BRIEF

Audit. An independent review for assessing compliance with software requirements, specifications, baselines, standards, or procedures.
Auditee. Person who is receiving the audit on behalf of the supplier.
Auditor. Person representing the pharmaceutical and healthcare manufacturer and who conducts the audit. The auditor may be a third party sanctioned by the pharmaceutical and healthcare manufacturer to act on his behalf.
Quality. The totality of features and characteristics of a product or service that have a direct bearing on its ability to satisfy given needs.
Validation. Establishing documented evidence to provide a high degree of assurance that a specific process will consistently produce a safe product, and continuously meet predetermined specifications and quality attributes.

REFERENCES

FDA. "Glossary of Computerized System and Software Development Terminology," issued by U.S. Food and Drug Administration, 1995.

GAMP Forum. "GAMP Guide for Validation of Automated Systems in Pharmaceutical and Healthcare Manufacture," GAMP 4, distributed by ISPE. 2001.

Garston-Smith, H. *Software Quality Assurance: A Guide for Developers and Auditors*, Interpharm Press, Denver, CO, 1998.

Wingate, G.A.S. *Validating Automated Manufacturing and Laboratory Applications: Putting Principles into Practice*, Interpharm Press, Buffalo Grove, IL, 1997.

Wingate, G.A.S. *Computer System Validation: Quality Assurance, Risk Management and Regulatory Compliance for Pharmaceutical and Healthcare Companies*, CRC Press, Boca Raton, FL, 2003.

APPENDIX A: ISO 9000 CLAUSES

- Management responsibility.
- Quality system.
- Contract review.
- Design control.

- Document and data control.
- Purchasing.
- Control of customer-supplied product.
- Product identification and traceability.
- Process control.
- Inspection and testing.
- Control of inspection, measuring, and test equipment.
- Inspection and test status.
- Control of nonconforming product.
- Corrective and preventative action.
- Handling, storage, packaging, preservation, and delivery.
- Control of quality records.
- Internal quality audits.
- Training.
- Services.
- Statistical techniques.

APPENDIX B: SUPPLIER AUDIT POSTAL QUESTIONNAIRE

Audit Details

- What is the name and address of the firm undergoing audit?
- Who is the contact at the firm?
- What are the names and qualifications of the auditors?
- What is the date of the audit?
- Is this an initial or followup (surveillance) audit?

Business

- How long has the company existed?
- How is the company organized?
- How many pharmaceutical and allied industry users does the company have?
- Do they have any user citations for good work?
- Is the company's pharmaceutical and healthcare related business profitable?
- What is the long-term pharmaceutical and healthcare related business plan?
- Is the company in any litigation?
- Does the company hold a recognized quality certification?

Organization

- Has a quality control system been established? Is it documented?

- Who is responsible for quality management?
- Is there a quality assurance management structure?
- Is there a project management structure?
- Are project work practices documented?
- How does project work conform to quality standards?
- Has accreditation and registration been achieved? (ISO 9000, specify other.)
- Is the quality system audited on a regular basis?

Employees

- How many permanent, contract, or temporary staff does the company employ?
- How long, on average, do employees stay with the company?
- What is the company's training policy? Are there any records?

Planning

- Are project and quality plans produced for projects? Who approves them?
- Does planning include a contract review?
- Is there a defined project life cycle? What is it?
- How are project documents controlled?
- How is conformance to user GxP requirements ensured?

System Design and Development

- Do design considerations cover
  - Reliability?
  - Maintainability?
  - Safety?
- Do design considerations cover standardization?
- Interchangeability?
- Are design reviews carried out? Are they minuted?
- Are users invited to attend design review meetings?
- Are design changes proposed, approved, implemented, and properly controlled?

System Build

- Are there guidelines or standards for software programing and hardware assembly?
- How does the company ensure they conform to current industry requirements?
- Are records available to show which projects conform to company practices?

- What third-party hardware or software is used?
- Is software and hardware supplied by reputable firms?
- How would changes to third party products affect the user's end product?

Predelivery Testing

- Are test specifications produced? Are expected results defined?
- Who performs the tests? How is testing organized?
- Are versions of hardware and software inspected?
- Is software "black-box" (functional) testing conducted?
- Is software "white-box" (structural) testing conducted?
- How rigorous is testing? Are abnormal situations tested?
- How are failed tests documented and corrected?
- Are test results recorded, signed, and dated? Are these records maintained?
- Who signs for overall acceptance of testing?

Project Completion

- What is the mechanism for deciding a project is complete?
- Is there a certificate of conformity? Is there a warrantee?
- Are project documents handed-over to the user?
- Are project documents archived?
- Is there an access agreement for regulatory inspections (e.g., an escrow account)?

Control Procedures and Activities

- Is there configuration and version control within projects?
- Does the quality system provide for the prompt detection of failures?
- Are all failures analyzed? Are corrective actions promptly taken?
- Are regular internal audits carried out? Are auditing procedures documented?
- Are audits planned? Are corrective actions taken?
- Are audit records stored and available?
- Are responsibilities for document review assigned?
- Are responsibilities for change control assigned?
- Are obsolete documents withdrawn?
- Are changes notified to the user?
- Are subcontractors audited? How are they managed?
- Are subcontract documentation standards audited?

General and Housekeeping

- Are users solicited for feedback?
- How are user responses folded into development plans?
- Are users kept informed of development plans?
- Is there a list of users provided with a similar service or product that is the subject of this audit?
- Are users advised of problems found by other users?
- Who is responsible for ongoing user support?
- Is there a support fee?
- What are the response mechanisms and timings for user problems?

APPENDIX C: FULL SUPPLIER AUDIT CHECKLIST

This list is intended as a guide only and there may be other factors which require consideration when auditing. References to other sections of GAMP Guide are given where relevant (charts, company history).

A. Company overview

A.1 Audit details (address, audit team, supplier representatives).
A.2 Company size, structure, and summary of history (number of sites, staff, organizational).
A.3 Product or service history (main markets, how many sold, use in pharmaceutical and healthcare sector).
A.4 Summary of product/service under audit (product literature).
A.5 Product or service development plans.
A.6 Tour of facility (to verify housekeeping, general working environment, working conditions).

B. Organization and quality management

B.1 Management structure (roles, responsibilities).
B.2 Method of assuring quality in product or service (quality system, responsibilities for quality).
B.3 Use of documented quality management system (QMS) (e.g., policy, manual, procedures, and standards).
B.4 Maturity of QMS (relevance to product or service under audit).
B.5 Control of QMS documentation (reviews, approvals, distribution, updates).
B.6 Maintenance of QMS documentation (regularly updated).
B.7 QMS certified to a recognized standard (e.g., ISO 9001).
B.8 Method of checking compliance with QMS (internal audits, reviews).
B.9 Qualification and suitability of staff.
B.10 Independence of auditors, inspectors, testers, reviewers.

B.11 Staff training (general, QMS, product or service-related, new staff, changes to QMS, regulatory issues, training records).

B.12 Use of subcontractors (individuals, companies).

- Method of selection.
- Subcontractor qualifications and training records.
- Specification of technical and quality requirements in orders placed.
- Method of accepting product delivered by subcontractor.

B.13 Experience of validation process (with other users, previous supplier audits, services provided by supplier, involvement in regulatory inspections).

B.14 Awareness of pharmaceutical and healthcare regulatory requirements (knowledge of regulations, subscription to publications, attendance of relevant events, involvement in industry groups).

B.15 Continuous improvement program (use of metrics to evaluate and improve effectiveness of QMS).

C. Planning and product or project management

C.1 Use of quality and project plans (per project or product, defining activities, controlling procedures, responsibilities, timescales).

C.2 Status of planning documentation (reviews, approvals, distribution, maintenance, update).

C.3 Documentation of user and supplier responsibilities.

C.4 Use of validation plan where supplied by pharmaceutical and healthcare manufacturer.

C.5 Project management and monitoring (mechanism, tools, progress reports).

C.6 Accuracy of, and conformance to, planning and management procedures.

C.7 Use of formal development lifecycle.

C.8 Evidence of formal contract reviews where applicable.

D. Specifications

D.1 User requirements specifications.

D.2 Functional specifications.

D.3 Software design specifications.

D.4 Hardware design specification.

D.5 Relationship between specifications (together forming a complete specification for the system that can be tested objectively).

D.6 Traceability through specifications (e.g., for a given requirement).

D.7 Status of specifications (reviews, approvals, distribution, maintenance, update).

D.8 Accuracy of, and conformance to, relevant procedures.

D.9 Use and control of design methodologies (CASE tools).

E. Implementation

E.1 Specification of standards covering use of programming languages (e.g., naming and coding conventions, commenting rules).

E.2 Standards for software identification and traceability (e.g., for each software item unique name and reference, version, project and product reference, module description, list of build files, change history, traceability to design document).

E.3 Standards for file and directory naming.

E.4 Use of command files (e.g., make) for build management, to compile and link software.

E.5 Use of development tools (e.g., compilers, linkers, debuggers).

E.6 Evidence of source code reviews prior to formal testing (checking design, adherence to coding standards, logic, redundant code, critical algorithms).

E.7 Independence and qualifications of reviewers.

E.8 Source code reviews recorded, indexed, followed-up, and closed off (with supporting evidence). Evidence of management action where reviews not closed off satisfactorily.

E.9 Listings and other documents used during source code reviews retained with review reports.

F. Testing

F.1 Explanation of test strategy employed at each level of development (e.g., module testing, integration testing, system acceptance testing, or alpha or beta testing).

F.2 Software test specifications.

F.3 Hardware test specifications.

F.4 Integration test specifications.

F.5 System acceptance test specifications.

F.6 Structure and content of each test script (unique reference, unambiguous description of test, acceptance criteria and expected results, cross reference to controlling specification).

F.7 Relationship between test specifications and controlling specifications (demonstrating system has been tested thoroughly).

F.8 Evidence that test specifications cover:

- Both structural and functional testing.
- All requirements.
- Each function of the system.
- Stress testing (repeat testing under different conditions).
- Performance testing (e.g., adequacy of system performance).
- Abnormal conditions.

F.9 Test specification status (reviews, approvals, distribution, maintenance, update).

F.10 Formal testing procedure to execute test specifications (method of recording test results, use of pass or fail, retaining raw data, reviewing test results, progressing and resolving test failures).

F.11 Status of test results and associated review records (indexed, organized, maintained, followed-up on failure).

F.12 Involvement of QA function (as witnesses or reviewers).
F.13 Independence and qualifications of testers and reviewers.
F.14 Accuracy of, and conformance to, relevant test procedures.
F.15 Control of test software, test data, simulators.
F.16 Use of testing tools (documented, controlled).

G. Completion and release

G.1 Documented responsibility for release of product, such as certificate of conformity, authorization to ship (including evidence that testing has been accepted with or without reservations).
G.2 Handover of project material in accordance with quality plan or contract (e.g., release notes, hardware, copies of documentation or software).
G.3 Provision of user documentation (user manuals, administration or technical manuals, update notice with each release).
G.4 Records of releases (i.e., which users have which version of system or software).
G.5 Warranties and guarantees.
G.6 Archiving of release (software, build files, supporting tools, documentation).
G.7 Availability of source code and documentation for regulatory inspection (use of escrow accounts for which releases).
G.8 Customer training (summary of courses, given by staff or third parties).
G.9 Accuracy of, and conformance to, release procedures.

H. Support and maintenance

H.1 Explanation of support services (agreements, scope, procedures, support organization, responsibilities, provision locally or internationally, use of third parties, maintenance of support agreements).
H.2 Duration of guaranteed support (number of versions, minimum periods).
H.3 Provision of help desk (levels of service, hours of operation).
H.4 Fault reporting mechanism (logging, analyzing, categorizing, resolving, informing, closing, documenting, distribution, notification of other users with or without support agreement).
H.5 Link between fault reporting mechanism and change control.
H.6 Method of handling user complaints.
H.7 Accuracy of, and conformance to, support procedures.

I. Supporting procedures and activities

I.1 Documentation management (covering QMS and product or project documents):

- In accordance with QMS or quality plan.
- Following documentation standards.
- Indexed, organized.
- Reviews carried out prior to approval and issue.

- Reviews recorded, indexed, followed-up and closed off (with supporting evidence).
- Evidence of management action where reviews not closed off satisfactorily.
- Formal approvals recorded, meaning of approvals defined, distribution controlled.
- Document history maintained.
- Removal of superseded or obsolete documents.

I.2 Software configuration management:
- System for identifying, controlling and tracking every version of each software item.
- System for recording configuration of each release (which items and versions).
- Identification of point at which change control is applied to each software item.
- Control of build tools and layered software products, including introduction of new versions.

I.3 Change control covering software, hardware, documentation:
- All change requests formally logged, indexed, assessed.
- Rejected requests identified as such, reasons documented, signed by those responsible, originator informed.
- Changes authorized, documented, tested, and approved prior to implementation (except emergencies).
- Emergency procedure documented, covering reviewing, testing, approving, recording.
- Impact of each change (on other items and on requirements for retest) assessed and documented.

I.4 Security procedures (physical access, logical access to accounts and software, virus controls).

I.5 Backup and recovery procedures (secure storage and handling of media, onsite, offsite, recovery procedure exercised).

I.6 Disaster recovery procedure (tried).

I.7 Control of purchased items bought on behalf of user (e.g., computer hardware, layered software products), including associated packaging, user documentation, and warranties.

I.8 Accuracy of, and conformance to, relevant procedures.

APPENDIX D: CHECKLIST FOR CUSTOMER AUDITS

Preparation Work	**Comments**
• Prepare internal ISO 9000 mapping report.	
• Prepare internal GAMP audit report.	

- Prepare confidentiality agreement proforma.
- Train supplier personnel responsible for receiving.
- User audits in ISO 10011 audit process.

Invitation to audit

- Send out and sign confidentiality agreement.
- Agree upon scope and method of audit.
- Get auditor contact details for communications.
- Agree upon response time for postal questionnaire.
- Agree upon date, duration, and participation for full supplier audit.
- Agree upon supplier review and approval of audit report.

Quality review

- Consider issue of internal ISO 9000 mapping report.

Postal audit

- Complete postal questionnaire, retain own copy.
- Consider issue of internal ISO 9000 mapping report.
- Consider issue of internal GAMP audit report.

Full supplier audit comments

- Agree upon audit schedule in advance of audit.
- Facilitate audit logistics.
- Consider issue of internal ISO 9000 mapping report.
- Consider issue of internal GAMP audit report.
- Prepare and issue audit presentation slides.
- Take own notes during audit.
- Have summary at closeout of audit.

Audit follow-up

- Review draft audit report.
- Retain your comments.
- Retain copy of draft and final audit report.
- Agree in full, follow-up actions and timescales.

Chapter 6

Developing Good Specifications

Mark Cherry

CONTENTS

There are varying levels of specification covering computer systems. This chapter focuses on the development of the user requirements specification (URS). As the first link in the chain between the customer and supplier, the overall quality and delivery of the final system is highly dependant on the quality, accuracy, and understanding of this key document.

GENERAL CONSIDERATIONS

There are some common attributes that apply regardless of the specification type. Specifications should be defined in advance of any development activity or production of lower level specification to which they pertain. Specifications are essentially defining what you want. Where specifications are not predefined, then retrospective production is essentially a reporting activity of what you (think you) got.

The intended audience for specifications should be clear, the level of detail and technical content should be consistent, and appropriate to the audience and intended specification use.

Specifications should be readable and individual requirements or functions should be clearly identified and structured in a manner that will aid traceability. Multiple requirements or functions should not be combined and certainly not defined together in long narratives. GAMP 4 recommends that individual requirement statements are no longer than 250 words.

The status of the document content should be clear. For example, information that is in draft form, illustrative examples, and any assumptions should be clearly stated.

The customer should write the URS, and the author must have a thorough understanding of the (business) process that the system is to support. The use of diagrams or flowcharts here can be helpful in illustrating the logic and flow of the process.

Responsibility for developing user requirements should not be delegated to technical or development staff. Technical or development staff involvement is required, indeed valuable in terms of technical review and feasibility of the requirements and advice as to available technologies, solutions or suppliers, but they are generally not experts on business processes. Where the responsibility for authoring a requirements specification is delegated to a potential systems supplier, then there is clearly potential for a conflict of interest; the requirements specification may be biased towards the suppliers products or preferred technology, and not the needs of the user.

The purpose of the URS is to clearly define what functions the user requires to support the associated business processes. Prospective system suppliers use the document to establish the adequacy of their system in meeting the requirements, and usually as the basis of cost and time estimates for implementing the system. It is essential that both the customer and prospective suppliers have a clear and common understanding of the requirements. Terminology is often a stumbling block, and the URS presents the user with the opportunity to provide clear definitions of terms to potential suppliers.

The URS should not generally be written as a document specific to a particular system. It must contain sufficient detail for the customer to evaluate the suitability of proposed systems functionality against the requirements.

Simply reflecting existing business processes and ways of working within the URS without challenge should be avoided. This can result in overly complex systems, replication of workarounds, expensive development of bespoke functionality (rather than utilization of standard system functions) and crucially misses a golden opportunity to make the processes more efficient.

Time spent at the outset critically analyzing, challenging, and simplifying requirements and associated processes should result in better requirements and a simpler system that is likely to take less time to implement, test, and support.

Users should also consider the degree of flexibility they are prepared to accept in implementing requirements. If it is possible to make a minor change to a business process, which results in acceptance of a standard system, this may outweigh the development and support costs of bespoke system development effort.

For larger projects, and particularly those involving process automation systems, the scope of the project is likely to be wider than the computer system alone, often including process equipment and facilities. Where this is the case consideration should be given to whether individual (but related) URS should be produced, or a single document.

The decision is likely to be based on a number of factors. Where the project is delivering packaged equipment (i.e., process equipment with embedded computerized process control), then it makes sense to have a single specification. For a project to deliver a batch plant with a complex distributed process control system and process equipment from a variety of suppliers then individual specifications are probably more appropriate. Where multiple specifications are used, it is however, important to understand the relationship between the specifications and the impact that a change within one document may have to others.

When preparing a URS, the balance of detail must be considered. It may be tempting to include great detail on requirements that are well understood and defined. Too much detail, however, may mean that the requirements stray into defining functional requirements (i.e., delivery of a requirement rather than just defining what is to be delivered). By doing so, it is likely that the system or supplier selection will be constrained at a very early stage. This may mean that full benefit from the supplier's experience of how to most efficiently and effectively implement its solution cannot be obtained.

There may be areas where the requirements are not well understood, are poorly defined, or likely to be subject to change. It is important that such areas of ambiguity are identified as such; in many cases prospective suppliers may have sufficient experience or knowledge to assist the customer in better defining these areas.

Often requirements development involves both the customer and supplier, and in such cases joint workshops, prototyping exercises, and reference site visits can contribute to gaining clear requirements definition.

Where partnering type agreements are established with suppliers, then the scope for collaborative working to refine the requirements is much greater than situations where the URS is the basis for competitive tendering. Where suppliers have tendered competitive bids on the basis of the URS, then subsequent changes to the scope of requirements are almost certain to incur additional costs. The pricing of scope changes should be agreed between the customer and supplier prior to placing the order with the supplier.

The user requirements should be maintained and reflect the operational system. This document can then be used to support design and performance qualifications and the maintenance of the system in the future.

Care should be taken to avoid duplication and particularly contradiction of any requirements statements. Also duplication of information contained within other project or system documentation should be avoided if possible to reduce the chances of documentation not being updated following changes made during the project, and also subsequently during the operational life of the system.

GXP CONSIDERATIONS

For quality related GxP applications, quality assurance or regulatory input, review and approval of the URS should be obtained. This is primarily to ensure that all quality related requirements have been identified and included, and any associated regulatory requirements addressed (for example relevance and requirements of electronic records, electronic signatures requirements).

Requirements should be individually identifiable, and categorization into "must, should, and like" is worthwhile. An assessment of each requirement in terms of GxP and business criticality should also be performed, and the outcome documented. The method of recording this may be within the URS itself, or separately, for example within a requirements trace matrix.

A fundamental validation requirement is the ability to trace individual user requirements from the URS through functional or design specifications, testing, and through to user acceptance testing. This needs to be considered at an early stage in the project as the structure and style of the URS content can significantly hinder or assist subsequent efforts to provide traceability.

Traceability can be achieved by means of a requirements trace matrix, these can be produced manually or with the use of computer-based tools. Computer-based tools are particularly useful for large or complex systems or projects, and generally provide electronic document management functionality in addition to requirements traceability. For smaller projects or systems often a relatively simple spreadsheet based system can be devised. Regardless of the traceability method selected, the key considerations are the complexity of the system, the likely scale of changes and the level of effort required to maintain the documentation and traceability.

Figure 6.1 illustrates GxP areas that typically may be supported by computerized systems.

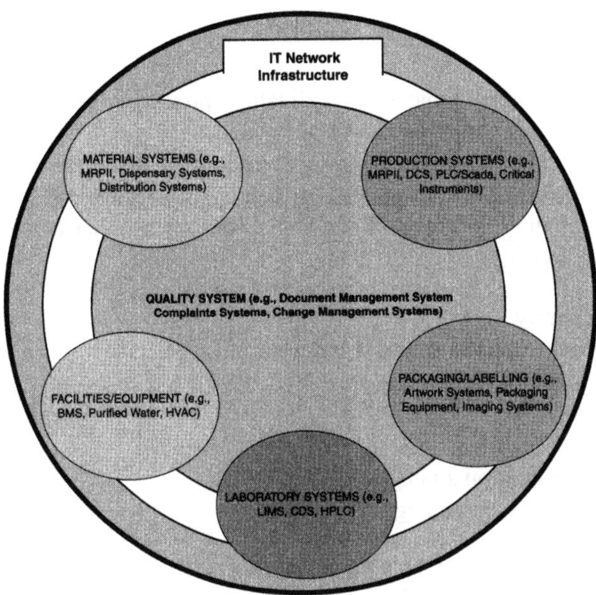

Figure 6.1 Classes of typical GxP related computerized systems and examples.

Within the user requirements, functions should be classified with regard to their GxP or business criticality. High, medium, low, or none are the suggested classifications.

It is also recommended that records and data that the systems will collect or store should also be classified.

Systems may be direct or indirect quality impact systems. For example, manufacturing, labelling or packaging systems are direct quality impact systems, whereas document management or training systems would still be considered as GxP, but are indirect quality impact.

USER REQUIREMENT SPECIFICATION SECTIONS

The following section provides an overview of some typical sections to be considered for inclusion within an URS.

Introduction

Provide a high level overview of the required system, its purpose and a brief summary of the key requirements.

Detail the locations and departments involved in the project and the business stakeholders. Include stakeholders from the project, quality assurance, and support teams.

Refer to any related projects or validation programs, provide a high level description of the overall project and background.

Include a high level statement regarding required quality attributes of the system and adherence to relevant GxP pharmaceutical agency regulations.

Consider including an indication of key system or supplier attributes that will influence selection such as:

- Product maturity.
- Installed base in pharmaceutical industry.
- Technical support.
- Training.
- Staff experience.
- Upgrade or migration strategy.
- Product development strategy.

Include a statement to make the contractual status of the URS clear to the supplier.

System Overview

Provide an overview focusing on the key elements of the required system, including a description of the business process that the system is to support. Where possible include diagrams or flowchart representations to aid understanding. Where business processes are described ensure that people aspects (roles, responsibilities) are also included.

It is recommended that the existing systems and technology are detailed when describing the business process, and in particular indicate which of these are likely to require modifying or replacing (and hence decommissioning) as part of the project.

System Interfaces

Include a summary of any other systems with which the system must interface, if the interfaces are manual or automatic, and also highlight interfaces that include the transmission of GxP relevant information and instructions.

Highlight system interfaces that will be modified, removed or decommissioned, or are new — particularly where the new interfaces are to existing systems.

Functional Requirements

Detail the operational functional requirements that the system is required to address, consider also the data and interfaces associated with required functions. It is important within this section to maintain focus on "what is required" rather than "how the function is to be delivered."

Although the focus of the URS is on user requirements, also consider within this section any requirements for system administration functions. For example, system performance monitoring, user account administration, system maintenance functions, etc.

Each requirement should be ranked in terms of business and GxP or quality criticality to the product or process or data. In particular records/data and functionality involving electronic signatures that are considered as GxP should be clearly identified to ensure, where applicable, compliance with pharmaceutical agency electronic record and electronic signature requirements is specified. For systems with safety, health or environmental (SHE) impact, consider whether each function needs to be individually ranked as to SHE impact.

For GxP records and signatures provide an indication of the required record retention period, and the regulation applicable to the record (i.e., GMP, GCP, GLP). As record retention periods will often be in excess of the likely system lifetime, consider requirements regarding record retrieval or migration as part of eventual system decommissioning.

Note that only providing suppliers with a blanket statement regarding electronic record or electronic signature compliance is unlikely to be helpful. It is the customer, not the supplier that has the detailed understanding of the system aspects that will have direct or indirect quality or regulatory impact, and this information needs to be clearly relayed to the supplier.

In some cases it may be prudent to separate out all business or quality critical requirements into separate sections of the user requirements.

The following list provides some examples of areas to consider when assessing the direct or indirect GxP impact of the system requirements.

- Product composition (manufacturing process).
- Raw materials (identify, quantity).
- Packaging materials.
- Product recall.
- Lot traceability.
- Product labelling.
- Environmental and storage conditions.
- Analytical results.
- Batch status (records, approvals).
- Regulatory submission records.

To aid subsequent requirements traceability, each function should be individually identified and numbered. This can be facilitated by laying out the section in tabular form. This will aid identification, allows columns to be added (for example for GxP impact, criticality and electronic record or signature relevance), and deters the author from including excessive narrative and combining requirements.

The following attributes should be considered with regard to each function.

- User access levels, login and logout, and security of interfaces to other systems.
- Operating modes — for example manual, automatic, stop, start, hold, shutdown, action in event of hardware or software failure, etc.
- Alarm conditions including communication of status, recovery routines, interlocks, and any associated safety requirements.
- User interface requirements (including graphical user interface, data input, and detection of invalid input data or instructions).
- Interfaces to other systems or functions (including detection of invalid or corrupted input data).
- Performance, timing, and response requirements. For example, relating to input or output scanning times, report generation, fast control loops.
- Calculations and any critical algorithms.
- Reporting requirements — include data and description of reports, frequency of reporting and types of reports. For example standard, *ad hoc* reports, on-line or batched reports, report formats.
- Capacity requirements (for example concurrent users, maximum number of batches in process, etc.).
- Sequencing of process steps or transactions (and how to ensure these are enforced for systems with electronic record or signature requirements). Consider the most appropriate method of documenting these for example via flowcharts or in structured English format.

Examples of how to define a functional requirement using tabular format are illustrated here.

<table>
<tr><td>Reference:</td><td>3.1</td><td>Description: (include capacity and performance requirements)</td></tr>
<tr><td>Criticality: (must, should, like)</td><td>Must</td><td rowspan="3">The system must allow user configurable batch recipes, and the recipe structure must comply with requirements of S88.01. The system should support at least 100 types of batch recipe, 50 unit types and 100 generic phases.</td></tr>
<tr><td>GxP: (direct, indirect, none)</td><td>Indirect</td></tr>
<tr><td>ER,ES,N/A:</td><td>ER, ES</td></tr>
<tr><td>Related Refs:</td><td colspan="2">3.1.1, 3.1.2</td></tr>
</table>

Ref:	3.1.1	Description: (include capacity and performance requirements)
Criticality: (must, should, like)	Must	Batch recipes must only be changeable by authorized users, changes must be tracked and approved by electronic signature.
GxP: (direct, indirect, none)	Indirect	
ER,ES,N/A:	ER, ES	
Related Refs:	3.1, 3.1.2	

Ref:	3.1.2	Description: (include capacity and performance requirements)
Criticality: (must, should, like)	Must	The system must be capable of clearly indicating to users the status of live batches within the system, and must allow for a maximum of 15 live batches in plant concurrently.
GxP: (direct, indirect, none)	Indirect	
ER,ES,N/A:	NA	
Related Refs:	3.1, 3.1.3	

Ref:	3.1.3	Description: (include capacity and performance requirements)
Criticality: (must, should, like)		The system should have a trace or step mode available to aid fault finding when testing recipes.
GxP: (direct, indirect, none)	None	
ER,ES,N/A:	NA	
Related Refs:	3.1, 3.1.2	

Data Requirements

The data and records requirements should be considered in conjunction with the functional requirements, and the following points should be considered.

- Has all required data been described, including the format, required field length and precision where relevant?

- Data and records confidentiality and security — is the status of records and data clear in terms of confidentiality, are the requirements of the Data Protection Act addressed, who should have access to records and data?
- What are the storage and capacity requirements for data — ensure that capacity for future expansion is taken into consideration.
- What requirements are there for data archiving and retrieval (how frequently is data likely to require restoring, what time frame is acceptable for retrieval)?
- What requirements are there for validation or input check of data?
- Manual data loading — what are the requirements, how will they be achieved, how will data be verified?
- What requirements are there regarding migration of data from legacy systems — what is the expectation regarding validation of any migration tools?

System Requirements

The following sections outline some general system requirements that need to be taken into account within the URS, such as system security, electronic record or signature controls, and any environmental factors.

SYSTEM SECURITY

The following security requirements should be considered particularly for systems that include GxP electronic signatures and records. Note that there is a strong case in terms of basic good practice for applying these controls to any GxP computerized system.

- Detection and reporting of unauthorized access attempts.
- Configurable automatic user logouts after periods of inactivity.
- System access must be limited to authorized users.
- Restrictions on reuse of previously assigned user IDs and passwords.
- System function access provided according to predefined user profiles.
- Password expiry applied by the system according to configurable parameters.

Any corporate or local standards regarding the compatibility and installation of antivirus software or other security controls such as firewalls should be specified.

ELECTRONIC RECORD (ER) CONTROLS

For systems where the requirements specify storage of GxP electronic records, the following requirements should be considered (based on US FDA 21 CFR Part 11).

- Electronic records must be accurately and completely reproducible in electronic and paper form.
- Records must be retrievable throughout the specified retention period for the record (which may be beyond the system lifetime).
- Include a human readable secure audit trail that includes the date and details of record or data creation, update or modification, and deletion.

ELECTRONIC SIGNATURE REQUIREMENTS

For systems that include GxP electronic signature functionality, the following requirements should be considered (based on US FDA 21 CFR Part 11).

- The name of the signer, date and time stamp, and purpose of the signing must be captured and available for the signed record.
- The signature must be applied at the time of the transaction or operation to which it relates, and the system must clearly identify the individual signing at the time of application.
- The signature components must consist of a user identification code and password as a minimum, and must be traceable to an individual.
- The signature must be linked to the electronic record, and must not be able to be cut, deleted, or copied either from or onto records other than by the act of signing.
- The system must require reentry of at least one signature component for each subsequent signing within a single session.

ENVIRONMENTAL FACTORS

Detail any special requirements that relate to the physical environment in which the system (or parts of the system, for example, plant-based user terminals) is to be located and used. Examples could be temperature, humidity requirements, and any applicable hazardous area (ATEX) constraints or regulations. Also consider other aspects such as sterile, dirty, wet, or dusty environments and any required ingress protection (IP) ratings for equipment. Consider any surface finish or cleaning requirements for equipment based in manufacturing facilities, and any requirements for any parts of the equipment that may be in contact with process materials.

Consider any constraints or corporate standards regarding the IT infrastructure and network environment in which the system may be installed, and in particular any standards or known compatibility issues with regard to equipment selection or use of existing infrastructure.

Include any requirements where the physical layout of the equipment within the plant or workplace may be an issue. For example, with process control system there may be constraints regarding the physical length of cabling between controllers and associated input or output racks or devices. Also consider physical space limitations which may have an impact in terms of forced cooling requirements within equipment cabinets.

OPERATING PROCEDURES AND TRAINING REQUIREMENTS

Specify who and what are responsible for the development of operating and support procedures for the system, and the timing for their development.

Procedures must be considered for:

- System access and security administration.
- System backup and restoration (including disaster recovery).
- Contingency plans for system downtime.
- Data archive and restoration.
- Change control.
- Configuration management.
- Incident reporting.

Ensure that any training requirements for technical, development, support, and operational staff are considered and where necessary included. Consider whether bespoke or standard courses are likely to be appropriate and the level of competency required.

HEALTH AND SAFETY

State whether the system has an impact with regard to safety, health, or environment. Describe the process to be used for detailed evaluation of the system or functions with regard to SHE. For example, HAZOP, CHAZOP, display screen evaluations, etc.

PROCESS EQUIPMENT

Where the user requirements are a combined document for both process equipment and the associated computerized system, include details of the equipment. Include, for example, capacity, performance, maintenance, surface finishes, durability, materials of construction, cleaning requirements, etc.

SYSTEM INTERFACES

For each function consider and define what interfaces apply. Consider interfaces in terms of manual, end user interfaces, interfaces with other computerized systems, and those with plant or equipment. When considering interfaces consider elements such as the frequency of update, volume of information transferred, security of transfer, and compatibility with existing systems or equipment.

SYSTEM MAINTENANCE AND AVAILABILITY

Include the requirements for system reliability, and the expected availability. Specify maximum allowable periods of downtime, both in terms of scheduled and unscheduled maintenance and support.

Consider any specific maintenance requirements, including the development or supply of relevant procedures and the requirements for any support agreements. Within the scope of support agreements consider if remote access is acceptable and what constraints the supplier would need to agree to in order to grant such access. Consider the required supplier response time to system problems, and whether 24 hour support is required.

PROJECT REQUIREMENTS

Include project-related requirements such as supplier assessment, communication, documentation, frequency of project meetings, project plan and milestones, project audits, quality systems approach, the approach to acceptance testing, and consider any specific contractual requirements.

The process for performing supplier assessment should be outlined to the supplier, particularly where a detailed (site based), supplier audit is required. The fact that the scope of validation activities will be influenced by the audit results should also be made clear to suppliers.

Communication:

- Who are the key points of contact between the supplier and customer?
- What is the expected frequency and method of communication?
- How will decisions be formally recorded and communicated?
- Where there are multiple suppliers, how will they be coordinated?

Project plan:

- How will the plan be developed, and by whom?
- How will changes be agreed?

- How will project delays be communicated and handled?
- How will the project and validation plans be maintained and synchronized?

Documentation and electronic media:

- What level of documentation is required?
- What documentation standards are agreed?
- Do GMP standards apply to all, some, or no system documentation?
- How many copies are required?
- Is documentation required in hard copy or electronic format?
- What is the review and approval process for documentation?
- How many copies of software will be provided, and in what format?

Acceptance testing:

- What level of testing is expected from the supplier?
- Will acceptance testing be performed at the supplier's premises, the customer's, or both?
- Who will provide resources for testing?
- Are simulation packages permitted during testing?
- What level of documentation, witnessing, and collection of evidence is required at each stage of testing?

QUALITY SYSTEM REQUIREMENTS

State the requirements with regard to the quality management system to be used during system development.

Detail and expectations with regard to the customer and supplier quality systems, in particular consider any requirements with regard to change control and configuration management during the project.

REVISION HISTORY

Provide detail of revision dates, version numbers, overview of revision details, and who was responsible.

APPENDICES AND REFERENCES

Include references to associated project documentation for example P&IDs, input and output schedules, internal and external quality standards, etc.

Chapter 7

Traceability of Requirements Throughout the Life Cycle

*Keith Collyer and Jeremy Dick**

CONTENTS

---

*Some of the information presented here has appeared in different forms in training courses produced by Telelogic UK Ltd. and *Requirements Engineering.* [4]

INTRODUCTION

In this chapter, we introduce the concept of traceability. Traceability is the recording of relationships. Traditionally, it is concerned with relationships between requirements and development information. However, we can, and should, record relationships to qualification and risk information.

Before we can discuss traceability, we need to provide a brief overview of systems engineering, requirements management, processes, and information models.

We will also place traceability into context, describing how we use models in requirements management and providing a generic process for systems engineering.

SYSTEMS ENGINEERING AND REQUIREMENTS MANAGEMENT

Introduction

"Systems engineering is about creating effective solutions to problems, and managing the technical complexity of the resulting developments" [1]. The Channel Tunnel Rail Link is a good example of such a project. It is complex, involves many disciplines, has significant safety issues, and multiple contractors. Clearly, for such a project to have any chance of success, those involved must know what they are doing. Therefore, effective requirements management is vital.

So what does the Channel Tunnel Rail Link have to do with the pharmaceutical industry? Any project of significance in the industry will share these characteristics.

In this chapter, we will be introducing requirements management, in particular concentrating on the importance of maintaining traceability through the life cycle of the system. In this context, "life cycle" means the whole life of the system, not just its development.

Projects Are Tough

You are probably familiar with the statistic (or at least you have heard similar) that in the year 2000 only 28% of projects involving software succeeded. Here we define success as on time, on budget, and with all required features. This compares to 16% in 1994. We can attribute this improvement at least partly to two significant changes: increased tool use and process improvement activities. Neither on its own is sufficient. Tools remove a lot of the need for tedious, error-prone, manual work. However, without good processes, there is little benefit in implementing tools.

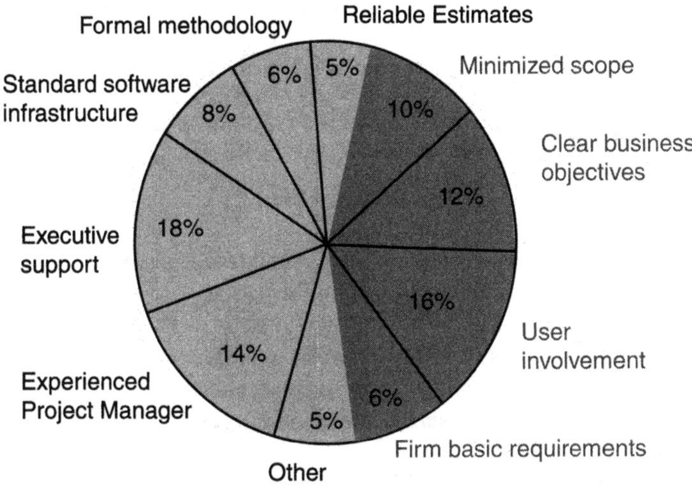

Figure 7.1 Reasons for Project Success

The Standish report "Extreme Chaos" [2] is an example of an industry report produced by independent analysts. Figure 7.1 shows some results from this survey. When project managers were asked what contributes to project success, 44% gave reasons related directly to requirements. That is nearly half the reasons for success directly related to one single discipline: requirements management — a discipline, which, based on these numbers, we cannot afford to do half-heartedly.

Requirements Are Vital

A good set of requirements provides a clear statement of objectives. They describe the set of acceptable solutions and provide guidance in the selection of the most appropriate solution. The greater the complexity of the system that we are acquiring or supplying, the greater is the need for us to manage the requirements well.

For effective requirements management to be effective, we must remember that it is not just a front-end activity. It forms the backbone of the *whole* life cycle, not just during development but also through to disposal — and beyond. It enables us to focus on the most important objectives, not all requirements are equal in cost, risk, or benefit.

If we manage our requirements effectively, two benefits result.

- Fewer defects are introduced.
- Those defects that are introduced are detected earlier.

Early detection of defects is vital. The longer a defect goes undetected, the greater the amount of rework needed. Thus effective requirements management can reduce the overall cost of development. This is the basis of the famous quote "Quality is free" by Philip Crosby [3].

TRACEABILITY

Traceability is an essential part of requirements management. It documents the relationships between different types of information, for example:

- System requirements *satisfy* stakeholder requirements.
- Architectural design *satisfies* system requirements.
- Acceptance tests *qualify* stakeholder requirements.

The availability of traceability information means that we can carry out various analyses.

- *Impact analysis*: what is affected by a change?
- *Traceability analysis*: what gives rise to a particular development artefact? For example, what is the purpose of a particular test?
- *Coverage analysis*: have all requirements been met and are all features necessary? For example, do the system tests cover all the system requirements?

These analyses are extremely useful, if not essential, in giving customers confidence that they will get everything that they do want and are not being asked to pay for anything they do not want. From the development viewpoint, they give a way of responding to change requests by pointing out the potential impact of changes.

Information Models

In order to understand traceability, we need to understand information models. Information models are best created by considering the processes that we use in developing systems. Figure 7.2 shows one form of the classic "V-Model" for systems development. In this figure, the relationships are shown by labelled arrows.

We can make the fact that we are concerned with information relationships more explicit by redrawing this diagram using more representative terms. Figure 7.3 shows an example of this.

What does it mean to carry out an analysis? Figure 7.4 shows the use of this model to carry out an impact analysis. Essentially, we are asking, "What if this was to change?" Before agreeing to a change, we use impact analysis to understand how

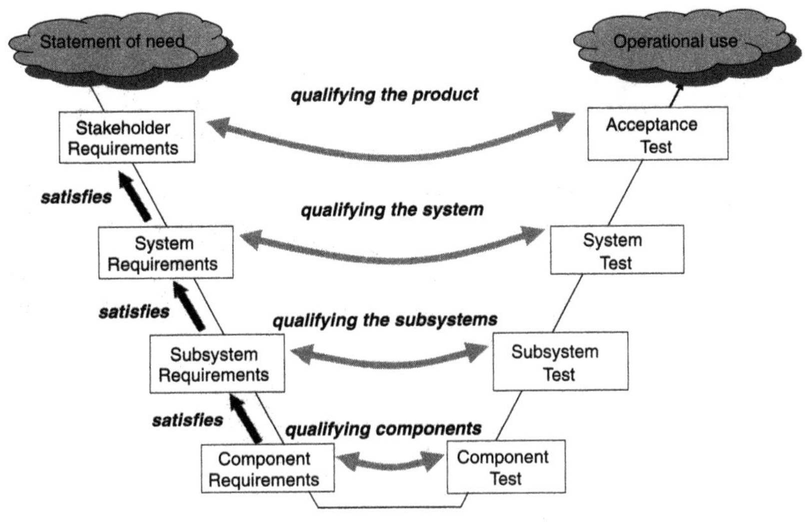

Figure 7.2 V-model.

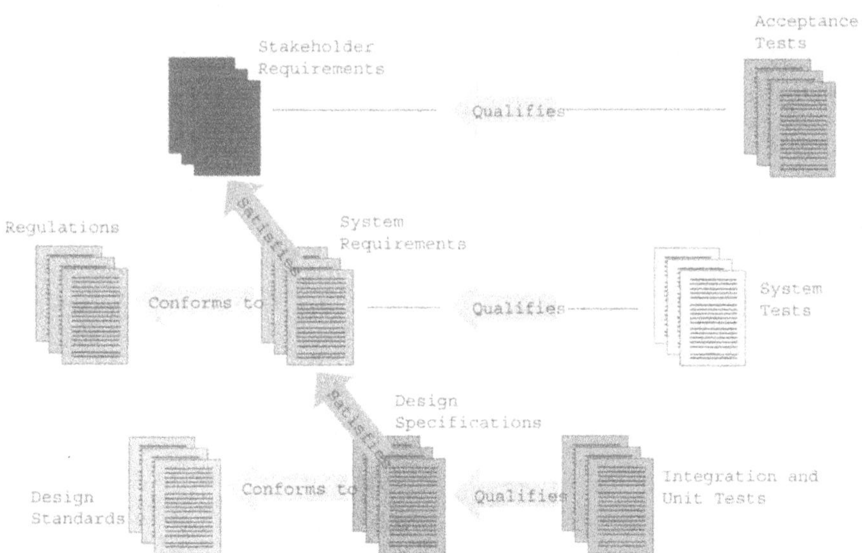

Figure 7.3 V-model as information model.

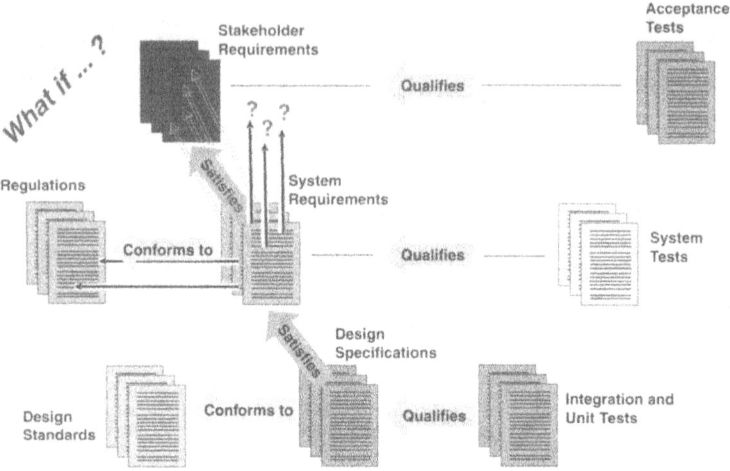

Figure 7.4 Impact analysis.

the effects of that change ripple through the development layers. For instance, we can see which tests we may need to rerun or rewrite in response to changing a requirement.

We can also follow relationships in the other direction. Figure 7.5 shows an example where we are trying to find out if we can trace all the requirements in the system requirements specification back to stakeholder requirements or to regulations.

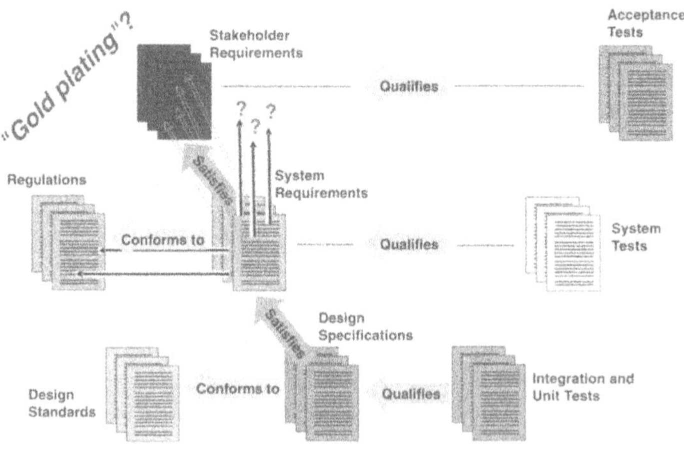

Figure 7.5 Derivation coverage analysis.

If we cannot find such a trace for a system requirement, we must ask if the requirement is necessary. Adding items to a specification that do not trace to a higher level is commonly referred to as gold plating, as it adds to cost without necessarily producing any benefit for the stakeholders.

3.2 Rich Traceability

A vital part of the systems approach is to know what the system is supposed to achieve and why — to understand how programs, projects, and subsystems cooperate to achieve it. In order to do this, we need to be able to annotate the relationships. It is not sufficient just to state that two items are related and give the relationship a name; we also need to explain the relationship. Figure 7.6 shows an example, where the relationships between the subrequirements and the original requirement are annotated with information about *how* the derived requirements satisfy the original.

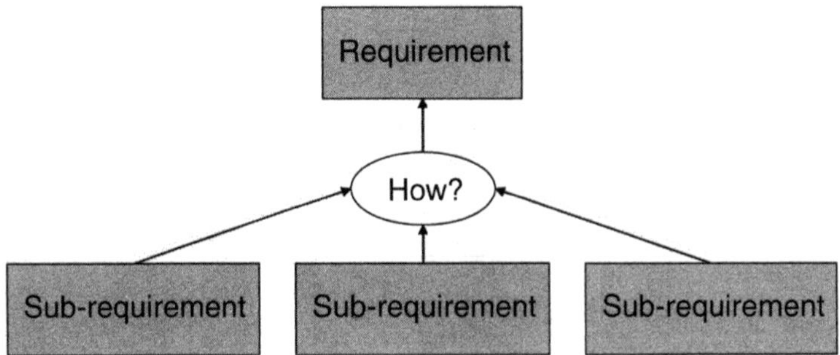

Figure 7.6 Rich traceability.

In terms of relationships between requirements at different levels, we refer to the annotation as the *rationale*. Two types of rationale information are useful.

- *Satisfaction*, which explains how higher-level requirements are met.
- *Justification*, which explains how a lower-level requirement contributes to higher level requirements.

Figure 7.7 shows an example where satisfaction information is used. These are called *satisfaction arguments*. This approach is frequently used where the owner of the higher-level requirements can provide additional information to guide the authors of the lower-level requirements.

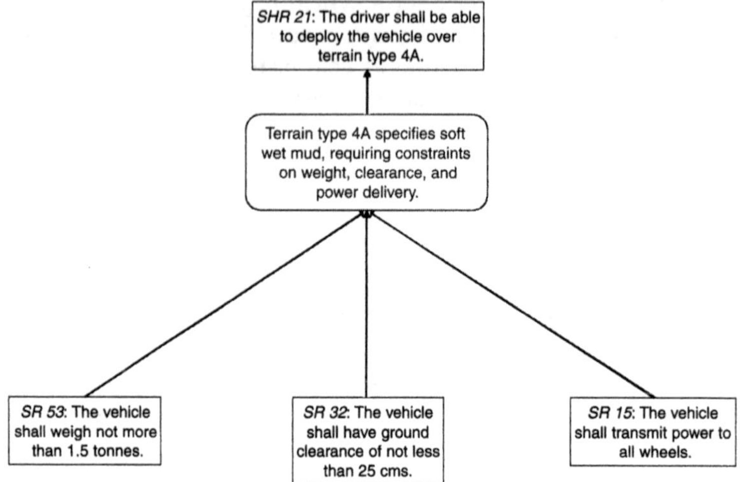

Figure 7.7 Satisfaction arguments.

Figure 7.8 shows the use of *justification arguments*. Here, the authors of the lower-level requirements have provided additional information to *justify* their choices.

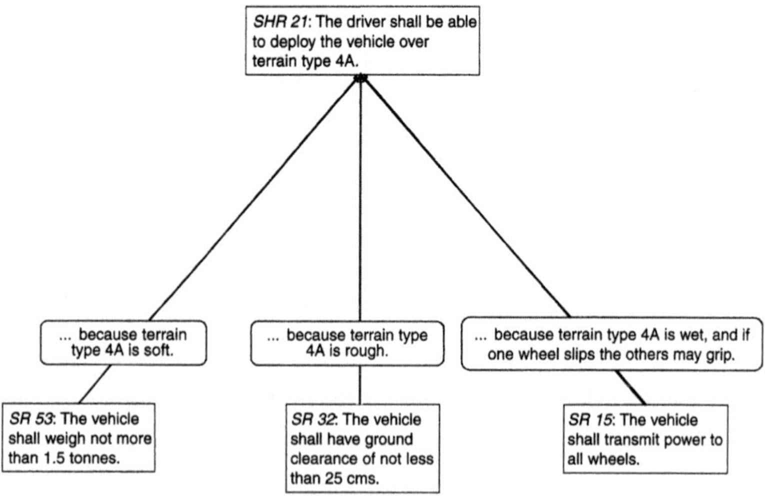

Figure 7.8 Justification arguments.

Of course, we can use rich traceability for any kind of relationship, satisfaction as in Figures 7.6 to 7.8; for validation, as shown in Figure 7.9 where the argument on the validation relationships actually shows the *validation strategy*; for safety, where the argument explains how the safety case arises, etc.

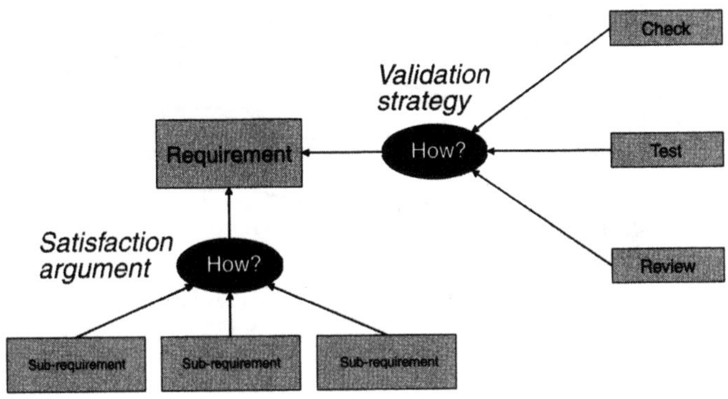

Figure 7.9 Multidimensional rich traceability.

THE ROLE OF MODELS

We model to understand and analyze a problem. Modeling provides a basis for reasoning about the problem, potential solutions, etc. Modeling therefore complements requirements engineering.

The models required depend upon the application domain, the disciplines involved (e.g., electronics, hydraulics) and the level of development (e.g., stakeholder requirements, system requirements, system architecture).

As examples of domain specific models, consider:

- *Aircraft industry*: aerodynamic models, three-dimensional spatial models, weight distribution models, flight simulators.
- *Rail industry*: timetable simulation, safety, reliability, and maintainability models.
- *Car industry*: styling models, dashboard models, aerodynamic models.

So how do models and requirements relate to one another in a development process? Figure 7.10 shows an example. Here we start with a statement of need, and then we do model usage to help us to derive the stakeholder requirements. We use functional modeling based on the information in the system requirements to help us to create the system requirements. Finally, we use a variety of performance models to help us to create the appropriate architecture to meet the system requirements.

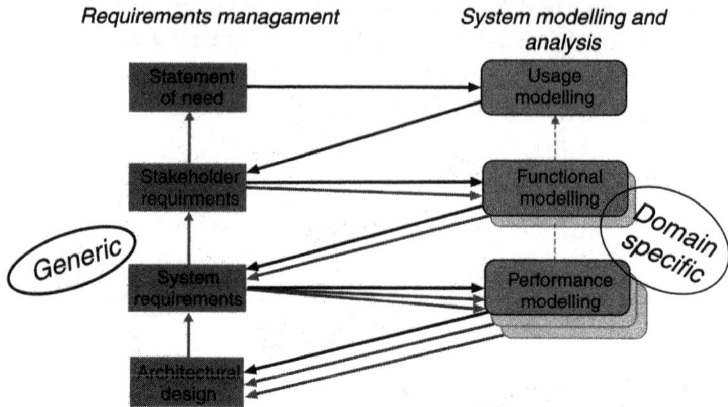

Figure 7.10 The role of system models.

From this, we can see that modelling is vital throughout the development of a system, and one of its uses is in supporting the requirements derivation. Interestingly, the further development progresses, and the closer to implementation, the more the requirements support the building of models, rather than the other way round.

GENERIC OR SPECIFIC?

Overview

The idea of a generic process for requirements, applicable wherever requirements were written, first occurred to us in Telelogic some time ago [4]. We asked ourselves the following questions:

- Are all the system development processes different?
- Are they all the same?
- What makes them differ?

Our answers are, first, there are many common aspects; second, it is worthwhile separating out the similarities and the differences.

Let us first remind ourselves of the V-model, but this time highlight the levels, as shown in Figure 7.11, where we can clearly see that we have to deal with requirements at every level.

At every layer of the V-model, we have a process of creating artefacts. We call this process *engineer product*. Also at every level, we have to produce these

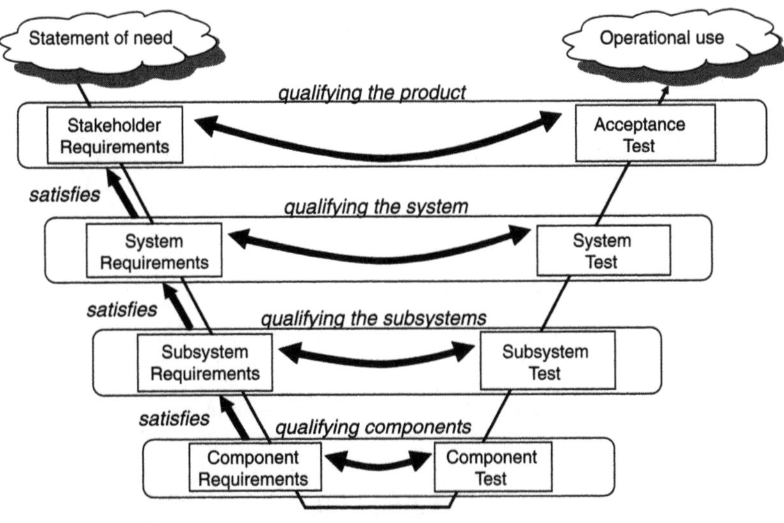

Figure 7.11 V-model — requirements at every level.

requirements and their matching qualification strategy from existing material. We have also seen, in Figure 7.10, the importance of models. We can draw this all together into a picture of a single layer, as we show in Figure 7.12.

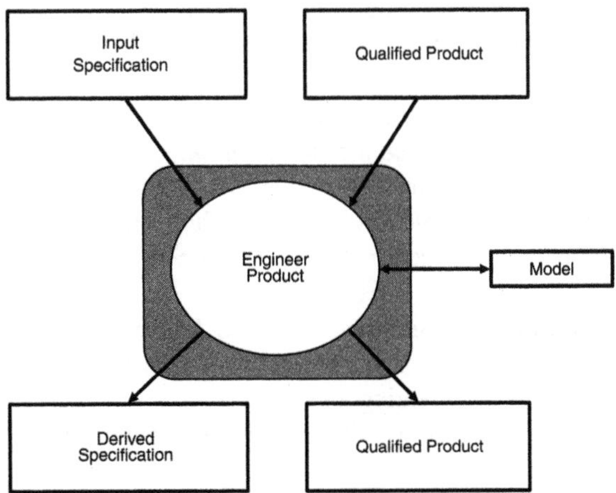

Figure 7.12 Engineer product in context.

If we expand the contents of the *engineer product* process, we have the activities and work products that we show in Figure 7.13.

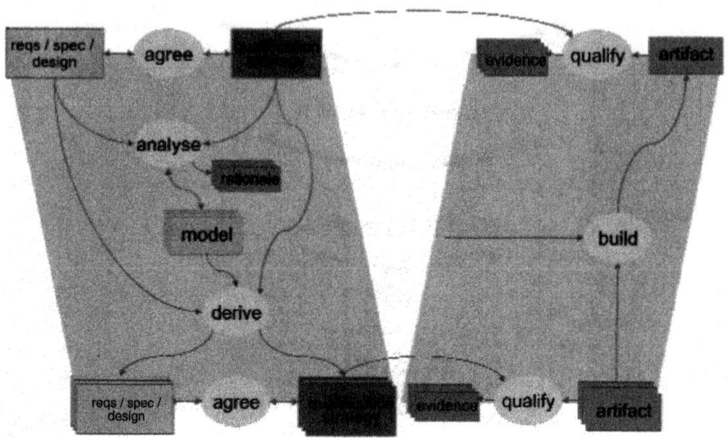

Figure 7.13 Engineer product in detail.

Figure 7.13 introduces some significant topics.

- The idea that it is necessary to *agree* upon the source requirements, specification, or design* and the derived specification.
- The need to produce the *qualification strategy* in tandem with producing specifications.
- The production of *models* during the analysis activity.
- The separation of the process on the left-hand side of the "V" into *analysis* and *derivation*.
- Recording the *rationale* for analysis.
- The production of *evidence* for *qualification.*
- A reminder that the purpose of the whole process is to produce *artefacts* through *building* multiple lower-level artefacts into higher-level items.
- The *build* activity is based on (some of) the *models* produced during *analysis*.

Of course, even this is a simplified picture. In particular, we have omitted any mention of change. However, it clearly shows the principal activities and work products that go towards creating a system.

In the following sections, we discuss these topics in detail.

---

*For simplicity, we refer to requirements, specifications, and designs jointly or separately as *specifications*.

Agreement

Whenever any person or organization requests some third party to solve a problem, typically by producing some system, the two need to agree on the definition of the problem. Therefore this is the first activity in engineering a product. We must also agree on the qualification strategy, not just the specification. Ideally, these occur in parallel, since there is little value in agreeing upon what we must do if we have no idea how we are going to prove that it has been done.

Analysis

We analyze the provided specifications, using appropriate models, first to help us to understand their places in the context of the problem; second to help us to understand how they relate to one another; and third to extract information from them. This activity may include decomposing specification items for more detail, though this more typically happens during derivation. The exact nature of the analysis will vary considerably, depending mostly on the nature of the problem and the current level of abstraction.

One of the key results of the analysis activity is an agreed understanding of the *scope* of the problem between the customer and the supplier.

Derivation

Derivation is the process of creating the next level of specification and qualification strategy from the input material. In this, we use the models and analysis results we have created.

The process that we use for deriving requirements depends on both the relationship between the input requirements and the derived requirements, and where we are in the life cycle. There are four things that we can do when deriving requirements:

1. Converting vague statements into rigorous requirements. For example, taking a statement of need and deriving stakeholder requirements.
2. Converting problem-oriented statements into solution-oriented statements. For example, taking stakeholder requirements and deriving system requirements.
3. Allocating requirements to lower-level artefacts. For example, taking system requirements and deriving requirements for specific subsystems.
4. Decomposing requirements into more detail — this is often part of the first three items.

Although we cannot start derivation until we have done some analysis, we do not have to wait to start until we have finished analysis.

Qualification

There are two aspects to qualification. One is to check the progress of building; the other is to check the progress of specification. In the first, more common usage, we check that the current level of build of the artefacts satisfies the appropriate level of specification. In the second, we check that the specifications produced at each level jointly satisfy the specifications from which they were derived.

Build

The *build* activity is where we bring together artefacts from lower levels and construct higher-level items from them. Building is outside the scope of the current discussion, but we must recognize that information used and generated during building is related to information generated and used during specification. It is important that we maintain these relationships.

RISKS, ISSUES, AND ASSUMPTIONS

Overview

In an ideal world, we have perfect knowledge of everything that can affect the solution to the problems with which we are presented, together with their likelihood and possible effects. In addition, we would know exactly how to overcome those problems. In the real world, this is simply not true. We need to consider three areas, risks, assumptions, and issues.

Risks

Risks are essentially unknown events. Our lack of knowledge is either ignorance of the event itself or about its likelihood. There is little that we can do to plan for unknown events*, but we can attempt to make some assessment of the likelihood and likely effect of known events. Knowing this, we can then assess what we could and should do about them. Although we use the term "risk," it is, of course, possible that an event could have positive effects. Risks can be internal or external to an organization. Typical types of risk include:

- Political.

---

*Hand me that crystal ball!

- Economic.
- Technical.
- Managerial.

If the negative effects of a risk are high enough, we must decide what to do about it. We can adopt one of two approaches (or a combination). We can try to prevent the risk occurring (mitigation) or we can provide some fallback if the risk should occur.

Whatever the risk and whatever we choose to do about it, we need to link it to those requirements it affects. After all, if an event will not prevent us from meeting our requirements, then, no matter how serious it may be outside the scope of the project, it is of little interest to the project.

When we have identified risks, we will probably generate additional requirements to manage mitigation and fallback.

Issues and Assumptions

Issues and assumptions can be managed in a similar way to risks. Issues are known, whereas risks are unknown. For example, if we know we do not have enough capacity, this is an issue. We make assumptions where there are unknowns, but we need to make progress. For example, we might assume that we can show conformance to a specific protocol that is not yet fully defined.

SUMMARY AND CONCLUSIONS

In this chapter we have presented requirements management as an essential topic for engineers. Key items we have discussed include:

- The importance of controlling requirements.
- The use of traceability to understand relationships.
- The use of traceability analysis to check satisfaction, qualification, ...

Change management is needed in any process; in particular, we must not let changes happen in an uncontrolled way.

Risk management is also essential. We must understand our risks, understand mitigation and fallback, and not forget issues and assumptions.

REFERENCES

1. Stevens, R., Brook, P., Jackson K., Arnold, S. *Systems Engineering: Coping with Complexity*. Prentice Hall Europe, 1998.

2. Standish Group, The. *Extreme Chaos*, www.standishgroup.com, 2001.
3. Crosby, P. B. *Quality Is Free*. New York, McGraw-Hill, 1979.
4. Hull, E.C., Jackson, K., Dick, J. *Requirements Engineering*. Springer, New York, 2002.

Chapter 8

Good Documentation in Practice

Michael L. Wyrick

CONTENTS

INTRODUCTION

One of the areas that continue to challenge project teams at project initiation is documentation. The following documentation issues often lead to "project paralysis."

- What documents need to be generated?
- Who is responsible for document generation?
- What is the format for documentation?
- What is the document approval process?
- Where are documents stored during the development phase of the project?
- What is the document "change management" process during the development phase of the project?

Experience has shown that implementing the following three steps mitigates this documentation dilemma.

1. Write a policy or procedure for each compliance domain defining the deliverables and who is responsible for creating each.
   - Determine which deliverables need to be consistent, and provide templates and forms. Templates comprise standardized documents used as a framework for the creation of other documents. Forms are standardized documents with blank areas to be filled in by the user for the creation of records. Both these are enablers designed to encourage compliance with policies, procedures, or standards.
     - The templates and forms should be referenced within the appropriate policy, procedure, or standard.
     - Use version control and change control to maintain templates and forms.
     - Maintain electronic copies of templates and forms in a controlled environment, similar to maintaining application software.

2. Create a corporate documentation standard that deals with creation and maintenance of controlled documents. The remainder of this chapter is designed as examples of documentation standards.
3. Develop a separate change management procedure for the development phase of the project. Change management is often referred to as "change control lite." The change management procedure is a less stringent "change control" process that maintains up-to-date project documentation without significantly slowing down the development phase. At project implementation or project acceptance time, change management stops and change control begins.

Purpose

Documentation standards cover the format, content, and attributes of documentation produced during the development and maintenance phases of application software validation and platform qualification projects. To identify additional practices regarding documents and record management.

The standards do not include format attributes such as fonts, type size, tabs, justification, etc. Corporations should develop templates that support the documentation standards and the templates should contain document format attributes.

Scope

Documentation standards should be applied to all formally reviewed and approved documents. Documentation standards are applicable to both manually and electronically generated documents, regardless of the application software used for their generation. It is expected that the majority of these documents will be created using a word processor (e.g., Microsoft Word); therefore, specific standards within this document may only apply to documents created using this product.

Documentation standards do not apply to:

- GxP standard operating procedures (SOPs) that will be created or revised according to applicable corporate, divisional or site SOPs.
- Informal types of communication such as memos or e-mail.

Rationale

It is expected that the majority of formal, approved documents will be used to support application software validation and platform qualification. Validation of systems, facilities, equipment, and processes is a requirement of current good manufacturing practices.

Both ISO 9000 quality standards and current good manufacturing practices require a system for document control. ISO 9001 and 9002 include sections regarding document control that support five basic requirements for documents.

- They must be reviewed and approved prior to issue.
- They must be distributed or made available to locations where they are used.
- Obsolete documents must be removed from points of use.
- Changes to documents must be authorized and approved.
- There must be a system (a master list or equivalent) to identify the current revision of documents.

DOCUMENT MANAGEMENT TASKS

The tasks associated with documentation standards include:

- Creating initial documents.
- Revising, editing, and annotating draft copies of documents.
- Approving documents.
- Handling paper copies, including obtaining handwritten signatures and management of approved documents.
- Moving documents to and from a secured storage location.
- Verifying of compliance to documentation standards.

DOCUMENT STANDARDS

Assumptions

All electronically generated documentation will be created using approved corporate standard software.

Tools or systems that self-generate project documentation should adhere to documentation standards as closely as possible. Where a deviation to standards occurs, the missing information should be included or referenced in the quality assurance review (QAR) form or signature page.

A validated electronic document management system may be used providing it is compliant with 21 CFR Part 11, Electronic Records; Electronic Signatures. Parts of a documentation standard may not be applicable when utilizing an electronic document management system (e.g., managing hardcopy documents).

Content

Each document should contain the following information:

- Title.
- Document approval.
- Revision history.
- Table of contents (for documents more than five pages long).
- Definitions and acronyms.
- Reference documents (including title and location of document).
- Document information and attributes (defined in section 3.2.7).

Title

The title of each document should be unique, and summarize the content or purpose of the document.

Document Approval

Approval may be documented on a signature page within the document itself or on a separate QAR form. All documents that support application software validation and platform qualification require signatures to demonstrate review or approval. These documents include, but are not limited, to:

- Plans (validation, qualification, configuration management, security, test, training, business continuity).
- Specifications (requirements, design).
- Standards (documentation, programing, naming convention).
- Testing (cases, scripts).

Note: The applicable application software validation and platform qualification plan will identify the required persons, by position and title, who will be expected to sign-off on specific documents.

Major changes to documents need to be reviewed and approved by people in the same roles as those who gave approval to the original document. A document owner can accumulate changes until periodic review time or until a future change request occurs for that document in order to bundle changes together into a single revision.

For all documents requiring signatures the following must be included:

- A signature page or QAR form.
- Revision number.
- Revision history.

Where signatures are not recorded on the document itself, use the QAR form template. For example, when multiple documents used as a set (e.g., design documents, test cases, or scripts) are reviewed and approved together, a QAR form may be more appropriate. Consult with your local quality representative (i.e., validation coordinator, qualification advocate, or QA/QC) if further clarification is needed.

A review and approval is not required for documents such as:

- Meeting minutes.
- Presentations that are not part of approved training material.
- Project administration information unrelated to application software validation and platform qualification.
- Lists (e.g., master document list).

Signature Page

A signature page template includes some examples of boilerplate signature descriptions that may be used. Portions of the signature description are expected to vary depending upon the purpose of the document itself.

It is recommended, but not required to have the author, reviewer, and approver names preprinted on the document. Include a place to print the name in addition to the signature, if pre-printed names are not included.

QAR Form

The QAR form is used to record reviewer comments and signatures. Make sure that document title, revision number, change request number, and the purpose of the review are included on the form. Completed QARs should be retained as documentation that the document is acceptable.

Revision History

Include a revision history following the signature page in all approved documents. The revision history will include the revision number, revision date, reasons for revision, and person revising the document (typically originator). Identify the change request number in the reasons for revision section. Only revisions that are approved must be listed in the revision history table.

The explanation of the revision-numbering scheme is located in section 3.2.7.

Table of Contents

Include a table of contents for documents over five pages in length.

Definitions and Acronyms

Include a table listing any acronyms and definitions needed to understand the content of the document. If a term is defined in an existing glossary, list the glossary in the reference section instead of including the definition.

References

For reference documents that are part of an application software validation or platform qualification package, list the name of the document as it appears in the master document list (MDL), including section or page number if relevant, and include the location of the MDL instead of listing the location of each document.

For other reference documents list the document name, including section or page number if relevant, and provide a URL, path or physical location of the document.

Document Information and Attributes

It is recommended that templates are developed for all documents created using Microsoft Word, Excel, and PowerPoint. These templates should include all required attributes.

Detailed requirements and tips for including the attributes in Microsoft Word are included in Table 8.1.

Other Document Formats

Tools or systems which self-generate project documentation should adhere to the following standards. The following information must be added to the QAR or signature page if not included in the document itself.

- Title.
- Electronic file name.
- Revision number.
- Originator.
- Revision date.

Document Appendices

Information that requires frequent updates (e.g., specific names, phone numbers) may be included in an appendix document that can be revised with an abbreviated

Table 8.1 Document attributes

Document Information and Attributes	Description and Usage
Title	Use the Microsoft Word field code {title} to place the title description from the File Properties Summary dialog box into the document.
Electronic file name	Use the Microsoft Word field code {filename} to place the file name into the document.
Page numbers	Use the Microsoft Word field codes to place the page number {page} and total number of pages {numpages}, respectively, into the document.
Revision number	Use the following revision numbering scheme for identifying formal documents: N.N or N.NN Always start original draft revisions with revision 0.1. Each time a document has completed the approval process, increment the number preceding the decimal point by 1. Thus the first time a document is routed for signatures, assign it revision 1.0. Subsequent approved revisions will be 2.0, 3.0. etc. The numbers following the decimal point may be used for tracking iterations during a change cycle. Thus, iterations may be 0.1, 0.2, etc. or 0.01, 0.02, etc. Where a review is conducted for multiple electronic files, only those files that were actually modified will get a new revision number. Each file's revision number will be recorded in the master document list. Note: The revision number must be manually incremented in the footer and in the revision history table.
Originator	Use the Microsoft Word field code {author} to place the author description from the File Properties Summary dialog box into the revision history table of the document.
Date of last revision	Use the Microsoft Word field code {savedate} to place the last date that the document was saved into the document. Include descriptive identifier "last save date." Specify the month using alphabet characters to avoid ambiguity between North American (mm/dd/yyyy) and European (dd/mm/yyyy) formats. Field-specific switches within field codes may be used for this purpose.
Print date	Use the Microsoft Word field code {printdate} to place the date the document was printed. Include descriptive identifier "print date." Specify the month using alphabet characters to avoid ambiguity between North American (mm/dd/yyyy) and European (dd/mm/yyyy) formats. Field-specific switches within field codes may be used for this purpose. The print date may appear either on the first page or on each page.
Document number	*Optional* Some areas assign unique document numbers for identification purposes.

approval process. The required approvers for this abbreviated process must be specified in the document. In addition, when the appendix is revised, the revision history for the appendix must reflect the reasons for revision and the appendix revision number must be incremented.

Document and Record Management

Most of this section is applicable to a manual document or record management process and does not apply when using an electronic document management system.

Creating and Modifying Documents

Table 8.2 Recommendations for creating and modifying documents

Topic	Recommendation
Drafting originals	Require that the standard document template be used when creating original Word documents unless more specific document templates have been approved. By completing the File Properties Summary dialog box, the revision number is the only information in the footer that will require manual updating for each revision.
Annotations or Revisions	When reviewing draft or interim revisions of Word documents the reviewer can use either annotations or revisions to record comments in the document. However, authors should either lock the document for annotations so that only the author can directly edit the document or lock the document for revisions, so that they can be tracked and accepted or rejected later. (Use the Tools Protect Document dialog box to activate or deactivate these features.)
Revision marks	Revision marks may be used for highlighting draft or interim Word documents, however, remove all revision marking when printing a document for formal signoff. The comparison of versions to previously approved versions is greatly facilitated by using this feature. (Use the Revisions dialog box from the Tools menu.)

Signature Routing

The sequence for collecting signatures is:

1. Originator.
2. Reviewers.
3. Approvers.

Collect signatures such that the author and reviewer signatures are obtained prior to approvers. It is possible to route documents in parallel, i.e., obtaining signatures at multiple sites using separate signature pages.

Generally speaking, documents that require both reviewers and approvers are plans that require execution (e.g., validation plan, configuration management plan, security plan). The reviewers are technical experts responsible for assuring that the content of the document is complete and accurate. The approvers are area management (e.g., project leaders, managers) responsible for assuring that the document was reviewed by the appropriate technical experts and acknowledging the responsibility of their area during execution of the plan. A QA or QC approver is also required for certain application software validation and platform qualification documents related to GxP systems. If required, the QA or QC approver must be the final document approver.

Faxed signatures are acceptable as a temporary placeholder for the original signatures and documents can become approved and effective based on faxed signatures, but original signatures must be collected and maintained as the official record.

Checking in Documents

When all required signatures have been obtained, the signed off hard copy is forwarded to the document owner.

When receiving the approved document, the document owner will file the hard copy in the appropriate section of the application software validation and platform qualification library. The document owner will also copy the electronic file from the working directory to the secure, approved document directory and delete the file in the working directory. It is recommended that the document owner set the read-only file attribute prior to filing the document in approved document library. Only finalized, approved records will be placed in the secure approved document library.

Master Document List (MDL)

The project manager will assign an individual with responsibility for maintaining a MDL of all project and application software validation and platform qualification documents. This list will be updated when a new document, or revision to an existing document is stored in the secure approved document library. The MDL file itself will also be stored in the secure approved document library. The MDL should contain, but may not be limited to, the following information about the document:

- Title.
- Primary electronic path and filename.
- Primary hardcopy location, if applicable.
- Revision number.
- Originator.
- Effective date.
- Retention category (e.g., batch history, product history, department, division, and site history).
- Live or historical designation.

Document Retention

The hardcopy signatures along with the hardcopy document need to be retained unless a document management system that meets the requirements of 21 CFR Part 11 Electronic Signatures; Electronic Records is used.

If the document management system utilized is compliant with the electronic record requirements, but does not include electronic signature functionality, then the signature page must be linked to the electronic record with which it is associated (e.g., by including the unique record number on the signature page). In this case, only the signature page needs to be retained.

Revising Documents

If an approved document needs revision, the file is copied from the secure approved library to a working directory where the Read Only attribute is reset.

Caution: Documents that previously existed in other libraries or on workstation hard disks must not be used as starting points for new revisions.

Distribution

The hard copy documents need not be distributed if the electronic copies are accessible by the users. The approval or effective date of documents should be communicated to the project team. Only the current, approved version of the document should be available to the users. Notification will consist of an electronic mail message or other communication that will detail the location of the electronic copy as well as any self-study or training materials.

Note: When hard copies are maintained, it is the user's responsibility to ensure that they are replaced when a new revision is released.

HANDWRITTEN RECORD ENTRIES

Assumptions

This entire section is applicable to handwritten records or documents.

Signatures and Entries

- Use only permanent, preferably black, ballpoint ink for signing or for manual entries.

- Always accompany a signature with the date of signing (use four-digit year).
- Complete all information blanks on the document. If a field requiring input does not have any entry, use "N/A" to indicate that the field was not skipped or forgotten.

Corrections

Never erase an entry or make it illegible. If a correction to an entry error is necessary, the person who made the entry error will be the one who corrects it. Where this is not possible, then the corrector must be a member of supervision or a member of quality assurance or quality control.

Using a black ink pen, correct an error by drawing a single line through the incorrect entry. Write the correct entry as near as possible to the original entry, the reason for the correction and then initial and date the revision.

Changes or Additions to Records

If additional information or instruction is needed and can be made in the space available, make the change by hand, initial and date it.

Otherwise, add a full-page insert, according to the following instructions:

- The text of the change must be handwritten legibly in black ballpoint ink, or typed, onto a blank series of pages.
- In the upper right hand corner of the insert page, record the page number and title of the original record, the entry number of the change (if applicable); the signature of the person (the writer) composing the insert and the date; and the signature of a second person may be either a member of supervision or quality assurance or quality control.
- Attach the insert to the original record.
- Never remove any portion of an original record or document. Void nonapplicable portions of a record by marking a boxed "X" across the entire nonapplicable section. Initial and date the voided area.

Signature and Initial Logs

The project manager will ensure that an up-to-date log of signatures and initials for all project team members who may sign or initial records is maintained. For all other personnel signing or dating records, individual departmental management has the responsibility of maintaining signature logs within their own departments.

SECURITY AND ACCESS

Electronic Document Security

Validation and qualification documents must be located either on a secured, managed server or in a validated electronic document management system.

When using a secured server, update access to the approved document library must be limited to designated personnel and assigned by project management. Backup and recovery procedures must be in place in accordance with the applicable corporate policies or procedures.

Folders should be labeled to clearly distinguish between in-process documents and approved documents.

For example, a common scheme is to use three folder types:

- Working — documents under development.
- Review — documents currently in the review or approval cycle.
- Approved — documents that have been approved.

Hard Copy Document Security

Access to the application software validation and platform qualification library containing approved copies of qualification or validation documents must be limited to appropriate personnel as determined by project management.

GLOSSARY AND REFERENCES

Definitions and Acronyms

Table 8.3 contains definitions of terms used in this document.

Table 8.3 Definitions

Term	Meaning
Document	An instruction or plan containing information on how a company functions, how specific tasks are carried out, and how to build specific products or services. e.g., a form to be used in an inspection report is a document. "The ABCs of Document Control" PI Quality July/Aug 1993 Jack Kanholm pp.48–49.
Electronic signature	The entry in the form of a computer data compilation of any symbol or series of symbols executed, adopted, or authorized by an individual to be the legally binding equivalent of the individual's handwritten signature. (21CFR Part 11)

Table 8.3 continued

Term	Meaning
Form	A standardized document with blank areas to be filled in by the user for the creation of records.
GxP	A term that combines good manufacturing practices (GMP), good laboratory practices (GLP), and good clinical practices (GCP).
Handwritten signature	Handwritten signature means the scripted name or legal mark of an individual handwritten by that individual and executed or adopted with the present intention to authenticate a writing in a permanent form. The act of signing with writing or marking instrument such as a pen or stylus is preserved. The scripted name or legal mark, while conventionally applied to paper, may also be applied to other devices that capture the name or mark. (21CFR Part 11)
Historical document	Documents maintained during the system development life cycle (i.e., throughout the implementation phase) and then retired.
QAR	Quality assurance review. This is a stand-alone form used to record the peer review of a document or set of documents to assure that the content is accurate and correct and that the content complies with applicable standards. The term "quality assurance" is used in the generic sense and does not imply the corporate quality assurance group.
Living document	Documents maintained throughout the entire system life cycle (i.e., until the retirement life cycle phase).
Major change	Any change that impacts the scope or intent of the document or results in changes to the scope or intent of other documents. Note: A major change to a document will impact associated training material and requires retraining.
Minor change	Changes to documentation that have little or no impact upon the scope or intent of the document. These kinds of changes do not require an approval. Rather, another team member may verify that the impact of the change request has been evaluated. The changes do need to be documented. Examples: • Correcting typographical errors. • Changing format or style. • Adding or changing authors, reviewers, approvers. Note: Minor changes do not require retraining.
Record	A written statement of data or facts pertaining to a specific event, person, process, or product, e.g., a completed (filled out) form in an inspection report is a record, Jack Kanholm, "The ABCs of Document Control" *PI Quality* July/Aug 1993, pp.48–49.
Signature or signs	The name of the operator, writer, checker, quality control representative, etc., handwritten by the individual with permanent black ink or other authorized ink color. Initials are acceptable if they are properly included on the current departmental log of authorized names, signatures, and initials. A typewritten signature or a signature stamp is not acceptable.
System documentation	Written or pictorial information describing, specifying, reporting or certifying activities, requirements, procedures or results of a computerized system's performance, development, operation, support, and maintenance.
Template	A standardized document to be used as a framework for the creation of other documents.

Reference Documents

Table 8.4 Reference Documents

Title	Location
Current Good Manufacturing Practice for Finished Pharmaceuticals, 21 CFR Parts 210 & 211	http://www.fda.gov:80/cder/dmpq/
ISO 9001 and 9002	Available through International Organization for Standardization (http://www.iso.ch/iso/en/ISOOnline.frontpage)
ANSI/ASQC Standard Q91–1987 American National Standard, Quality Systems — Model for Quality Assurance Model for Quality Assurance in Design/Development, Production, Installation, and Servicing	Available through American Society for Quality (http://www.asq.org/) or American National Standards Institute (http://web.ansi.org/default.htm)
Electronic Records; Electronic Signatures, 21 CFR, Part 11	http://www.fda.gov/ora/compliance_ref/part11/
GAMP4	Available through ISPE (http://www.ispe.org/gamp/)
GMP Documentation Requirements for Automated Systems: Parts I and II	Ronald F. Tetzlaff, *Pharmaceutical Technology*, March and April 1992
Documentation Revisited	Barbara Immel, *BioPharm*, January 1997

Chapter 9

Good Testing Practice: Part 1

David Stokes

CONTENTS

INTRODUCTION

There is myriad testing "best practice" guidance available within the general computer systems and IT industry. This has been developed since the dawn of the computer systems age, where the value of testing software prior to use was first realized.

Some of this best practice guidance has specifically been written for use within heavily regulated industries such as the aerospace and nuclear industries, where a potential software failure can have immediate and fatal effects.

Many of these principles can apply equally within the life sciences industry where it is also true that software problems can have (and have had) fatal consequences for patients. When such software problems do arise and the consequences are widespread these are deemed equally newsworthy of any plane crash or a nuclear incident.

However, the reality is that most of the potential problems are discovered before the health or safety of patients is affected. What is therefore needed is practical guidance that can be applied in a pragmatic and cost-effective manner by those involved in testing GxP critical systems or software.

This chapter, along with Chapter 19, aim to build upon basic testing "best practice." There are plenty of examples of test specifications, templates for test cases, mappings of testing within the overall life cycle, discussions of test coverage, test objectives, etc. and repeating these add nothing new (although references are given to such guidance).

The intention here is to provide useful and pragmatic advice on how to apply those principles in practice, with specific focus on current regulatory trends such as risk assessment and cost effective validation. The approach recommended is to leverage existing test planning, execution, and reporting activities and to build support for the validation case into test documentation that would already be developed by the implementation team.

This has the following advantages:

- It reduces the validation costs by minimizing separate "validation" activities.
- It ensures that the test team are responsible for, and take ownership of, the system verification through appropriate testing, and for the overall validation of the system.
- It ensures that testing activities are appropriate to the risks associated with the system.

It should be noted that although this chapter describes an integrated approach with an integrated set of test documentation, this is not meant to be in any way proscriptive. As with any validation activities, the approach can be simplified and documents combined for smaller or simpler systems or pieces of software, and the principles described scaled as appropriate.

DEFINITIONS

General Testing Terms

Before embarking upon any program of testing (or indeed any computer systems implementation or validation project), it is essential that a common set of terms and definitions are defined, understood, and used.

These may be standard terms within an organization or they may be specific to the project. While a user or supplier organization may have their own consistent set of terms and definitions, problems often arise when users and suppliers work together on a project, and each has a slightly different understanding of the various terms, document titles, and acronyms used by the other.

This can often lead to a great deal of confusion during the specification and execution of tests and in the worst cases these may invalidate some tests or require certain tests to be rewritten or reexecuted. While the users and the suppliers technical teams may be "on the same page" with respect to what they are doing, the users IT or IS quality group, or the users validation group may have a completely different understanding of what testing is taking place, and why.

In order to successfully plan, specify, and execute tests, it is therefore essential that:

- A common set of testing terms, definitions, and acronyms are defined.
- That these are communicated to all of the project team members involved in testing.
- That these are not only read, but understood by all involved.

Following our own advice, this chapter and Chapter 19 will use a common set of testing terminology, in this case the terminology defined by the U.S. Food and Drug Administration (FDA) in its *Glossary of Computerized System and Software Development Terminology* [1].

TESTING, VERIFICATION, AND VALIDATION

Within the general world of computer systems there is sometimes confusion between software quality, validation, and testing. Many experienced testers believe themselves to be computer systems validation experts based solely upon in-depth testing experience, while other experts in the overall process of computer systems validation believe themselves to be experts in the field of software testing.

While there are various definitions for each of these, there is certainly a difference between software (computer systems) validation and testing.

The U.S. FDA adopts the IEEE definition of "testing" and the NBS definition of "software validation" as follows:

> "testing. (IEEE) (1) The process of operating a system or component under specified conditions, observing or recording the results, and making an evaluation of some aspect of the system or component. (2) The process of analyzing a software item to detect the differences between existing and required conditions, i.e., bugs, and to evaluate the features of the software items" [1].
>
> "validation, software. (NBS) Determination of the correctness of the final program or software produced from a development project with respect to the user needs and requirements. Validation is usually accomplished by verifying each stage of the software development life cycle" [1].

Within these and most other definitions, the testing of a computer system or software is just part of the overall validation process. A more useful definition from the FDA [2] classifies software testing as one of a number of software verification activities, that collectively contribute to the process of software (or computer systems) validation.

The testing of a computer system (or software) is a key activity in the overall process of validation. Those wishing to successfully validate a computer system (or software) certainly need to understand a good deal about the reason for and the process of testing, but need not necessarily be experts.

Likewise, software testing experts sometimes fail to see the "big picture" with respect to the overall process of validation, or to understand that testing by itself is of little use with respect to system validation.

WHY TEST?

"On the Road Again..."

"One, two. One, two. Testing, testing..."

At some time or another we have probably all heard a band or a sound technician checking out a sound system. However, there is a big difference between a simple sound check in a local bar, and a full sound test conducted by a major rock band on an international tour.

In the case of our jazz trio in the local bar it is usually a simple sound check. Make sure the amplifier is working, that the people at the back can hear and some check of sound quality if you are lucky. There is no written procedure, no checklist, no record of the check.

There is no definition of the test criteria (no script for something as simple as "One, two," no specification of how fast or slow to say the words, who should say the words or how often they should be repeated). Without these it is possible that two people could conduct the same check, and that one person could get the check to "pass" and another (with a quieter or louder voice) could get the check to fail.

There is also nothing to specify what should be done if the check fails. Turn up the amplification if people at the back cannot hear, or turn it down if there is feedback. Turn down the treble if there is a "hiss" on certain sounds...

In the case of the rock band on tour it is a much more complicated process. There are checks to make sure that everything is connected properly (there are a lot of cables), checks to make sure that the computerized light show is working correctly, sound checks for each instrument and each vocalist, overall sound checks for balance, volume, sound quality, and so on.

Because of the increased complexity there will be many more checklists and a clear order in which the checks should be done. Without these it would be virtually impossible to complete the checks in the time allowed. However, not all of the checks will be specified in detailed procedures, and not all of the results will be recorded.

As uncertain as these checks may appear to professionals in the life sciences industry, they are fit for purpose and ensure that the "show goes on." There is less of a requirement for repeatability when the show is held in a different venue every night and the risks are fewer.

Or are they? What about local legislation defining the maximum sound levels during a show? If these are exceeded, a venue could lose its license, and musicians, technicians or fans could lose their hearing in the long term. What about a badly made electrical connection? We have all heard stories about guitarists being electrocuted, but what if a problem puts the audience at risk? Is there not a moral duty to ensure that basic safety tests are conducted?

Perhaps insurers should require that certain tests are documented, to ensure that there is documentary evidence that proves that no one was negligent during the "sound check?" Perhaps the technicians should start making notes of the set-up for their own sake?

Perhaps most importantly, both the jazz trio and the rock band should make sure that they only purchase their equipment from a reputable source. They should make sure that they know all the equipment is compatible and that they know how it all goes together. Ideally this should be documented, saving time on tour and finally that they have checked that it all works and is safe before they go out on the road. Even then, there are a lot of cables, and every venue is different, so it never hurts to check.

Testing in Life Sciences

Stories of the road aside, the same principles apply to the whys and wherefores of testing in the life sciences industry.

Although we tend to focus on regulatory compliance, there are a number of reasons why we test computer systems.

- To save money (it is more cost effective to uncover and correct problems prior to going live with a system).
- To assure ourselves that they are fit for purpose (meet the specified requirements).
- To assure ourselves that they are safe (with respect to final product quality and

patient safety, but also with respect to immediate health and safety issues for employees and environmental requirements).

- Because our internal auditors and external regulators require us to.

As with the sound check analogy, although testing is important, it is only part of an overall process that assures fitness for purpose and all of the reasons listed above.

Just as testing a sound system *in situ* can uncover problems, these cannot be resolved if the problem is down to a basic incompatibility between pieces of equipment, or if a U.S. band takes its show to Europe, forgetting that the power supply is not 110V!

The overall process is called "validation," and no amount of testing can compensate for a flawed validation process. While other validation activities are covered elsewhere in this book, it is worth considering how testing relates to the overall validation process.

TESTING WITHIN THE VALIDATION LIFECYCLE

Although just one of the verification activities that make up the process of validation, testing cannot be considered to be a standalone task if it is to be successful. While it is true that testing can often be managed a separate activity (and in many large and complex projects it must be considered as a separate stream of work), the interrelation between testing and other verification activities must be understood.

Start "Testing" Early

One of the key problems associated with testing is that the testing activities do not start early enough in the project. Pressure of project timescales mean the testing is squeezed into too short a period, resulting in testing that is inappropriately justified, poorly specified, badly executed, and inadequately recorded.

One of the major problems associated with the implementation of computer systems projects is that the go-ahead (budgetary approval) is often given later than expected, while the end date of the project seldom moves. This puts time pressure on a project from day one, and the natural reaction is to "get started."

This temptation leads to a host of problems from a validation perspective, but focus is usually applied to building the system, and properly specifying the system if the project team is lucky. In such circumstances, when everyone is keen to show progress, and the project may not be fully staffed, it is difficult to plan ahead for the testing.

However, thinking about testing from day one can save a great deal of pain in the long term, and a good project manager should always be thinking at least a couple of steps ahead.

Specifications and Requirements

The GAMP Guide [3] provides guidance on writing documents for the specification of computer based systems. At various levels of design deconstruction these document what the system should do, how the system will implement such functionality, and the detailed design of the software and hardware.

There are various questions to be answered when reviewing requirements given in such specification documents, but one of the basic questions is often overlooked: "How can I test this requirement?"

All requirements should be testable, or if not testable, compliance with the requirement should be verifiable by other means (such as visual inspection, comparing performance reports with specifications, confirming the availability of support from a help desk during specified hours and so on).

While some requirements can only be verified by other means, for most of the functional and detailed design requirements, testing is the preferred method of verifying that the requirement has been met, and that the system is fit for its intended use.

However, some requirements are so poorly defined or written that the effective and objective testing of the requirement is rendered virtually impossible.

This may be for several reasons.

- The basic requirement is poorly defined, either by users who do not really understand what they want the system to be able to do, or by developers who fail to correctly interpret the users requirements when preparing functional or detail design specifications.
- Although understood, the use of poor grammar renders the requirement vague and ambiguous. Unless clearly stated, a requirement can not be adequately tested in objective terms.
- Requirements are jumbled, one with another, making it difficult to understand where an absolute requirement ends and a "nice-to-have" starts. When multiple needs are stated in a single "requirement," this makes testing difficult in terms of understanding the objective of a test, and interpreting whether a test has "passed" or "failed" with respect to meeting the test objective.

For these and other reasons, requirements should be unambiguous, widely understood, traceable, and singly stated. One of the most useful questions to ask when reviewing a requirement at any level is "How can I test this requirement?"

On most projects, the majority of people included in a specification review will have insufficient experience to be able to answer this question in detail. Many will have no practical experience of testing computer systems or software, and even developers may have little real experience of developing and executing tests.

It is always useful to have at least one experienced tester review such requirements as part of the verification of the specification document. This will help:

- Identify poorly written requirements at an early stage, thereby minimizing the cost and inconvenience of rewriting at a later stage of the project.
- The test team to understand at an early stage what it is that will need to be tested.

While specifications are written and reviewed, the test strategy and plan can be prepared.

TEST STRATEGY

As with many validation activities, testing can best be planned by asking the six questions that journalists often use to get to the heart of an issue: Who? What? Where? When? Why? How?

By asking and answering these questions, a comprehensive and appropriate test program can be developed, executed, and reported. While many of the contents of a test strategy are included in the FDA definition of a test plan [1], the FDA definition does not list a rationale within the scope of a test plan.

Given the importance of this rationale in supporting the validation of the system or software, a separate test strategy highlights this rationale and helps answer the key question of "what testing was done, and why."

This may of course be included in a test plan document (or even within the validation plan, for smaller, simpler projects).

The Test Strategy

The test strategy answers some of the most critical of these questions, certainly from the perspective of supporting the system validation. When considering the appropriateness of any test program the key questions to answer are: what testing was done, and why?

At a time when life science organizations are looking to reduce the cost of validation it is tempting to reduce the scope of testing. This can be achieved but it should only be done where there is a sensible rationale for so doing.

By considering what testing needs to be done, the underlying rationale, and documenting this in the test strategy, the user should be able to focus testing activities where required, and "relax" testing in other areas. If questions arise at a later date ("Why did you not test this? Why did you focus on testing this area of the system?") they can be answered by referencing a documented, logical and consistent rationale.

Testing and Risk Assessment

There is a commonly held belief that the use of risk assessment during the validation process will help reduce the scope and complexity of testing, and that this will help to deliver cost savings.

While this is true at the simplest level, a more detailed examination of risk assessment during the validation process reveals that what is actually accomplished is that risks are identified at an earlier stage, and mitigated by less expensive verification activities.

In a typical project that does not use risk assessment, risks are often highlighted for the first time when a test fails due to some "unexpected" test error. This may be due to a poorly understood or documented requirement, poor detailed design, badly developed software, and so on. In many instances, the reason for the failure is quickly understood, resolved, and the test re-executed.

However, this is a relatively expensive way to go about uncovering risks and the fact that the risks are quickly understood highlights the fact that a formally documented risk assessment should have uncovered them.

The GAMP Guide [3] describes a risk assessment process that can be used throughout the implementation and validation process. This has the advantage of using a relatively simple risk assessment model, but although it highlights the need for risk assessment throughout the life of the system, it does not provide detailed insight into the use of how risk is mitigated by different verification activities throughout the validation life cycle.

A better description of this process is perhaps given by the FDA in its guidance on the use of off-the-shelf software for use in medical devices. [4] This describes a process where risks ("hazards" in medical device terminology) are mitigated by a number of different activities. While these may not be specifically applicable to a pharmaceutical organization developing a new computer-based system, it should be recognized that risks can be mitigated by a number of activities, including:

- Changes in requirements to avoid risk.
- Design or redesign to reduce the risk probability, or increase the likelihood of detecting the problem.
- Providing users with appropriate warnings and appropriate training.
- Additional measures, external to the system.

As can be seen from this list, testing does not figure in the list of activities designed to reduce risk. Testing alone can not reduce risk probability or improve the likelihood of detection, but can be used to provide assurance that identified risks have been mitigated, or to attempt to identify risks that have not been identified to date.

Simply testing a system, no matter how comprehensively, cannot address all of the risks associated with a computer system or piece of software. Using a risk assessment process can help to effectively address risk by a combination of verification activities and identify an appropriate test strategy.

By using residual risks (those risks remaining following mitigation by earlier

Table 9.1 Example of test types, descriptions, and purpose

Test Type Name	Description	Purpose
User acceptance testing	Functional testing of the main system requirements. Does not include any challenge testing.	Designed to demonstrate that the user requirements have been met. When all user acceptance testing successfully passes, the system is deemed fit for purposes (assuming full test coverage of user requirements).
Software module testing	Detailed testing of the lowest software component in the system. May include challenge tests.	Designed to demonstrate that the "as-built" software module correctly executes, as defined in the appropriate software module design specification.
Challenge tests	Tests designed to challenge the component or function under test. A general term used to describe boundary testing, performance testing, invalid case testing, and so on.	To demonstrate that the component or function under test is repeatable, reliable, and robust under both normal and abnormal operating conditions.
Performance tests	Tests designed to show that a component or function under test meets to specified performance criteria (e.g., number of users, bandwidth, speed of response).	Tests designed to show that the component or function under test meets the specified performance criteria, or to establish upper limits at which performance starts to degrade.

verification activities) to guide the nature and scope of testing we can focus testing on areas of greatest risk and optimize the cost and benefit of testing activities.

The Nature and Scope of Testing

In order to be able to answer the "what" and "why" of testing it is necessary to define and document both the nature and scope of the testing to be performed, and to provide a supporting rationale.

The nature of the testing defines what types of test we intend to execute, and why. The scope defines how much of the system or software we intend to test, to what extent we intend to test it, and what type of tests we intend to conduct.

The Nature of Testing

Before considering how much testing to conduct, we must consider what types of testing we may wish to conduct, and why.

The GAMP Guide [3] defines different types of test, and maps each of these against an appropriate type of specification (acceptance tests against user requirements specifications, software module tests against software module design specifications and so on). The GAMP Guide [3] also references various types of test such as white box testing, black box testing, etc.

Whatever terminology is agreed for an organization or project, the most important thing to consider is what types of test will need to be conducted, and why. Tests may be conducted for a variety of reasons and it is important that each of these test types is defined, and a rationale given for conducting each type of test. This can be documented in a simple table (Table 9.1).

For a fuller list of test types and their description refer to the FDA glossary [1]. Which of these are applicable to any specific computer system or piece of software will, of course, depend on the nature of the software.

Clearly documenting the different types of test, and providing a description and purpose for conducting the different types of test, will help project team members to determine the appropriate level of testing for each function or component within test scope.

Testing Scope

The testing scope can be considered as having two dimensions, for which we will use the terms testing breadth and testing depth.

The breadth of the testing determines how much of the system (or software) we intend to test. Most systems are composed of a number of different types of software, and different functionality.

Table 9.2 Example of rationale for testing breadth

Software Function	GAMP Software Category	Within Testing Scope?	Rationale (Y/N)	Alternative Verification Activity
UNIX operating system	1	N	Tested by developer and in widespread industry use. Fitness for purpose to be demonstrated as part of general test activities.	Record version and manage under change control and configuration management.
Oracle 9i database	3	N	Tested by developer and in industry use. Fitness for purpose to be demonstrated as part of general test activities.	Record version and manage under change control and configuration management.
Purchasing functions	4	N	Tested as part of Phase 1. No interaction with Phase 2 functionality.	To be included as part of Phase 2 user acceptance test.
Training records	4 and 5	Y	Implemented for the first time in Phase 2.	
Quality management	4 and 5	Y	Tested as part of Phase 1, but has interaction with training records.	

The type of software can be categorized using the existing five software categories from the GAMP Guide [3].

Other factors to consider may include the extent of testing previously performed, either on previous projects or by the supplier. While some would like to rationalize away the need to test all software functions (or "routes through the software"), the fact is that all software functions that are GxP critical (or may interact with GxP critical functions) need to be tested.

However, where software has been adequately tested before, and where traceability can be shown to this testing (by adequate change control of version numbers, reference to adequate test records, and so on), there is no need to repeat this detailed testing as part of a new project (although acceptance testing will still be required).

Users should therefore request suppliers (software developers) to make available details of all standard testing performed on a product, and this should specifically be requested during the audit of a potential supplier. Where possible, suppliers should ensure that all test documentation is appropriately managed and should offer to share the details of testing (under suitable nondisclosure agreements) with their clients.

Based upon all of the above, a decision can then be made as to which software components will be tested by the user, and why. This can be documented in the form of a simple table (Table 9.2).

Even in the largest and most complex of systems, it is possible to test every software function and route through the software — all that is needed is a virtually infinite level of resources and period of time.

In the real world, decisions need to be made as to what level of detail testing is appropriate for each of the areas of a system under test. Once the breadth of testing has been determined, the depth can be determined for each of the functional areas or software components.

Based upon the outcome of a documented risk assessment (assuming risk mitigation has been included in previous verification activities), each function or software component will have a documented risk priority. While testing will not change the risk priority, rigorous testing will help to provide assurance that:

- Previous risk mitigation activities such as redesign have been successful.
- The software is reliable, robust and repeatable, and is fit for purpose with respect to the risk priority.

When determining how much testing is "appropriate" it is important to remember that some software functions or components have more residual risk associated with them than others. It is therefore sensible to focus testing activities on those functions and components that represent the highest risk and for which reliability, robustness, and repeatability is most critical.

Based upon the documented risk assessment, various risk scenarios will have been identified for each software component or function. Having also described the

Table 9.3 Example table documenting testing depth

Testing Scope	GxP Risk Priority			Business Risk Priority		
	High	Medium	Low	High	Medium	Low
Unit Testing (GAMP software category 5 only)						
Unit challenge testing	Yes	Yes	Yes	Yes	No	No
Unit acceptance testing	Yes	Yes	Yes	Yes	Yes	No
Software Module Testing (GAMP software category 4 only — configured as standard)						
Software module challenge testing	Yes	No	No	No	No	No
Software module acceptance testing	Yes	Yes	No	Yes	No	No
Software Module Testing (GAMP software category 4 only — reconfigured)						
Software module challenge testing	Yes	Yes	No	Yes	No	No
Software module acceptance testing	Yes	Yes	Yes	Yes	Yes	No
Software Integration Testing						
Software integration challenge testing	No	No	No	No	No	No
Software integration acceptance testing	Yes	No	No	No	No	No
System Acceptance Testing	Yes	Yes	Yes	Yes	Yes	Yes

purpose of each type of test (including boundary value testing, branch testing, compatibility testing, structural testing, functional testing, invalid case testing, interface testing, and so on) appropriate types of test can then be determined for each software component or function, based upon the risk priority and the identified risk scenarios.

These can then be documented in the test strategy.

A table such as Table 9.3 can be used to document the basic principles to be applied when determining the nature and depth of testing to be conducted on various software functions and components.

However, these principles will need to be reviewed for each function or component, based upon the documented risk scenarios. For some functions or components the nature of the risk scenario may require exceptions to the general principles documented in the test strategy, and these should be highlighted in the test plan.

How Much Testing Is Enough?

Ask most software developers how much testing they perform and the usual answer is "enough." Most are hard pressed to give an answer when asked: "How much is enough?", but this is a crucial question to answer with large and complex computer-based systems.

One of the best answers (in principle) to the "How much is enough?" question was "Enough to prove that the function under test works, and that we didn't break anything else at the same time."

Given the complexity and size of many modern systems, and the interrelated functioning between various components and functions, even the software developers (suppliers) are hard-pressed to justify the necessary scope of regression testing when a new software version or "bug-fix" is released.

The answer to this will obviously vary depending upon the scale of the new release or the nature of the bug fix. But when answering the question "How much testing is enough?" the following points should be borne in mind.

- What other functions or components are this function or component designed to interact with?
- What functions or components share common database tables, utilities, files, or tools with the this function or component?
- What unexpected interactions between functions or components have been reported (during testing, by users, and so on)?

Answering these questions (supported by the use of comprehensive configuration management records identifying such inter-relationships), combined with the use of documented risk scenarios and test types will help to answer the question, "How much testing is enough?"

Where available, test metrics and other statistics from previous projects can be used to support the test rationale. Techniques such as six-sigma can be used to capture statistics regarding the number of "errors" uncovered at each stage in the validation of the system. For example, how many errors were detected by various verification activities such as:

- Review of user requirements.
- Review of functional requirements.
- Review of detailed design requirements.
- Source code review.
- Testing.
- Incident reporting during the operational phase of the system.

Collection of such statistics removes the sole emphasis of "bug finding and fixing" away from testing. Moreover, where risk assessment and testing is being used appropriately it should be possible to prove that:

- Most errors are detected and corrected prior to testing.
- Testing is appropriate, because very few critical errors are detected in the operational phase of the system.
- A trend of continuous improvement in both respects.

While this may still require comprehensive regression testing to be performed for new software releases, bug fixes or planned change control, documenting all of the above will at least provide a rationale for not conducting any additional tests, thus justifying a move away from the trend to "test everything again, just in case."

THE TEST PLAN

The test plan is defined by the FDA [1] as a document including the "scope, approach, resources, and schedule of intended testing activities," and that it should identify "test items, the features to be tested, the testing tasks, responsibilities, required resources, and any risks requiring contingency planning."

As suggested above, the scope and approach could be included in a separate test strategy document, clearly highlighting the "what and why" in terms of an overall rationale.

This leaves the test plan to focus on the more pragmatic aspects of testing such as:

- The grouping and ordering of the tests (there may be prerequisites which determine the order of certain tests).
- The expected duration of the testing activities.
- The resources required.

- Roles and responsibilities.
- Risks associated with test execution.

These items are adequately covered in existing reference material, and are well understood by professional or experienced testers, and will not be discussed in detail here.

The test plan may also build on the rationale developed in the test strategy, to provide specific rationale for conducting individual tests, and by linking these to risk scenarios.

This can again be done in the form of a table focusing on documenting the rationale for conducting individual test cases (Table 9.4). Guided by the general rationale included in the test strategy this can be used to identify which tests will be conducted for each software function or component, and which of the residual risks each test is intended to address.

In a normal test plan these will be supported by additional tables or documents describing roles and responsibilities for executing individual tests, target dates, and so on. The test plan therefore addresses the important practical questions of "who, where, and when" of testing.

Test Objectives

One of the areas where many test case authors struggle is with defining the test objective. This is usually because the "what and why" have not been adequately described in a test strategy and test plan.

In the rush to proceed with most projects, test case authors very often attempt to develop test cases against early drafts of the appropriate specifications, without really thinking about the purpose of the testing. The end result is often a set of test cases that do little more that "walk through" the standard functionality, and do not adequately address the risks associated with the system or software

Once the "what and why" have been properly thought through and documented, the objective of individual tests becomes much clearer. Examination of the entries in the "test type" and "test case description" columns in Table 9.4 shows that the test objective can be derived with relative ease once the reason for conducting the test is understood.

While this may appear to be "late in the day" with respect the development of test cases, there is no reason why drafts of the test strategy, test plan, and test cases cannot be prepared against draft specifications, as long as these also bear in mind the output from initial risk assessments.

Table 9.4 Examples of test plans showing test types and associated risk references

Test Set	Test Case ID	Software Function or Component	Test Type	Test Case Description	Risk Mitigation Reference
TS_001	TC_001_001	Batch end-point controller (BC_0013)	Software module test — functional test	Tests normal operation of software module.	None
	TC_001_02		Software module test — boundary value test	Tests operation of software module at boundary conditions, specifically focusing on low values of pH.	HA_02_013_02
	TC_001_03, TC_001_04, TC_001_05, TC_001_06, TC_001_07		Software module test — branch testing	Series of tests to check all branches of the software module used for error handling (alarms and logs).	HA_02_013_03
	TC_001_08		Software integration test	Tests integration of batch end point controller with associated software modules (batch mixing [MX_0032] and batch discharge [TX_0009]).	HA_02_013_04
or					
TS-A-003	TC-A-003-001	Maintain inspection catalog codes (QMMD03-01-01)	Detailed functional test	Tests basic ability to maintain inspection catalogue codes.	None
	TC-A-003-002		Abnormal input testing	Tests that the software rejects users entries in illegal formats.	RA-QM-22-01
	TC-A-003-003		Abnormal input testing	Tests that the software rejects a duplicate code.	RA-QM-22-02
	TC-A-003-004		User acceptance testing	Functional walkthrough by user to demonstrate fitness for use.	None

Test Coverage and Traceability

While it should be common practice and should not need emphasizing here, while the test plan is being developed the requirements traceability should be maintained in order to ensure that every requirement is tested (or otherwise verified).

Each requirement should be traceable to one or more test cases, to ensure that every requirement has been tested (or otherwise verified).

Where risk-based testing is used, the traceability can also be extended to cover risks (or at least the priority of risks that should be proactively mitigated — it is common not to mitigate low priority risks). By ensuring that all residual risks are traceable to test cases it can be demonstrated that the testing is appropriate to the risks associated with the system or software, and are not just a set of random tests thought up in isolation.

TEST PROCEDURES AND TRAINING

The test strategy and test plan have covered the what, why, who, where, and when. All that remains to answer is the how?

Many well-planned test programs are undermined by poor execution, largely because the "testers" were unfamiliar with testing in a regulated environment and made simple mistakes such as:

- Preparing poor quality test cases.
- Continuing with test that was fatally compromised and should have been aborted.
- Aborting a test that could have been continued once a test incident had been reported.
- Failing to capture sufficient test evidence.
- Recording results incorrectly.
- Improperly managing test documentation.
- Forgetting to sign and date test records.

In the worst cases, these minor errors can build to such a level as to call the quality of the whole test program in to doubt, and there have been examples of complete test programs having to be repeated, or projects cancelled because of the poor quality of testing.

Best practice for all of these issues are again covered in the referenced literature, but the point to make is that all of these mistakes can largely be avoided if test procedures are developed, and if project team members are trained in them.

These may be developed as organization, department or project and product specific procedures and should cover:

- How to prepare a test case, with annotated "best practice" examples covering issues such as writing clear test objectives, expected results, review, and approval.
- How to execute test cases, with annotated examples of a completed test case, including the recording of results and attaching test evidence.
- How to report test incidents, including how to suspend and subsequently continue with a test, or how to abort a test.
- How to review executed tests, including the link between the test objective, expected and recorded results and any attached evidence.
- How to manage all test documentation.
- How to manage test incidents, including the link to configuration management and change control.

Inexperienced members of the test team should be trained in these procedures, and should ideally be "walked through" their first few activities to ensure that they understand the principles and will not undermine the test program.

IN SUMMARY

To summarize, planning for a successful test program requires some relatively simple processes to be followed.

First, do you have a clear picture in your mind as to how testing fits into the overall validation process?

- Ensure that the requirements are testable.
- Identify test types appropriate to the category type of software under test and appropriate to the risks.
- Develop a test strategy appropriate to the type of software and nature of the risks (leveraging supplier testing and validation metrics where possible).
- Identify the specific residual risks remaining from earlier verification activities.
- Develop a test plan and test cases to address the residual risks.

Second, have you answered all of the basic questions in the relevant documents?

What? Why?	Test strategy (and details in the test plan).
Who? Where, When?	Test plan.
How?	Test procedures and training.

For those who prefer to think in terms of pictures see Figure 9.1.

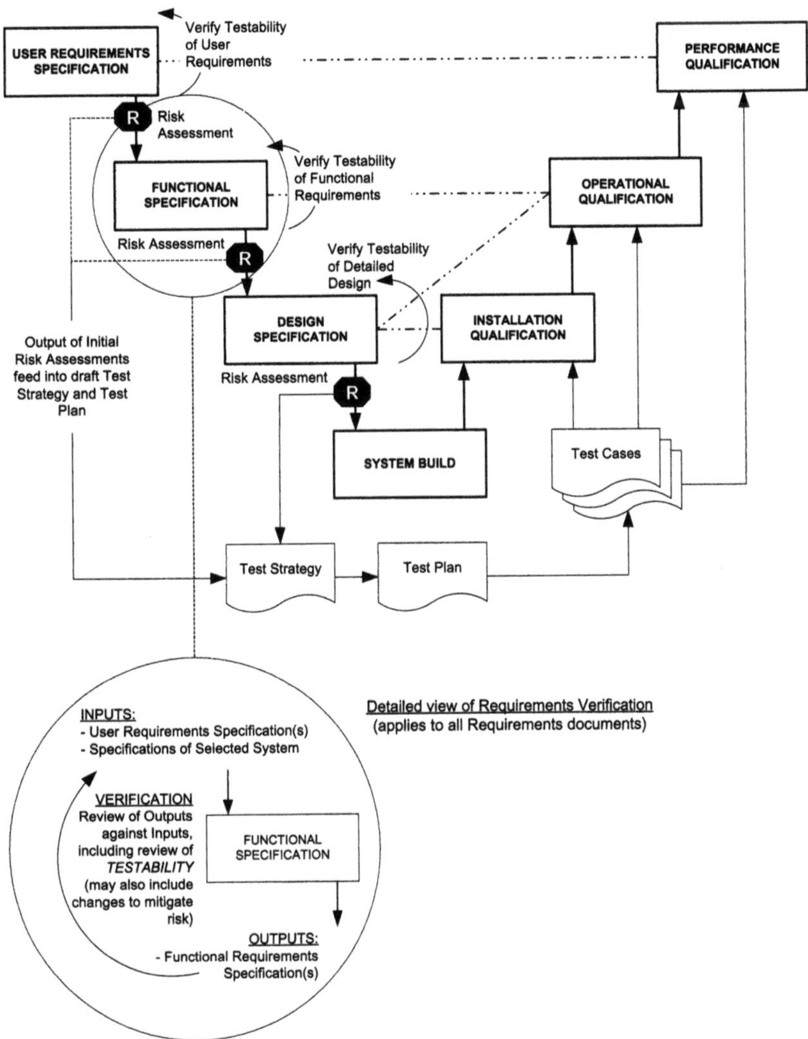

Figure 9.1 Overview of testing within the validation life cycle.

REFERENCES

1 FDA. *Glossary Of Computerized System and Software Development Terminology.*

2 FDA. "General Principles of Software Validation; Final Guidance for Industry and FDA Staff," page 6, January 11, 2002.
3 Good Automated Manufacturing Practice (GAMP) Guide, version 4. ISPE.
4 FDA, "Guidance for Industry, FDA Reviewers and Compliance on Off-The-Shelf Software Use in Medical Devices," September 9, 1999.

Chapter 10

Enterprise Resource Planning Systems — Aligning Business and Validation Requirements

A. Nobibux, Julien Peters, Steve Sharp, and James Stafford

CONTENTS

Implementing an enterprise resource planning (ERP) system is almost certainly going to be the largest and most expensive software project undertaken by a company in the medium to long term. Third party organizations are normally contracted to manage the implementation of such systems.

However, the practice of software implementers to market rapid or accelerated implementation methodologies in order to keep the projected costs and implementation timescales competitive in the marketplace may compromise an ERP implementation for regulated organizations. The implementation could be compromised if software partner organizations are unfamiliar with the additional project success criteria required by regulated organizations and associated semantics; namely, delivery of a validated or validatable system into production and the necessary documentary evidence to support the validity of the implemented system and operational usage.

In addition, a company's information systems group, familiar with managing the support of legacy business applications and systems, is unlikely to have the necessary infrastructure and skills to support a new ERP implementation and will be reliant upon the third party for project management skills and technology transfer.

Furthermore, the experience of a company's quality assurance group, though well versed in process validation, qualification of computer-based equipment and instrumentation and associated semantics, may be less versed in validation requirements of pure software systems.

Adopting a systematic, risk-based approach that follows a documented project methodology designed to satisfy these additional quality criteria will increase the likelihood of a successful outcome. The methodology must add value, should leverage available project management processes and not only include the adopted software development life cycle, but also supporting processes, e.g., quality assurance, configuration management, and change control. These processes must be carried over to support the system's operational use.

This chapter will seek to outline good working practices associated with deploying ERP systems assuming a combined approach to business, technical, and validation implementation considerations is adopted. The authors highlight variations from good working practice during the ERP deployment life cycle, which typically result from a disconnect between traditional technical implementation methodology and demands of the validation life cycle. The following sections discuss in more detail practical insights gained during successful implementations of ERP systems in a regulated environment. The discussion is structured according to a generic phased project approach as outlined here.

- Key differences in ERP system usage within regulated organizations.
- Optimizing the methodology.
- Initial engagement.
- Project initiation.
- Solution design.
- Solution build.
- Solution migration.
- Go live.
- Operational support.

KEY DIFFERENCES IN ERP SYSTEM USAGE WITHIN REGULATED ORGANIZATIONS

ERP business solutions are designed to manage and integrate the business processes of diverse organizations that create value for stakeholder communities, and are employed by the majority of large organizations to run their businesses. The manner in which ERP solutions are applied to meet each sector's requirements dictates flexibility in the way the solutions are developed by application vendors. The cost and time involved in implementing ERP business solutions varies between a few months to many years, and from tens of thousands to many millions of dollars or pounds.

Organizations implement ERP solutions for a variety of business reasons, which all seek to deliver business benefit. The potential coverage of an ERP system is summarized in Figure 10.1 which depicts a virtual model of a company identifying typical functional responsibilities. Physically these activities can be carried out at different sites.

An ERP system is simply a transactional engine that enables automation of data flow associated with execution of business processes. Initially, focus and business drivers were on improving flow of data associated with managing "make to order"

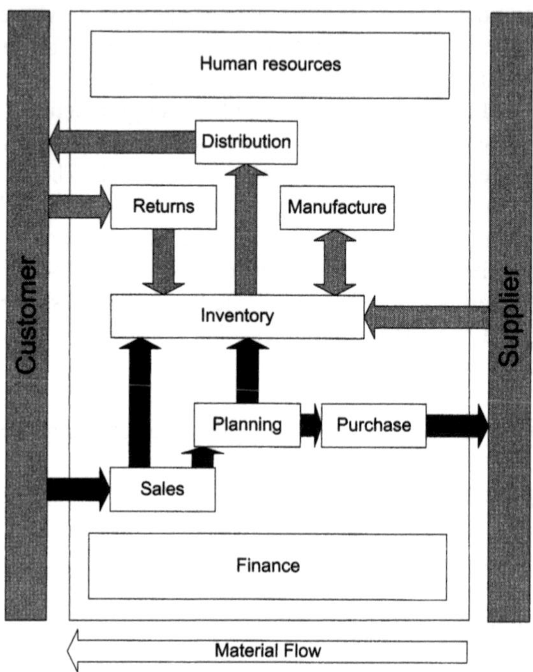

Figure 10.1 ERP scope.

processes and associated financial services (depicted as solid arrows in Figure 10.1). While it was quickly recognized that potential automation efficiencies could be extended to data flows associated with product material flows (depicted as dotted arrows in Figure 10.1) the regulatory implications were often not appreciated. The regulators not only required validation of computer systems used to support manufacture of regulated products in the life science sector, but also that they are maintained in a validated state. The underlying predicate rules supporting GMP processes and the evolving regulatory landscape, which includes compliance with financial regulations such as the Sarbanes-Oxley Act of 2002 [1] and IAS regulatory requirements [2], can increase the complexity associated with delivering *regulatory compliant business efficient* solutions.

Compliance with the regulations is enforced through inspections, which place great weight on the existence of documentation to demonstrate appropriate control of GMP processes. This requirement extends to the implementation of computer systems supporting GMP processes. Organizations should adopt a risk-based approach to determine how to approach the implementation, documentation, degree of testing, and associated traceability throughout the implementation life cycle. This approach should extend into the operational life cycle of the deployed business solution.

The adoption of a risk-based approach will enable organizations to demonstrate compliance with regulatory drivers, while ensuring mandated requirements are combined with those of the business community. This combined approach reduces the total cost of compliance while ensuring delivery of the desired business benefit associated with an ERP system.

OPTIMIZING THE METHODOLOGY

ERP implementations are normally carried out using the methodologies of the implementation partners, which are generally not tailored to the regulated life science sector. These methodologies are designed to drive and manage implementations using time and fiscal constraints, and do not take into consideration the key deliverable of regulatory compliant business efficient solutions. In order to increase the likelihood of a successful outcome, the applied project methodology must be designed or adapted in order to reduce the risk that additional validation goals required by regulated organizations will not be met. This is best achieved through development of additional quality procedures managed separately using a project quality plan. The additional procedures should focus on ensuring the documented quality of the project hardware, software and documentation *deliverables*.

Implementer's Methodology May Be Incomplete

An implementer's methodology may be incomplete for a number of reasons. Incomplete or undocumented procedures will result in lack of suitable evidence to support the controlled development and validated status of the implemented system.

Software Project Management Methodology Not Certified

Ideally, an implementer should have a documented quality management system (QMS) for implementing software systems certified by an independent third party. For example, a TickIT certified scheme implies the existence of and adherence to a documented QMS for software project management that meets ISO9001 requirements subject to ISO9000-3 [3]. The scope and suitability of the system for meeting the extra requirements of regulated organizations can be readily established by review and audit.

The QMS should cover all the requirements for meeting an implementation project's success criteria. The scheme's continuous improvement requirement should ensure that gaps in the processes are identified and resolved.

Methodology Has Undue Focus on Project Management or Not Fully Documented

Disastrous reports of runaway costs associated with implementation of ERP systems has forced implementers and customers alike to look very closely at managing project costs. Rapid or accelerated implementation approaches have been designed to reduce the risk of runaway costs, and appropriate project controls are documented and implemented in order to support phased approaches to software implementation. Typical phased approaches are summarized in Figure 10.2. Nevertheless, the implementation processes are often adaptations of the software manufacturer's methodology and may only be documented at high level in the form of a letter of intent, project management plan, roadmap, or project charter.

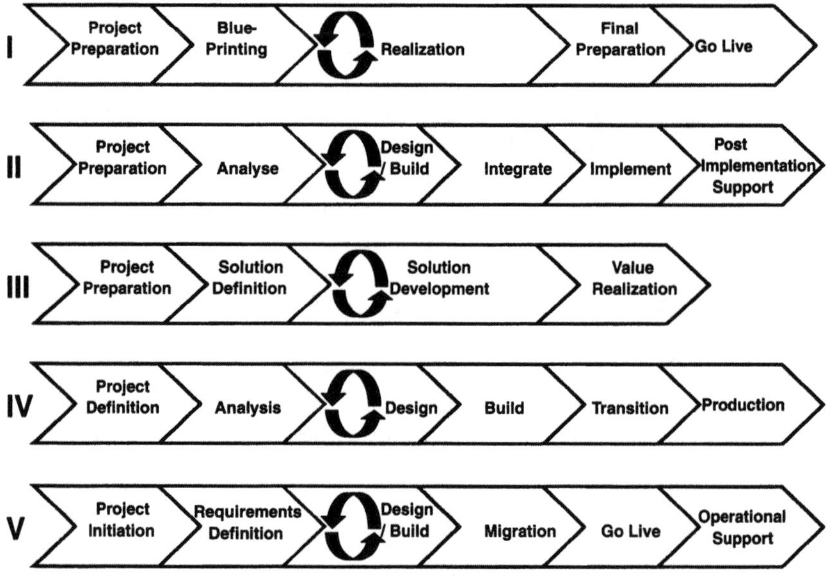

Figure 10.2 Examples of phased implementation approaches.

Much emphasis is placed on the existence of tools and templates to support deliverable development. However, the use of the tools and evaluation of the deliverable itself is less often documented.

Essential supporting processes such as document control, configuration management, and other quality assurance activities, e.g., review and audit may be executed on an informal basis, but the processes are not documented. Consequently, their execution and associated records are uneven.

Risk Management Processes Are Focused on In-Project Risks and Project Residual Risks Not Fully Identified for Mitigation

Risk management is a standard component of project methodology and the prime focus tends to be associated with mitigation of risks to project delivery on time and within budget. However, implementation projects in regulated environments have significant project residual risks associated with regulatory compliance. The risks must be identified at the initiation of the project for timely mitigation. Often risks are informally identified, but a standard approach will increase the probability of a successful outcome.

Disconnect between Technical and Validation Work Streams

The traditional focus of the partner has been on the technical and project management work streams, and the system sponsor organization on the validation work stream. This approach leads to a disconnect between these complementary work streams to the detriment of the project quality objectives.

Software Development Life Cycle Geared toward Prototyping Approach

The increased availability of configurable applications and the need to involve the user community more closely in defining and refining the system requirements has encouraged the use of prototyping, i.e., using conference room pilots (CRP) to validate the proposed or envisioned business solutions and identify gaps in requirements. Typically, the gathering of requirements for the initial set up and the first CRP sessions are highly interactive (signified by the arrows in Figure 10.2). As a result, processes and documentation tend to be poorly defined. User requirements are encompassed in the application's configuration and there may be no traceability to documented needs.

Organizations' Computer Validation Methodology Inappropriate

Organizations' computer validation semantics tend to reflect the waterfall model for a software development life cycle (SDLC) wherein custom-built software systems were specified to control or support manufacturing systems, e.g., GAMP 4. [4]

Concepts and Terminology Based on Process Validation

The predicated requirement for validating manufacturing processes and the increased use of computers to control manufacturing operations naturally led to the

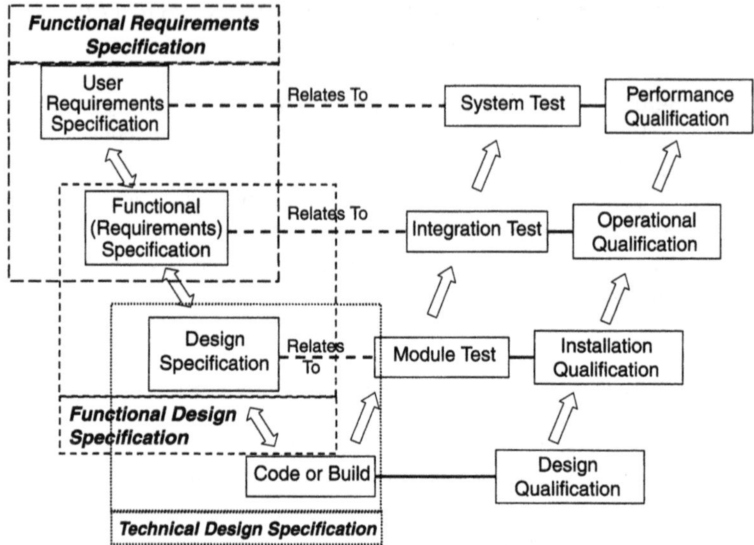

Figure 10.3 Waterfall SDLC and validation framework.

need to demonstrate that the computerized equipment itself was fit for purpose. A validation framework based on the waterfall SDLC model is used to facilitate communication between pharmaceutical manufacturing engineers and software manufacturers (e.g., GAMP 4). An adapted model is summarized in Figure 10.3 as the elements within solid-lined boxes.

However, the use of prototyping development techniques, configurable software applications and phased implementation models has led to the combination of sequential waterfall SDLC specification phases yielding collapsed models, e.g., functional design specifications and technical design specifications (identified within dashed-line boxes), all adding to the semantic confusion.

Procedures written to support the waterfall model may not have the flexibility to reflect the implementer's SDLC. Consequently, the implementer's SDLC and its relationship to the standard validation model must be explicitly described as part of the project methodology, supported by the appropriate documented procedures.

Validation Plans

Validation plans are the standard mechanism for internally defining and managing the tactical approach to validation of computer systems and are the responsibility of the sponsor organization. These plans will also define the required quality attributes for the validated system and its development and reference appropriate procedures. However, validation plans are insufficient for tactical planning at a project level when a third party manages the implementation. An additional level of quality planning is required, which both the third party and sponsor can agree to as part of the contract.

Company's IS Organization and Processes Inappropriate

Even if an organization's IS department undertakes "in house" custom software development it is unlikely to have the necessary experience to effectively manage and resource an ERP implementation. Their experience will primarily be in system maintenance and any management (quality) structures will reflect this. Apart from change control, the support processes may be poorly documented or fragmented. Processes put in place to maintain validated systems tend to be inappropriate for major system development projects.

Quality Planning Component of Project Methodology Required

A distinct project quality plan is required to identify implementer and organization procedures for use on the project. New project procedures should be created where current ones are inappropriate, poorly defined, or missing. In some instances there will be a quality planning section in the project management plan or equivalent. The scope and use of procedures and practices described at this level must be clearly defined. In most cases, there will be insufficient detail to ensure their effectiveness in managing the quality of project deliverables.

Quality Plan

The form and content of quality plans is highly variable, but for the purpose under discussion they should consolidate the project and development practices of the implementer, the validation processes required of the sponsor, and any additional procedures to ensure that the implemented system is validated and there is documented evidence to support this premise.

As a minimum, the plan should identify all the formal project deliverables, procedures, quality records, and the procedures necessary to ensure that the quality records are generated.

In some cases, it may be possible to incorporate procedures within the plan, but the document should not become unwieldy to use or maintain. New or adopted procedures must add value to the project's objectives.

The following support procedures apply across the project phases and typical deficiencies are summarized.

Change Control

Project level change control is often not designed to manage project deliverable maintenance. Consequently there is a high risk that changes to documentation are not appropriately documented and tracked.

Configuration Management

Configuration management is rarely documented as a discrete project process and will appear in various guises, e.g., under change control, document management, instance or project environment management. As a result, there is no consistency in definition, naming, and management of configuration items or baselines for verification and validation activities. Consequently, there is a high risk that there is no controlled documented definition of what was validated at go-live.

Document Management

Given the dynamics of phased implementation methodologies, the number of documents and versions involved and the size of the implementation teams, it is essential that the most current documents are worked on and that it is clear when and how the documents are to be placed under change control. Surprisingly, document management is often poorly defined within a project environment yet it is the foundation on which validation evidence is based.

Problem Management

Also described as issue or incident management this process is aimed at managing issues at the project management level. The process is often not designed to cope with incidents or issues that have yet to impact on timely project delivery, e.g., deliverable quality or completeness.

Verification and Validation Management

Verification and validation management describe activities that ensure deliverables from one phase are fit for their purpose as input into following phases, and that the software deliverable meets its intended purpose as defined by the user requirements. These are critical activities and often poorly defined. Consequently, any evidence to support the premise that documented specifications and software meet their intended purpose will either be inconsistent or missing. Typically, deliverables from user requirement definition, code reviews, functional testing, and data migration activities are inappropriate.

Quality Assurance

Often short-sightedly perceived as a non-value-added activity, quality assurance procedures such as project audits are frequently overlooked in the effort to keep the project on schedule. The tendency for different parts of a project to move out of phase, as resources are juggled to keep the project on track, means that use of audits to control phase completion and entry may not be ideal. However, quality audits are essential in ensuring that agreed project procedures are adhered to and that project deliverables are of suitable quality. The use and purpose of the audits should be driven by the need to add value. In this case, the value lies in ensuring that the appropriate deliverables and quality records are generated during execution of normal project activities, and not as a catch-up at the end or after go-live.

Risk Management

Risk assessment and management procedures are used to formally establish controls and practices in the manufacture of pharmaceuticals and medical devices. Risk-based approaches to software development are advocated (e.g., GAMP, CDRH, [5]) but have yet to be widely adopted in implementation methodologies. Where adopted, they are focused on in-project risks. Adoption of a risk-based approach that also addresses residual project risk will facilitate the identification of value-added activities that will increase the probability of regulatory compliance and successful project outcome.

INITIAL ENGAGEMENT

Implementation engagements frequently commence following the receipt of an ITT (invitation to tender) or RFP (request for a proposal) defining the implementation requirements, the business processes that should be covered, and other extended functionality of the ERP system. This is all wrapped up in a bundle of "GMP compliance" and "validated system" without too much detail on how this is to be carried out. The onus is placed on the bidders to provide a response that will be compliant and attractively priced.

Implementation partners with little or no experience of implementing large ERP systems in a regulated environment typically underestimate the importance and work involved. They often, incorrectly, assume that they will be able to learn a great deal about validating systems by working with the client teams during the implementation, and that they can pick it up as they go along. This is a dangerous and incorrect assumption. This leads to one of two types of tender response.

- Promising what cannot be delivered, and trying to deliver what is not understood as part of the project.
- Responding with a partner who will be responsible for the validation and compliance of the project, but who will not have financial control, leading to pressures later in the project to cut corners around the quality element of delivery.

Both these approaches carry high risks of project failure.

These risks are mitigated from the sponsor's perspective by recognizing the need to fully understand the implications of current regulations on their business supported by the proposed ERP system, and using this knowledge to carefully select appropriately incentivized implementation partners based on their ability to deliver, in a cost effective manner, compliant business solutions by integrating technical and validation work streams.

Understanding the Project Context

Many companies include the definition of relevant predicate rules and project governance as one of the deliverables of the project, and then select an implementation partner inexperienced in this process. If this is not part of the initial engagement, the selected party needs to address how this process will be achieved, preferably as a prerequisite to issuing the final contract. An initial focus on defining the predicate rules and governance, along with the project policies and procedures, mitigates many of the risks described above. However, time and money pressures often push this activity into the main implementation project and the outputs are included as part of the project deliverables, increasing the risk of lower quality and lack of validation and regulatory (GMP and financial regulatory) compliance.

Cost-Effective Delivery

The failure to understand the implications of implementing a validated and GMP-compliant system leads to inappropriate selection of implementation methodology and lack of validation activities, e.g., deficient project procedures and documentation standards during the early part of the project. This leads to rework and retrospective validation later, both of which are expensive and could potentially miss vital areas that require validation.

In order to reduce costs later in the project the quality, typically validation and GMP compliance, elements are not given due consideration. Either with an inexperienced partner they are ignored and quality reduced, or when a third party is introduced, pressure is brought to reduce the implementation cost by reducing the level of validation, or carrying out validation at a later date and removing it from the scope of the project. Obviously a short-term financial gain, but in the long term much less cost-effective and unacceptable from a regulatory perspective.

Appropriately Incentivized Implementers

Few supplier selection or final negotiation processes end with the implementer targeted or incentivized by anything other than financial or time drivers. The quality of the delivery, or compliance of the system is often overlooked as a key implementation deliverable that will be measured and rewarded.

Vendor and Implementer Selection

The level of computer system, validation knowledge within life science organizations is variable and a successful ERP implementation typically requires a partner able to provide expert advice on integrating the validation requirements within the technical and business related activities. The choice of partner is greatly facilitated when activities are conducted within a "quality assurance" framework. The assessment of an implementer's capability is assessed through auditing their work practices. Ideally, the audit should be carried out prior to contract signing in order to agree on how any remedial actions will be effected and embodied in the project management and quality plan for control. Often, vendor audits are carried out retrospectively. Any ability for remediation of observations at this time is severely restricted and corrective actions expensive to execute.

PROJECT INITIATION

Several case studies of implementing mission critical systems such as ERP systems have shown that project initiation is a key activity in the project life cycle and is pivotal to the success of the implementation of a system. Planning resources, forming project teams with the right set of competencies and skills, defining an effective and efficient reporting structure and the definition of standards, controls and policies, are some of the issues that may bring challenges and, therefore, need adequate attention.

Considering that implementation of ERP systems in itself is a big challenge, the complexity of project activities will increase when the system is validated. This increase in complexity will be reflected in the planning of project initiation activities. Successful projects integrate the technical and validation work streams and ensure that team members are suitably trained and have ownership of the validation responsibilities.

Integration of Implementation and Validation Work Streams

Experience shows that when implementation and validation activities are performed without a formalized and well-defined plan describing *integration* of these activities, the probability of success reduces rapidly. Often the responsibilities for validation and implementation are divided between two work streams: one team responsible for validation and the other for implementation. Typically the disconnect between the two work streams highlights a couple of significant organizational issues.

- The validation work stream is often perceived as a bureaucratic regime that impedes system implementations, rather than adding value to the system implementation life cycle. The result is higher cost of compliance, duplication and in the worst case, reworking of deliverables due to misalignment of work stream activities.
- Implementation and validation efforts are not performed in a synchronized manner and incurred project risks difficult to mitigate. In many cases, validation activities fall behind schedule and sometimes are even carried out retrospectively. As a result, information needed to support critical decisions, e.g., project milestones or deviations, is unavailable or incomplete. Consequently, unnecessary project risks due to poor synchronization and compliance risks due to noncompliance with regulations or not conducting an activity are incurred. At this stage, the concept of "building quality into the system" is no longer applicable.

These situations can be prevented from happening by creating the required awareness in the earliest stages of the project. During project initiation, validation and implementation should be defined as *an integrated set of activities*. A common basis for interaction and communication throughout the project team is essential for success. By adopting this approach an open environment is created facilitating management of both validation as well as implementation.

This concept is summarized in Figure 10.4.

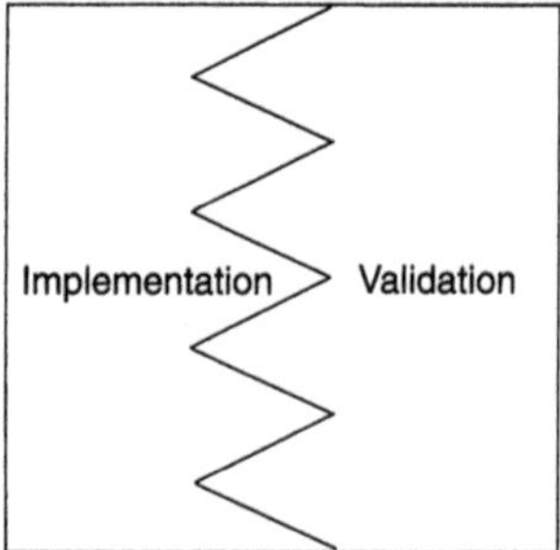

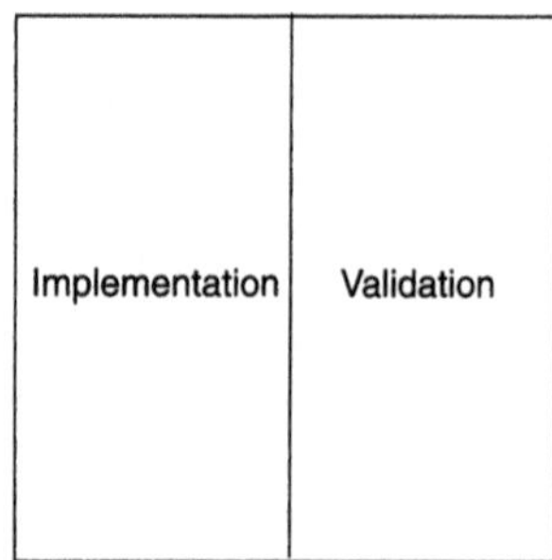

Figure 10.4 Integration of validation and implementation activities.

Aligning validation milestones with technical ones will ensure that validation requirements are designed into the program prior to commencing the project, thereby eliminating the need to retrofit standards, approaches, and validation prerequisites. Analyzing and addressing noncompliances as well as business issues from both the validation and the implementation perspective at the same time during the project life cycle will increase business efficiency and regulatory compliance. The ability of project management to base decisions on a complete and integrated set of information is thus more efficient.

Validation Awareness

One of the first requirements for a validated ERP implementation is often to carry out training for the whole project team, detailing the validation and GMP compliance requirements for IT system implementations together with the procedures that need to be followed to meet them. This training should extend to the sponsor's team members to ensure understanding of the implementer's methodology. The awareness resulting from training should reinforce the concept that the whole team has a role to play in delivering a compliant business solution.

Formalize Validation Ownership

In order to ensure that validation gets the required attention and emphasis, it is recommended that the committee with overall responsibility for the project appoint a member who will be responsible for monitoring validation activities.

Validation and implementation should also be integrated into the project team management function. Ideally this means that the project manager should be responsible for both validation and implementation activities. Since the implementing party generally appoints project managers, they may not have the knowledge or experience that is needed to manage validation activities. In order to solve this problem, the sponsor company should appoint a person to the team with enough validation experience to help the project manager identify and manage the validation activities. This person's role should not be equated with that of a second project manager. To do so would only have a negative effect on the team's cohesion.

SOLUTION DESIGN

Hindsight is a beautiful thing. It enables us to highlight the deficiencies and lack of detailed focus that often characterize the early stages of an ERP implementation with respect to solution design, policy and procedure definition, business interviews, and documentation of functional solutions.

User requirements specification (URS) and solution design are typically considered mutually exclusive, but interrelated activities. However, user communities have difficulty in articulating their business needs in a manner that is unequivocal and readily understood by the implementer or third party. Poorly described user requirements are often the root cause of improper validation of many systems. There have been examples where regulatory agencies have defined systems as noncompliant, based solely upon the scope, content, and quality of the URS. Opportunities afforded by the design of ERP systems for prototyping by configuration can be used to capture business processes and verify user requirements. This approach captures both business and regulatory requirements within the delivered design concept — designing compliance into the solution, rather than retrospectively linking URS and solution documents.

User Requirements Specification

Construction of the URS for an ERP implementation is arguably the most critical aspect of implementing a validated business solution that is both regulatory compliant and business efficient. During the 1980s and 1990s many implementations focused on technology delivery, force fitting business processes to the selected ERP application, with regulatory compliance considered as an afterthought. The net result of this approach characterized ERP projects as ineffective and high-cost ventures to ensure a validated system was eventually delivered.

Typically user requirements documents are generated by the business community in the format of a monologue, stating process or functional requirements that have been derived by review of "as is" processes supported by legacy applications, that may have varying degrees of regulatory compliance.

Common issues associated with users requirements are:

- Lack of clarity between the regulatory (validation) purpose and contractual focus of documents.
- Failure to consider predicate rule requirements.
- Failure to consider the impact of electronic records and electronic signatures (ERES) requirements in sufficient detail.
- Placing contracts prior to conducting a supplier assessment or audit.
- Failure to fully assess a package or solution against a clear URS.
- Failure to define requirements that are traceable through to solution design, mapped to applicable supporting technology.
- Failure to produce requirements specifications that are testable, singly stated and unambiguous.

Although the business community must drive user requirements articulation, consideration must be given to each of the following five dimensions: Organization, process, information, technology, and regulation. Taking a "to be" approach to requirements definition activities will enable organizations to deliver a solution that does not impede business efficiency, while satisfying the evolving business and regulatory landscape. User requirements need to be defined in a manner to reflect the latter five dimensions and must:

- Provide a clear overview of the system or process, that can clearly be understood by suppliers, and can also be used as a formal "system description" (required to be maintained as a "live" document by various regulatory agencies).
- Define specific user requirements that are clear and unambiguous.
- State user requirements that are "singly stated" (ensuring that multiple requirements are not combined in a single statement, thereby facilitating requirements traceability).
- State user requirements that are testable (in order to clearly demonstrate that the system fulfills the user requirements, an important regulatory and contractual obligation).

The Five Dimensions

The five-dimension solution model is summarized in Figure 10.5 and detailed below in the form of a series of questions.

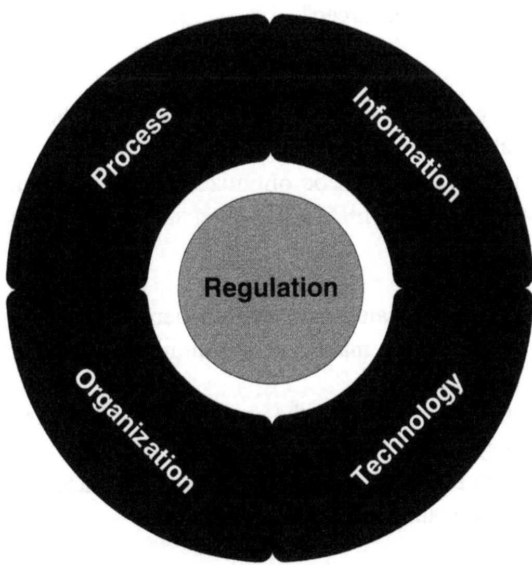

Figure 10.5 Solution dimensions.

Information:

- What records, audit trails, and signatures are required for compliance with applicable regulations, and what records are required in order for the business to function?
- In what format should information be available to enable financial results reporting to satisfy the U.S. Sarbanes-Oxley Act, international accounting standards (IAS), and other local country regulatory requirements?

Technology:

- What is the impact associated with using the ERP application in combination with e-mail, paper documents, computer notepad, and PDAs for example?
- How can technology be used to ensure that organizational performance is consolidated on a real time basis, rather than quarterly (hence minimizing risk and maximizing opportunities to enhance shareholder value)?

Organization:

- What rules and regulations must each site or department in an organization comply with?
- What financial controls, policies, and procedures apply at department, site, business unit, or corporate level, and to specific job profiles or even individuals?
- Who is performing the different roles within the organization? Have employees been trained? Should employees use different policies and procedures to satisfy the different regulatory demands in different countries?
- How do such controls apply to subcontracted organizations or individuals, and how are such controls enforced?

Process:

- What business processes are conducted and which of these fall within the scope of which regulatory requirements?
- How can business processes be optimized to satisfy regulatory demands and minimize business risk, while maximizing stakeholder value?

Regulations:

- Which regulations must an organization adhere to and how should variations in regulatory demands be managed to minimize the impact on operational efficiency?
- How are regulations created for the paper world to be interpreted and applied to computerized systems?
- Are all the paper records generated to support regulated processes still required once the process is automated?

Verification of User Functional Requirements

The initial draft of user requirements will be used to configure the business solution using standard ERP components. This initial configuration is evaluated and refined using business scenarios developed by the sponsor organization during what is called a conference room pilot (CRP). The CRP will also identify areas where there is a functional or reporting gap in a standard system.

Evolution of Solution Design

Depending upon the solution design strategy there may be several CRP iterations at this point, in order to evaluate alternate solutions. It is important to recognize that although the expression of the users' requirements is captured in the prototype configuration, this is not a substitute for a user requirements specification document. Full traceability between user requirement and associated system configuration setting must be maintained. This implies that CRP activities must be formalized and have identifiable goals.

Functional Requirements Specification

Functional and reporting gaps identified during CRP are evaluated and the necessary functional specifications developed. Traceability between user and technical requirements must be maintained.

Technical Requirements

Although the focus of the technical requirements is on the production system, a separate set of requirements should be developed for the project environment. This is necessary to ensure that there is appropriate support for the development and controlled test environments.

SOLUTION BUILD

Solution build is the phase wherein the hardware infrastructure and nonstandard software elements are designed, built, and integrated with the configured standard software, static and dynamic data to form the complete solution. Often overlooked is the need to include development of user operating procedures and test scripts. However, since these activities do not progress at the same rate, development and verification activities overlap and there is a high risk of unecessary task repetition due to poorly controlled development and test environments. Successful implementations ensure that the project environment can always be recovered to a known state, that software installation and data migration procedures and custom code are verified and that test scripts and user procedures are drafted and consistent with the solution design.

Design Qualification

Design qualification is the first qualification activity in a formal validation life cycle. However, given the dynamic nature of ERP implementations it is essential that this activity is managed to add value to the project. The qualification activity must reflect the dynamics between evolution of the solution design and build while ensuring that the necessary quality attributes have been considered.

Test Scripting and User Operating Procedures

Test script creation and user procedure writing is often left to the last minute: "We can't write the scripts if we don't know the solution," is typically quoted. Test scripts must be developed to verify the user requirements, and can therefore be derived directly from them, as they are not strictly dependant upon the technical solution. A risk-based testing strategy will determine whether more in depth testing is required at the technical level. Typically, higher risk is associated with custom functions and features.

Data Migration

All systems operate within the boundaries of data they are designed to manage and issues with static (master) and dynamic (transactional) data often arise following go live. Appropriate data cleansing, migration, and verification of the migration process and migrated data mitigate this risk. However, this activity is often subject to time and cost constraints. Failure to manage this activity effectively will have a major impact on the quality of the business solution delivered.

SOLUTION MIGRATION

Solution migration is the phase in which a documented and verified system configuration baseline is installed in a production-like controlled test environment for formal functional testing. The installed baseline configuration is verified by executing an installation qualification (IQ) and the configuration functionally verified by acceptance or operational qualification (OQ) testing. However, the solution should also be assessed for operational readiness, e.g., operation support procedures are in place and work and user procedures are available. This phase is often under severe time constraints resulting from late task completions earlier in the project and a seemingly immoveable go live date. The success and relevance of these qualification activities is entirely dependent upon the ability to infer functional equivalence in the production environment, based on a successful production IQ and having supporting documentary evidence of both IQ and functional testing activities. Consequently, the test environment should reflect the production environment as closely as possible in order to mitigate any risk associated with this inference, and testing should be formally documented and planned.

Test Planning and Execution

The planned execution of the test scripts should be carried out with enough time to ensure that all the user requirements have been met, and all the tests have been carried out to the satisfaction of the user community. Too often not enough time is allowed, or the project slips, and testing is curtailed to keep the project on track. Curtailing functional testing is not an option for regulated systems as much of the evidence required to support system validation is gathered at this point.

Test Procedure and Types

Testing must be conducted according to a defined procedure to ensure that there is consistency in the way testing is defined, executed, and recorded. Testing is discussed in more detail in another chapter in this book and only test types will be discussed further here.

Verification and Acceptance Testing

Verification tests are designed to demonstrate the correct operation of system functions, under normal (expected) operating conditions. The expected outcome of the test is usually the correct completion of that operation. In order to demonstrate correct operation a test may be applied against a single system function or multiple functions. Most system functions will be subject to verification tests at an appropriate level, although these may not be required for noncritical standard functions. This decision is based upon the outcome of the documented risk assessment and part of the testing strategy. Verification tests used to support acceptance of a system are often called acceptance tests.

Challenge Testing

Challenge tests are designed to specifically challenge operation of the system under abnormal (nonstandard), but definable, conditions. They are conducted to demonstrate that critical functions operate in a consistent, reliable, and predictable manner under abnormal conditions, and that unacceptable risks to product quality, patient safety, or data integrity are not caused by the system's response to abnormal conditions.

Stress Testing

Stress testing is meant to simulate the anticipated production environment and attempt to duplicate the types of demand which will be placed upon the system immediately after go live. This is performed in order to determine the limits at which system performance or data integrity is compromised, and set limits for subsequent performance monitoring in the operational phase of the system. Tests include having many users all accessing the system and data at the same time to assess system access, performance, and reliability.

Operational Readiness

Aside from verification activities that seek to provide documentary evidence that the designed business solution meets the user requirements, solution migration must also focus on supporting the business in its transitions between the legacy and new operating environment.

All too often, the transition phase is targeted towards delivering a technically efficient solution, rather than ensuring that each of the five dimensions within Figure 10.5 are balanced appropriately. The transition phase is an outcome of a process that commenced during the initial project engagement stages, and must be considered as a work stream in its own right, rather than simply educating the end users how to use and manage an ERP system.

Support Procedures

Appropriate project support procedures need to pass from the project life cycle to the operation life cycle, ensuring from day one in production that the system is supported in a controlled manner. Procedural controls must be established that relate to manual activities and application of the different technologies within the production environment, e.g., disaster recovery, backup, and restore. The point at which procedural verification is conducted will vary depending upon the velocity of a regulated organization. High velocity organizations that require product to be shipped immediately following go live should ensure that data, functional, and procedural verification is performed during the operational qualification stage of the project.

This approach will enable the user requirements, application, and applicable procedural controls to be verified as operationally acceptable and form the basis for qualified release of the business solution.

Qualification Reports

The results of each qualification activity are summarized and a consolidated report written. The consolidated report may act as an interim validation report summarizing the testing outcome from a regulatory perspective as defined in the validation plan. The decision to qualify the release of the system for production is based on this report.

GO LIVE

In order for an organization to move to the production environment, a go, no go decision is made. Traditional validation advocates often state that this decision or associated process is not required. If a robust validation life cycle is integrated into the technical implementation life cycle, release is based on an interim, validation summary report. However, a validated business solution may not be the only business requirement that needs to be met and a decision to go live will be based on due consideration of all business needs. Often regulated organizations will informally conduct a risk assessment to support the cut over to production. However, inadequate documentation, definition, and review of completed risk mitigation actions may result in regulatory bodies questioning the basis for decisions, such as the level of system acceptability prior to cut over to production. The go, no go decision should be considered as a documented risk assessment and mitigation activity that leads to a go live process that supports cut over to production. The vindication of the decision is established after conducting a system audit or review, also called the performance qualification.

Go Live Is a Process Not Solely a Decision

Once a decision to go live has been made, the business solution is installed in the production environment. This installation must be formally verified and include the balance of the static and dynamic data accrued after freezing the data load during the solution migration phase. Any residual risks associated with doubts concerning functional equivalence of test and production environments are mitigated by execution of additional functional tests.

It is important to be aware that the transition process from project to operational use continues after go live. Procedures and controls verified during solution migration must be handed over to the system owner. Typically, management of this transition state is very poor and can result in dips in performance, employee dissatisfaction, and high regulatory exposure due to short cuts taken to resolve system performance issues. Regulatory risks are mitigated through establishing robust operational procedures.

Vindication of Go-Live Decision

Vindication of the decision to move into production is formally established by conducting the final qualification activity whereby the operation of the business solution is assessed by carrying out a system-wide audit or review. The outcome of this audit should ensure closure of the validation plan and project activities by means of a final validation report to ensure a clean handover to operations. Typically, the performance qualification is executed some 2 to 3 months after the go live decision.

OPERATIONAL SUPPORT

Historically implementation methodologies place low emphasis on post go live support once the initial shakedown period is completed. Typically, issues arising during this period are managed on a "can do" basis, with an emphasis on keeping the system up and running. However, unless an appropriate support model is in place there is a high risk that changes are implemented in an uncontrolled manner. Life science sector companies must be able to demonstrate that the implemented ERP system continues to be maintained in a validated state and performs as specified. Uncontrolled changes jeopardize these requirements.

These risks are mitigated through establishment of a documented support model and quality assurance infrastructure that enforces a systematic approach to system and software maintenance, system and data security and performance monitoring with independent verification though audit.

Consolidation and Improvement

There is always a greater risk that something unexpectedly might happen immediately after go live rather than when the system has settled, e.g., system performance deteriorates, the system reports unexpected errors or users reporting incidents. Although users and application managers have had the necessary training, they will need time to get used to the system, and many unexpected errors or incidents may be user-induced. Other errors may be the consequence of undetected defects during earlier qualification testing or even incompletely defined requirements. During the shakedown period, the necessary controls and procedures must be able to distinguish, track, and manage these incidents and errors in order to keep the system at an acceptable operational and maintenance level.

At this stage, it is important to implement only those changes for which a workaround cannot be used. All changes implemented under emergency provisions of the change control procedure must be documented, and new or repaired functionality must be fully assessed for impact on the validated configuration. It is important to appreciate that an implemented system, though validated, is still subject to change, and measures must be in place to manage change.

Operations Governance

Many of the procedures used within the implementation project have their counterparts supporting the production system. However, they are not identical and a clear distinction must be made between support of the business solution in development and that in production. Often the project ethos spills over into maintaining the production system leading to confused reporting and decision structures and incomplete, inconsistent procedures.

Potential for inefficiencies are high in multinational companies where the business solution is deployed at several sites. Where IT or QA responsibilities are centralized and decisions concerning operational governance are communicated to local companies, we have observed that this process can be very slow and inefficient and in some cases can even lead to noncompliance. Companies should take a very pragmatic approach in order to speed up the process.

Additional procedures include a help desk that provides the user interface to the support model, system performance monitoring and periodic review.

Help Desk

The help desk is the point of contact for all users with system related issues and usually supports other business systems as well. It is the job of the help desk to deal efficiently with the issues to prevent them from becoming problems, by following a documented procedure. The sheer size of an ERP system and number of system users could swamp the help desk with ERP specific calls. Often companies will install a buffer between the help desk and the user in the form of a super user to filter calls. However, it is essential that the super user uses the same help desk process in order to capture appropriate call metrics. The use of a super user in this manner should be temporary. A continued need for this resource suggests an issue with training, either of the help desk or user community.

System Performance Monitoring

A system for monitoring system performance should be implemented at go live in order to collect information to support setting targets for production system responses. The frequency of performance monitoring should be relatively high during the shakedown period and immediately afterwards, in order to establish an accurate baseline for production system performance. During shakedown it is likely that the system performance will not meet expectations and implicitly indicates that there are problems. Performance issues are unlikely to be uncovered in preceding qualification phases unless severe and associated with system design issues. The probability of capturing performance issues will be higher during an intensified performance-monitoring program and corrective actions can be initiated in a more timely manner.

System Operation Monitoring

The operation of the system as a whole must be formally monitored and the records and outcome documented. This is achieved by periodic review whereby the operation of the system is audited. The purpose of the audit is to establish that the implemented system operates as specified, continues to do so, and that processes are under control. All quality records arising from system operation including support metrics are reviewed and compared against system specifications and current system configuration.

Typically, evidence generated during the first system audit or review will provide the basis for the final validation qualification activity.

Support Model

The development of a support model provides for a structured approach to identifying the service level agreements and support services that are required to support the production system and derive directly from nonfunctional user requirements. The support model will also include policies for system maintenance, e.g., database maintenance, backup and restore, data archiving and business continuity, and provide a framework for the associated work instructions or procedures.

The effectiveness of the support model may be ascertained by analysis of appropriate help desk performance metrics.

Quality Management

A formal quality management system comprising policies and procedures under which the ERP system is maintained provides a suitable framework for supporting audits and the evidence necessary to demonstrate that the system is under managed control. A loose collection of IT procedures and practices will not engender an environment for continual process improvement.

REFERENCES

1 Sarbanes-Oxley Act of 2002, U.S. GPO, January 2002.
2 IAS, International Accounting Standards.
3 ISO 9000-3:1997, Quality management and quality assurance standards — Part 3: Guidelines for the application of ISO 9001:1994 to the development, supply, installation and maintenance of computer software.
4 GAMP 4: GAMP Guide for Validation of Automated Systems, ISPE, December 2001.
5 General Principles of Software Validation: Final Guidance v2.0, CDRH/CBER FDA, 2002.

Chapter 11

Calibration in Practice

M.E. Foss

CONTENTS

INTRODUCTION

Calibration is a major part of validation in the healthcare manufacturing industries, pharmaceuticals in particular. It must be managed by those with good technical knowledge and a real understanding, as poor calibration practices can compromise product, plant, and economic success.

This chapter provides an experience-based overview of the practicalities of managing a calibration program, dealing with the definitions and fundamentals.

WHY CALIBRATION IS IMPORTANT TO VALIDATION

Over the years many organizations have pondered the question of quality assurance calibration, what, when, by who, and why? This chapter describes the principles and suggests a prioritized method for meeting the calibration need at the lowest cost.

The importance of control cannot be understated, after all, every day we make decisions based on information we have acquired. Whether we make the right decisions depends largely on whether the information we have acquired is correct. We often acquire information by way of measurement.

It is vitally important that any information provided is reliable and accurate. How would we feel if, when driving along a motorway at 70 mph, according to the speedometer, we are then pulled over by the police and informed that our speed was in fact 80 mph and then being receive a large fine and points on our license. We trust our speedometer because it comes with a high degree of assurance from the manufacturer, and the police apply an error factor usually about 10% worst case. We do not actually know the speedometer error but with a large band of certainty this is not necessary. However if this band of certainty was smaller we would probably be in receipt of a continuous supply of speeding tickets. Another factor for trust in this particular device is the simplicity of its design. Any drift in accuracy tends to be reduced to a minimum and therefore negates the need to recalibrate on a periodic basis thus allowing us to continue to motor on unhindered for years.

Process control instruments and devices are not completely stable after prolonged use and have a tendency to drift, also due to the complexity of their construction, and often the environmental conditions they may be operating under. This drift can be quite severe, over an unusually short period.

Generally the reaction regarding the periodic calibration of control devices or instruments is that it is seen, in most organizations, to be a costly and time-consuming activity to be avoided if at all possible.

What is needed is education in the importance of calibration and the need to prioritize. A complex statement for a complex subject but, does it have to be?

Put simply, if you do not measure it, you do not know if you are in control! The importance of the measurement error depends on what you are trying to measure. If you have a process that requires a temperature measurement to be taken at a critical step and the accuracy required is ±0.5°C, then the assurance of the accuracy of that measuring device is more important than someone measuring the temperature of an office when a ±3 degree error is common.

KEY REGULATORY REQUIREMENTS

The following statements are related to critical instruments. They outline the regulatory requirements that are key to a successfully managed instrument calibration program.

1. Each instrument should have a permanent master history record.
2. All instrumentation should be assigned a unique number and all product, process, and safety critical instruments physically tagged.
3. The calibration method should be defined by approved procedures.
4. Calibration frequency and process limits should be defined for each instrument.
5. There should be a means of readily determining the calibration status of each instrument.
6. Calibration records should be maintained.
7. All electronic systems used for calibration management for systems which affect products for supply to the U.S. must comply with the Food and Drug Administration's (FDA) regulation "21 CFR Part 11 — Electronic Records; Electronic Signatures."
8. Calibration measuring standards should be more accurate than the required accuracy of the equipment that is calibrated.
9. Each measuring standard should be traceable to a national or internationally recognized standard where one exists.
10. All instruments used should be fit for purpose.
11. There should be documented evidence of the training and competence of personnel involved in the calibration process.
12. A documented change management system should be in place.
13. These statements should be read in conjunction with the following documents:
    - 21 CFR Part 211 — "Current Good Manufacturing Practice for Finished Pharmaceuticals."

- 21 CFR Part 11 — "Electronic Records; Electronic Signatures."
- "Rules and Guidance for Pharmaceutical Manufacturers and Distributors 1997."

PRIORITIZATION

This therefore introduces the principle of assessment. Assessment of all your instrumentation into four main categories is the secret in keeping the costs of calibration to a minimum. Also what the company produces will determine the importance of the categories so, for the purpose of this example, let us look at this from a pharmaceutical company's perspective. The four main categories are:

- Product critical.
- Process critical.
- Safety critical.
- Noncritical.

A product critical process instrument is an instrument whose working accuracy may have a direct effect on *product quality*. This is a device whose operation has a direct effect on product quality, not yield or safety critical, e.g., weigh scales on an automatic check weighing system.

A temperature or pH control on a process whose product license specifies specific parameters for these measurements or control, i.e., new drug application (NDA) or drug manufacturing file (DMF). This may also have an effect on product yield but the product quality is deemed a high priority.

A process critical instrument is an instrument whose working accuracy may have a direct effect on *process yield*. These instruments would directly effect if incorrectly controlling or measuring the amount of product produced, e.g., a batch meter measuring water added to a process requiring the right amount of water to enable a process to react correctly. Too little and the process would die, too much and the yield would be small, but does not directly effect the quality or efficacy of the product.

A safety critical instrument is an instrument whose working accuracy may have a direct effect on plant and *personnel safety*. These might include boiler pressure relief system or controls. Safety cut out if a piece of equipment gets too hot.

Another example: a solvent recovery process shutdown system — if it fails there could potentially be a disaster and you could lose the site and injure or kill a lot of people.

A noncritical instrument is an instrument whose working accuracy is deemed to have *no effect on quality, yield, or safety*. An example for this type of device could be a pressure gauge whose primary function is as an indicator that pressure is present, not the specific value.

CRITICALITY ASSESSMENT

It is important to identify all the instruments associated with the process. If you do not know you have got them, what are they doing? What can they do? *Why have them?*

Once all the instruments have been identified, and formed into an instrument list, the process tolerances and limits will be required prior to a review meeting taking place.

A review meeting should take place during the installation or qualification phases of any project to define the calibration parameters. These should be reviewed again at the end of the project phase.

The *critical instrument review meeting* should comprise, as a minimum, the area or plant manager, plant engineer, and quality assurance representatives.

A suggested agenda for the meeting is:

1. Agreement of the potential impact of each instrument on product quality (direct, indirect, or none) and the significance of that affect. Agreement on which instruments are 'critical' and assign them reference numbers.
2. The acceptable process tolerance limits.
3. The required normal operating range.
4. The accuracy of each instrument.
5. The acceptable calibration frequency of each instrument.

The critical instrument review meeting, as well as producing a list of product critical instruments, will by default, also produce a list of process critical, safety critical, and noncritical instruments. The decisions taken at the critical instrument review meeting must be recorded and the instrument qualification document produced or updated. This should list the critical instruments for the process or plant, together with the process tolerance limits, normal instrument operating range, accuracy and frequency of calibration.

Examples of critical instruments are:

- Any instrument used to measure product quality.
- Any instrument used to control a parameter that could have a significant degrading effect on product quality if there is no measurement.
- Any instrument used to monitor or control the environmental conditions in areas where these are critical to product quality and the product is exposed to the environment.

The correct setting of calibration intervals is a vital activity for ensuring that the instrument continues to operate within its specified limits. The frequency should be set at the critical instrument review meeting.

When setting the calibration frequency the following should be considered:

- Manufacturer's recommendation.
- Duty of instrument if it differs from that recommended by the manufacturers.
- Relevant standards or regulation, e.g., HTM2010 (sterilizer guidelines).
- The consequences of a calibration "failure."
- Experience and knowledge.

These principles can still be applied to most other industries, but the priorities may shift. Once you have divided your list into the four categories then, what is next? Let us start with the noncitical systems. Here the principle of calibration should not be necessary. A calibration frequency is not important. In fact a check every now and then approach is properly best, to be fitted in with plant availability, or two-yearly maintenance schedules, or on a reported error basis.

Safety devices generally can be left to a yearly calibration regime or at a frequency dictated by risk assessment, legislation, or insurance specifications.

Process critical devices can be calibrated at a frequency deemed necessary. This should take account of the process accuracy required, the accuracy and reliability of the instruments, any historical data, what inaccuracy is likely to cost, etc. Basically it is down to you to determine when, but it can be planned to coincide with the main engineering activities at shutdowns, or the end of production campaigns, etc. This will help in reducing the cost.

Product critical devices must be calibrated at regular frequencies, initially a minimum of no less than twice a year. This must be rigorously followed and documented, until stability data can be collected that can form the basis of a justification for a wider frequency. The pharmaceutical regulator is looking for documented evidence that any process instrumentation deemed product critical is operating within the process criteria of the license.

Now that you have divided the instrument list into the four categories the calibration campaign is smaller and more targeted. If done correctly, it should be divided up to suit the plant availability with only the product critical instruments being dictated by date. However, even with these, you still have some leeway, as long as the twice-a-year principle is followed.

Calibration Interval

The accuracy of all analogue instruments will drift with time and usage. The extent of the drift is dependent on the type and quality of the equipment, and will be accelerated if the equipment is subjected to conditions beyond the manufacturer's specification. A digital display may be fitted with an analog sensor, an analog to digital converter, and therefore the system accuracy will drift with time.

The purpose of the calibration check is to detect the drift in equipment accuracy before it becomes unacceptable.

Initial Calibration Interval

The instrument assessment team will choose the initial calibration interval to ensure confidence in the measurement relative to the business risk and the reliability of the equipment.

The initial interval may use the interval specified for identical equipment used on similar applications.

If identical equipment is not used on site, then an interval no greater than the manufacturer's recommended interval may be used for PGMP applications.

Conditions that may increase the instrument drift and therefore need to be considered include:

- Temperature or pressure cycling.
- Conditions outside the equipment specification (equipment need not be operational).
- High humidity.
- Vibration.
- Dust.
- Corrosive atmosphere.

Adjustment of Calibration Interval

Increasing the Calibration Interval

It is essential that:

- Any lengthening of the interval between successive calibrations is supported by the history of the instrument performance.
- There is evidence to demonstrate that the instrument will operate satisfactorily over the new interval.

It is recommended that after three successive calibration checks without need for adjustment, a lengthening of the interval between successive calibrations is considered. If the interval is increased, it should not be more than doubled.

Reducing the Calibration Interval

Whenever a calibration check results in an unsatisfactory calibration, then the calibration interval should be assessed.

Criteria for reducing the interval are difficult to define as the instrument may have behaved in an unpredictable manner. Consequently the decision to reduce the interval (and to what extent) should remain based on the type of equipment, its performance history, the process criticality and the engineer's experience and assessment of the causes of failure. In extreme circumstances the instrument should be replaced with a more suitable one.

CALIBRATION

What is calibration? Calibration is a set of operations which establish, under specified conditions, the relationship between values indicated by a measuring instrument or system or values represented by a material measure, and corresponding known values of reference or standard.

Confusion again! In simple terms whatever it is you are trying to measure, somewhere there is a reference source for that measurement. Take the kilogram for example. The standard weight for a kilogram is housed in a room in Paris, France. For practical and financial reasons it is not possible to compare each measuring device directly with this primary standard in order to obtain tractability. In day-to-day practice secondary references are used. These reference weights are compared against the primary reference standard and housed by different countries as their national standard. In the U.K. the National Physical Laboratory holds this standard. This weight is then compared to individual calibration laboratories reference standards, who use their standard to compare to their working standards references and so on. Eventually someone calls at your site to calibrate your weigh scales with working reference standard weights. These are used to compare your working scales against these references and then determine if adjustment of the scales is necessary.

There is no objection to using these transferred standards as long as the chain leading to the primary standard is uninterrupted, reliable, and has been formally registered (see Figure 11.1).

UNCERTAINTY

However, it is not quite that simple! You also need to take account of:

- Errors of uncertainty from the measuring devices.
- The stated accuracy and range of the device calibrated.
- Your process accuracy required and the process operating range.
- The inherent errors introduced by the calibration activity.
- The environment where the calibration takes place.

To list but a few of the important ones.

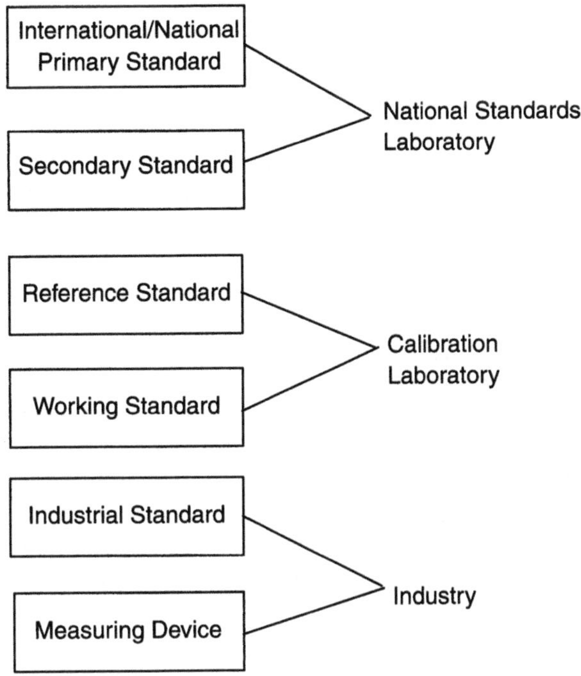

Figure 11.1 Calibration standards.

What are these issues and how do they impact on the calibration activity itself? To explain errors of uncertainty of the reference device, the following example needs to be considered.

Measure a length of wood and cut it. Then use the cut length to measure the next piece and so on. After you have cut a dozen or more lengths of wood, your last length of wood may be significantly different in length from your first.

The same is true of calibration except the lengths of wood may change on their own! Let us look at the issue of a reference source.

Regarding the reference source for the kg, the block of metal sitting in a basement in Paris. Every calibrated weight is referenced back to that reference — but it is important that there are not too many steps between the reference and the one used to calibrate production scales.

Like the piece of wood this is introducing *errors of uncertainty*. Most organizations providing a calibration service will pass on their estimates of the uncertainty error of their measuring devices. This enables you to take this into consideration or to estimate your own measurement errors of uncertainty.

Calibration activity measurement errors of uncertainty can take many forms, i.e., measuring equipment errors, human error, atmospheric pressure, temperature, etc., all of which need to be considered. Much can be dismissed as irrelevant, or eliminated following due consideration or factors applied to compensate for the result. What you can not do is completely ignore them as they require addressing to provide the *calibrated band of certainty.*

Most calibration engineers are aware of these errors. They should be easily capable of taking account of the different factors when setting up a calibration activity, and providing guidance about the consequence to any process. Estimating the calibrated band of certainty by mathematical extrapolation is also possible but requires a great deal of knowledge and skill.

When carrying out calibrations, the following rules must apply:

1. The calibration standard must have the right accuracy and be more accurate than the instrument under calibration.
2. The calibration must be performed under stable conditions; when the conditions are unstable the uncertainty increases.
3. The calibration must be traceable; the measured value must be derived from international standards.
4. Calibration procedures must be available and completely followed. To compare subsequent calibrations of the same instrument, the calibration procedure should be identical each time.

EQUIPMENT SELECTION

There is a very large selection of available instrument devices. When you are not an expert on instrumentation or calibration, it is difficult to tell the difference between the devices. You may be tempted to rely on the high accuracy claims of the supplier. You may think your worries are over. Unfortunately this is often not the case. Although the specifications may suggest a very high accuracy, a closer look may reveal that a number of important factors and influences have not been taken into account. When you add in all the possible errors such as non-linearity, hysteresis, temperature effects and repeatability, the accuracy can prove to be totally different from what you first expected.

The first important question to ask is: What do I want the instrumentation to do. What process accuracy is required, across what range. Then select a device that is ten times more accurate at best but, as this is not always an ideal world, at worst three times more accurate than the process requirements. It is important that all possible influential factors are considered at this stage.

Instrument Selection and Types

Instrumentation is a key part of pharmaceutical manufacturing operations. From laboratories to manufacturing plant, accurate measurements are an essential prerequisite to understanding and controlling the production process.

Instrumentation is the critical link between the manufacturing process and the control system. Instruments are the eyes (i.e., transmitters, sensors) and limbs (i.e., actuators, positioners) of a control system and able to perform the actions that were once performed by either operators or laboratory technicians. The number of instruments that can be involved with the operation of physical measurement in the pharmaceutical industry (both primary and secondary) can be large (2,000 to 5,000 units). In most cases, they are remotely installed from the control room environment and operate unsupervised except during routine maintenance work.

The correct operation of any computer control and data acquisition system is totally reliant on the information it receives from the instrumentation. If an instrument should malfunction, data integrity and the predefined control actions may be affected. Therefore it is essential that an instrument is carefully chosen fit for purpose, i.e., correct type, size, material, accuracy, repeatability, reliability, appropriate documentation etc. to enable confidence to be gained in its ability to perform its intended function [7, 14].

This chapter describes the process of specifying instrumentation for process duties, selecting an appropriate measurement technique, and specifying the instrument. The instrument design process is placed in the regulatory context in terms of the specific requirements for pharmaceutical plant.

A wide variety of techniques is available to meet the diverse nature of conditions encountered in pharmaceutical processes.

Supplier selection, predelivery testing, instrument handling, installation and instrument qualification are discussed in this chapter.

The Regulatory Context

Good manufacturing practice (GMP) is now a well established concept and affects all parts of the pharmaceutical manufacturing processes [1,2]. GMP regulations offer guidance related to the design, construction, location, and installation of equipment [3–6]. Measuring equipment is singled out in that the equipment must be suitable for its intended purpose and capable of producing repeatable, valid results [7].

We must also consider the life cycle of the instrumentation, and equipment must be installed in a manner to facilitate maintenance, adjustment, and cleaning. All those equipment parts in contact with the product should be inert with respect to that product [3].

The regulatory authorities seek to ensure components used in manufacture remain free from contamination and are stored and handled in a manner to prevent adverse effects [8,9]. The regulations go on to state the requirement for regular calibration and the retention of calibration records [5].

The Operating Environment

At the factory loop or in the clean room, instruments often operate in a harsh environment. Typically, instruments must contend with:

- Sterilization procedures within a clean room.
- High temperatures, humidity, and long running times.
- Dust build-up and chemical attack.
- Vibration and mechanical shock.
- Power disruptions and electromagnetic interference (EMI).

Construction

The regulatory authorities require that equipment must be constructed in such a way as to have no effect on safety, strength, quality, or purity of the drug product. Any part of an instrument that comes into contact with the product must not react to the product, so the materials of construction need to be carefully considered when selecting the instrument.

It is necessary to first define the process duty and physical phenomena requiring measurement before selecting a measurement technique and specifying the instrument.

Specifying the Process Duty

In order to allow the instrument specifier to specify the correct instrument details a definition of the process to be controlled is required. The process definition proceeds with the engineering line diagram (ELD) and the hazard study with either safety design review (SDR) or hazard and operability study (HAZOP).

The key process conditions and range require definition. Collaboration is required between the process or production disciplines and the engineering or calibration disciplines are needed to arrive at a final instrument definition. The split of responsibilities is normally:

- *Process*. Process duty, working, and maximum ranges, physical properties, engineering units, process function, e.g., control, measurement only, safety, control and alarm set points.
- *Instrument*. Instrument and installation details, manufacturers, instrument range, and accuracy.

It is important to carefully consider the accuracy requirements early in the instrument specification and to specify closely the actual operating range of the process.

Often the instrument is capable of reading a wider range than is required, so the calibration points need to be identified carefully, as opposed to a simple 0, 50, 100% of the instrument range. The personnel involved must have suitable training and experience to design the instrumentation system [1, 2, 10].

The specification conclusion involves an iterative approach where the stipulated instrument parameters are selected from standard manufacturer's products. A check is then required to ensure that no critical difference has arisen between the process definition and the available instruments, e.g., instrument range too large or too small.

Selecting the Instrument

With the process conditions specified, the appropriate instruments may be selected. Key parameters are:

- Instrumentation may be required to withstand sterilization by steam and 2.5 barg and 136°C without damage.
- Once sterilized, the instrument equipment must remain sterile.

The choice of instrument equipment needs to include consideration of the transmission system, e.g., connection to a control system, hazardous area requirements, the accuracy of measurement required, turn down range of measurement required electromagnetic compatibility (EMC) and RFI immunity. Equipment access for maintenance and calibration is a requirement, along with other considerations such as standardization on the plant or site and cost.

The following sections identify the typical selection criteria for measuring the majority of physical phenomena [11].

Temperature Instrument Selection

There are two common methods in general usage, resistance thermometers (RTs) and thermocouples. A comparison of RTs and thermocouples are shown in Table 11.1.

Table 11.1 Comparison of RT and thermocouple accuracy

		Platinum RT	Thermocouple type K
Span		–200 to +300°C	0 to 800°C
Tolerance	At 100°C	±0.8°C	±2.5°C
	At 30°C	±1.8°C	±2.5°C

RTs have the better accuracy for low temperatures and up to 350°C. Thermocouples are capable of reading continuously at greater than 350°C.

Thermometer pockets should generally be attached to pipelines and vessels by means of flanged branches meeting the pipeline specification. Vibration and length of immersion in a fluid are designed to prevent mechanical damage and the reception of a valid reading. Primarily heat transfer between the pocket and element determines speed of measurement response. Bare elements response is approximately 10 seconds, with time constants extending up to 60 seconds (longer for gas measurements). A long time constant can have serious consequences for control duties.

Head mounted transmitters must be subjected to no more than 60°C, to avoid stressing the electronic components.

Pressure Instruments

When selecting pressure instruments, the pressure characteristics of the duty need to be considered in terms of maximum working pressure, sudden pressure increases, or the presence of mechanical vibration. Whether the duty is clean or dirty influences the size of process connection. If any solids are likely to form at ambient temperatures winterization would be required.

Corrosive process materials require the use of exotic instrument materials. These materials need to be checked to ensure that they are inert with respect to the product. Pressure measurements within sterile areas should be made using pad type transmitters to avoid contamination of any dead spaces.

Process connections are generally 1 in for clean or dirty gases and liquids, 2 in for slurries and resins. Connections are generally 2 in for vessels.

Flow Meters

Often used flow meter measurement techniques are:

- Differential pressure.
- Orifice plate.
- Electromagnetic (EM).
- Vortex shedding.

Clearly for steam and gas duties, orifice or vortex shedders are options, whereas EM flow meters have negligible pressure loss over a very wide flow range. Orifice plate installations can trap material, avoided by vertical installation, and the design is critical. However you can choose the construction materials and a simple device with no moving parts.

EM flow meters operate with conductive materials (>5 micro Siemens/cm) are bidirectional and cope with pulsating flows. However, temperature can be a limitation and liners can be easily damaged, especially during installation. Gas entrainment is to be avoided.

Although low cost, vibration has a great affect on vortex shedders, and the advice is to install upside down to avoid the entrapment of air bubbles affecting the vortex detection. The choice is dependent on the process conditions, for which there is almost certainly a technique available for each duty.

Level Instruments

There are many techniques which may be employed to measure level.

- Vibrating fork.
- Pressure.
- Capacitance.
- Radar.
- Ultrasonic.
- Weight.
- Gamma radiation.

Certain common techniques are suitable for secondary pharmaceutical plant in that they may not withstand sterilization, e.g., the probe may harbor material following sterilization such as bubble tubes. However, some of these types may be considered for primary plants and "offsite" facilities.

Level measurement may be required — the range of material in a vessel, or as a level switch, the point at which a determined level is reached.

pH Instruments

pH instruments measure the effective concentration of hydrogen ions over a range of 0 to 14. A neutral solution has a pH of 7, with a pH of less than 7 representing an acid solution and more than 7 representing an alkaline solution. With a well maintained instrument, a reproducibility of better than ±0.01 pH may be attained, dropping to ± 0.1 with poorly buffered systems.

Buffer solutions, which undergo little pH change with the addition of acid or alkali, are used for calibrating pH-measuring equipment. An error of 10% volume of water in making up a buffer solution may be ignored if the accuracy required is less than 0.02 pH units.

The majority of pH units are manufactured using glass electrodes, the measured emf is relative to a reference electrode, corrected for temperature. These instruments can virtually cover the complete pH range while remaining unaffected by most chemicals and at the same time tolerate steam sterilization. Electrodes supplied dry should be conditioned before installation, e.g., using hydrochloric acid. Electrodes should be stored in distilled or demineralized water, or a buffer solution at temperatures close to those at which they will be used.

Installations constructed of stainless steel may be of a continuous flow with close coupled measurement of a sample loop, or immersion type where the electrode measures freely flowing material, e.g., in a tank. Care is required to reduce the effects of fouling and scaling. Self-cleaning techniques are available to counter these effects.

When installed in a tank, it is necessary to ensure the measurement is representative of the tank contents. Tank mixing is important. Avoid drying the electrode if the tank is drained.

The Instrument Specification

Once the process duty is known the instrument specification may proceed. This entails a statement of detailed requirements in terms of how the instrument application is to operate in the intended environment. The specification should clearly identify the following:

- Process to be controlled.
- Description of fluid involved.
- Power supply conditions.
- Operating range, e.g., 0–50°C, 1–10 barg.
- Accuracy.
- Output, i.e., 4–20 mA, 1–5 volts.
- Line size.
- Temperature range, working and maximum.
- Pressure range, working and maximum.
- Alarm, trip, interlock settings and direction (rising or falling).
- Communications with intelligent devices, e.g., Smart transmitter.
- Manufacturer.
- Part number.

A statement whether the instrument is performing a critical or noncritical duty assists in assessing the importance of the instrument. The allocation of critical category (product, process, safety, noncritical) enables the selection of the instrument as appropriate to the calibration regime [12].

Selecting of Safety Critical Instruments

Instruments installed for safety duties must be clearly identified as safety critical in the field. Configuration of Smart transmitters used for safety critical duties must be secured to prevent modification. Seals may be used to ensure that access is controlled to Smart transmitters used for conventional duties.

Intelligent Instruments

Smart transmitters contain embedded software driven by factory configured firmware [13]. For these types of devices it is necessary to record the configuration and ensure upgrades of firmware are handled under change control. *Networked devices require data transfer to be verified and secure.*

Analyzers

Analyzers are often computer controlled and are subject to the validation lifecycle of user requirements specification, functional design specification, installation and operation qualification. Sample loop design, data reports and communications with other systems all require specification and qualification for many analysis systems, e.g., total organic carbon (TOC) effluent monitoring systems.

Suppliers

The responsibility for the validation of process equipment rests with the pharmaceutical company. The selection of suppliers capable of delivering well-designed equipment and installations is carried out through the use of supplier audits [14].

Supplier Selection

Supplier selection is often based on site standards or technical evaluation. Supplier audits are generally used to ensure that the chosen company can supply the required instrument. Trained and qualified personnel should conduct supplier audits against the appropriate ISO 9000 standard. Reference should be made to software quality guidelines for instrument systems involving software (Smart instruments).

Predelivery Testing and Calibration

Prior to delivery, all instruments should undergo a factory test and calibration. All test equipment should be calibrated and a certificate issued (for example by NAMAS approved laboratory) and must have an accuracy and an order of magnitude better than the instrument to be tested. Factory testing should be carried out in accordance with written test procedures with the tests fully documented and results recorded. Where applicable, hazardous area certificates must also be supplied.

Factory calibration should be carried out against the specification sheets and address the following areas:

- Process operating ranges.
- Required accuracy.
- Repeatability.
- Hysteresis effects.
- Trip set points.
- Condition of switching (rising or falling).
- Trip action (open or close on fault condition).

Handling

Instruments require appropriate handling prior to installation. Care must be taken to ensure the storage of the instrument avoids damage to the materials of construction, electronics, and calibration.

Equipment Inspection and Storage

Careful unpacking and a visual inspection for superficial damage should be undertaken on equipment delivery. The equipment should be placed in a secure, dust-free store, suitably heated to avoid condensation forming on the electronic components. In order to minimize handling, larger items of equipment, such as control panels, should be installed directly in the final location. During the installation and construction phases of installation, the equipment needs to be suitably protected from other construction activities such as painting, welding, and scaffolding damage.

Installation

A good installation requires secure, vibration free, and accessible mounting of instruments. The instruments should have visible tags and labels and be located so that maintenance and calibration may be carried easily by maintenance staff.

Installation should be carried out according to the hook-up drawings showing process connection, mounting arrangements, and instrument loop diagrams. Air supplies should be clean and dry, distributed from a plant header, as shown on a pneumatic hook-up drawing. Pneumatic signals (3–15 psig) and tubing should be of short runs and suitably supported, e.g., on cable tray, and protected from mechanical damage.

Cable routes should be kept as short as possible and protected from chemical attack. Signals of different types should not be run in the same multicore, and intrinsically safe circuits should be installed in cables reserved for their use only.

Plant earthing systems should be segregated between instrument or "clean" earth, and factory earth with the loop impedance not exceeding 1 ohm. Intrinsically safe circuits must be tested in accordance with the manufacturers instructions. Each signal cable is to be tested for continuity.

Loop Testing

Prior to plant commissioning each instrument loop should be tested for correct operation, starting with a visual inspection of the loop, checking signal polarity, power supplies and fuses.

A checklist of points to note for instrument installations:

- Instrument installation:
  - Capable of sterilization.
  - IP rating.
  - Upstream and downstream lengths.
  - External influences minimized (RFI).
  - IS circuits.
  - Loop impedance <1 ohm.
  - Alarm, trip and interlocks.
  - Polarity checks and fuses.

- Signal tests:
  - Analogue and digital inputs and outputs.

- Earthing:
  - Instrument and factory earths.

- Power supply units (PSU):
  - Redundancy, supply filters, fed from different.
  - Transformers, PSU alarms.
  - UPS bypass for maintenance purposes.
  - Scope of UPS support and support time.

- Cable routes:
  - Secure route in factory.
  - Sealed entries into clean rooms.
  - Marshalling arrangements.

- Documentation:
  - Process definition, instrument specification.
  - Instrument loop drawings, factory test results, calibration certificates, process and pneumatic hook-ups, instrument arrangements, cable schedules.

- Service connections:
  - Air, nitrogen.

- Hardware failure modes:
  - State of signals on power fail burn out effects.

- Signal isolation:
  - Opto-isolation, galvanic isolators, barriers.

- Instrument location:
  - Access for maintenance and calibration.
  - Mechanical vibration protection.

- Measurement displays:
  - IPC, DCS, indicator, chart recorder.

- Communications:
  - Channels and interfaces.

Following the visual inspection, creating process conditions, or injecting 0, 50, 100 percent of range then test the instrument transmitters. Care must be taken to ensure at least one test point is within the process operating range. All test results should be recorded.

Alarm trip and interlock systems should be tested, along with the fail-safe and loss of power actions of the instrument loops.

Smart Instrumentation

Traditionally, operational errors in field devices can only be reported to control systems by setting the analogue value to a preset fail level defined in the transmitter's configuration. Since this means that the measurement value is no longer communicated, it cannot be used for "information" alarms or alerts, only catastrophic failure of the transmitter or sensor. Smart instrumentation with communication capabilities to host systems allows additional measurement and diagnostic information from the device to be made available.

However, the rapidly growing use of Smart instrumentation with these communication capabilities presents new opportunities and challenges in the areas of managing field instrument configuration, diagnosis, and calibration.

Instrumentation manufacturers are continually introducing new technologies and functionality. Much of the development is now focused on improving measurement stability and improving diagnostics, including calibration drift — both for the sensor and the transmitter. It has been a popular misconception since the advent of Smart instrumentation that there was no need to perform routine calibration checks, since the self diagnostics would alert the user to a problem.

While this is generally true for a complete sensor or electronics failure, it is not necessarily the case if there is a small shift in the operating parameters of the electronics or the sensor. The only way to definitively correct this is still with a conventional calibration check.

Automation

Instruments Needs

In order to utilize the functionality of Smart instrumentation providing predictive diagnostic alerts, the instruments need to communicate their status. Meter displays on the instrument itself are useful for local indication, however, a host system is needed to provide permanent monitoring capability.

Host systems can be hand held communicators, control systems, or dedicated instrument asset management systems (IAMS). Control system capabilities vary widely in their ability to support communications with intelligent instruments, and in the degree of data integration. The more advanced systems utilize a single database for control system and instrument configurations. This allows, for example, a change to a transmitter's range to be automatically replicated in the control system's configuration, thereby avoiding duplicate data entry and the risk of associated errors. Other systems, particularly older ones, are completely oblivious to intelligent instrument communications.

IAMS typically provide the following instrumentation management capabilities:

1. Management of configuration and specification data for both intelligent and conventional non-Smart instrumentation, including integration with mobile hand-held communicators and diagnostic tools.
2. Automatic recording of events for audit purposes of intelligent instrumentation configuration changes and diagnostic status changes.
3. Diagnostic interrogation of intelligent instruments.

4. A window for preventative or predictive maintenance alerts for intelligent instruments providing these capabilities.

The IAMS may include an integrated calibration management capability.

Diagnostic and Calibration Development Trends in Smart Instrumentation

One of the abilities of intelligent instrumentation is the capability to measure and process multiple variables in one instrument.

Measurement Integrity Validation and Self Calibration

Some intelligent transmitters can monitor their sensors, and signal a calibration drift condition to the user. The future trend is for this type of diagnostic information to increase as more processing power is added to commercially available intelligent devices. Typically, the user can configure how much drift is acceptable, and when that value is exceeded, a "calibration drift" alert is sent out to the instrument's meter, or communicated to a host system. By monitoring the sensor drift over time, the rate of future drift can be calculated. This enables predictions on how long it will take to reach the user preset calibration drift alert value, or even sensor failure. This capability does not prevent calibration drift, but monitors and informs accordingly. Periodic calibration using test equipment is still required, but test intervals can be extended, since monitoring drift status by a host system will provide a predictive alert, enabling action to be taken before operational limits are exceeded.

Once a calibration drift is detected, transmitters have the potential to automatically "self tune," or "self-calibrate" to correct for the drift. The use of such instrumentation may be used to justify the extension of calibration periodicity, but routine calibrations should still be made against test equipment.

Smart Calibrators and Test Equipment

The proven way to establish traceability to national standards is by the use of calibrators or buffer solutions, gases of known performance. The use of Smart documenting multifunction calibrators reduces the number of different calibrators required to perform tests on the many different measurements types. The documenting capabilities prevent transcription and other errors associated with the manual recording of calibration test results.

Even using documenting multifunction calibrators, performing calibrations on intelligent instrumentation still requires an additional communicator to perform trim adjustments to the instrument. However, some multifunction documenting calibrators are able to communicate digitally with intelligent instrumentation, allowing instrument testing and adjustment to be performed with one piece of equipment. Also, automatic capture of instrument manufacturer, model, tag ID, and serial number can help in reducing documentation errors and improve traceabilty.

Documenting multifunction calibrators help ensure accurate data collection, which can be the weakest link in the documentation chain. Eliminating manual data recording in the field significantly reduces the risk of transcription errors. Typically, the multifunction documenting calibrators capture the time, date and operator name, and if they communicate with the instrument, they can validate that the correct instrument is undergoing testing.

Third Party Calibration

Calibration may be carried out by third parties, e.g., contractors or instrument suppliers, but the responsibility for ensuring that calibration procedures have been correctly followed should remain with the instrument owner (i.e., the equipment user; the pharmaceutical manufacturer; the company subject to regulatory control).

The contract giver should assess the competence of the contractors (the contract acceptor), by performing an audit, or by other appropriate means, and should use only competent contractors approved in this way.

The contract acceptor should maintain suitable premises, equipment, knowledge, competent and experienced personnel. It may not pass to a subcontractor any of the work entrusted to him, or change any of the agreed tests, standards or limits, without the contract giver's prior evaluation and approval.

There should be a written contract covering the work to be done by the contract acceptor and any technical arrangements made concerning it. This contract should:

1. Specify the respective responsibilities of the contract giver and contract acceptor.
2. Describe (or reference) the tests to be done and the standards and limits to be applied.
3. Describe the quality system to be applied by the contract acceptor.
4. Specify the documentation to be used, produced, and retained by the contract acceptor, and to be supplied by the contract giver.
5. Permit the contract giver and specified regulatory authorities to visit the premises of the contract acceptor for the purposes of carrying out audits relevant to the calibration activities.
6. Specify the arrangements for handling, packing, and transporting the items to be calibrated, to minimize the potential for damage in transit.
7. Describe any hazards associated with the use or testing of the items.
8. Be drawn up with the involvement of suitably qualified and experienced personnel.
9. Determine the cleaning of product contact parts.

Documentation supplied by the contract acceptor to the contract giver on completion of calibration should clearly identify the items concerned, show the initial test results, indicate any adjustments made, and (where relevant) the test results after adjustment. Any raw data from the tests should be supplied to the contract giver (unless it has been specifically agreed that the contract acceptor should securely retain these). The documentation should record the test methods, standards and limits applied, or give references to these. There should be a clear statement, signed by a responsible person, indicating whether or not the items has been left in full working order.

When the contract giver receives the items returned from the contract acceptor, the items should be carefully examined for possible damage in transit. An appropriately qualified and trained person should review the documentation from the contract acceptor. If all is in order, this person should record in writing the acceptance of the items, with signature and date.

Instrument Qualification

Once the engineering design has been completed, the design qualification (DQ) may take place. The DQ checks the design documentation and audits the instrument package of design, construction, inspection reports, and test documents. Engineering drawings, operating and maintenance procedures, parts lists, and system descriptions are included in the DQ. The DQ offers the opportunity to ensure specified components are compatible with the target environment and meet EMC regulations.

Installation qualification (IQ) follows construction of the instrument loop and ensures the instrument and circuit components are in working order. The loop is subjected to a series of inspections, loop impedance and calibration tests, recorded on an instrument loop check sheet. Any reference documents, drawings, and instrument certificates should be included in the scope of the IQ.

Operational qualification (OQ) follows IQ and confirms the operation of the instrument loop as it is integrated with the overall control scheme, involving any computer functions operating the loop. Change control should be enforced to ensure changes are assessed for their potential impact on the system.

Conclusions

The selection of instrumentation relies on a detailed and accurate specification of the process duty and an early assessment of the instrument criticality in terms of the process operation. The wide variety of instruments available means that the instrument objectives and requirements of the pharmaceutical manufacturing environment need to be clearly borne in mind in order to make the correct choice of instrument technique.

Along with instrument selection, supplier selection is important to provide the information required ensuring technical success and regulatory compliance. Advice is required from suppliers regarding the instrument installation, materials of construction, factory testing procedures and documentation, handling and storage of the equipment. All this is needed in order that, once installed, the instrument is capable of producing valid results.

Instrument qualification, comprising DQ, IQ, and OQ ensures the documentary evidence is in place to demonstrate a well-engineered instrument has been installed meeting the regulatory requirements.

INSTRUMENT VALIDATION

When calibrating product critical instruments in a validation process it is imperative to consider the calibration against the process parameters.

The instrument list should include the process operating range and the required accuracy of the measurement. This accuracy must be realistic. If this stated accuracy is not attained a formal investigation and product recall will result. This list will also include device accuracy and instrument range.

The calibration activity will involve, as a minimum, a test point within the process range and one above and below the process range. It is good practice, however, to test five points.

- If maximum error recorded is within the device accuracy, and the process accuracy the device can be considered as passed its calibration, no action is necessary except to document the result. This will be useful data as part of a justification to extend the calibration frequency.
- If maximum error recorded is outside the device accuracy, but within the process accuracy, the device can be considered to have passed its calibration. But recalibrate the device to the instrument accuracy. Also document the results, as this may be useful data as part of a justification to extend the calibration frequency.
- If the maximum error recorded is outside the device and the process accuracy, then the device can be considered to have failed its calibration. However, if the results for the three measurements associated with the process range parameters are within the process accuracy then the device can be considered to have passed its calibration. If this is not the case, then an exception report must be raised and the consequences of the failure investigated.

If the device was selected correctly, and the periods between calibrations were realistic, a fail should not happen!

DOCUMENTATION

The proof of a validated instrument system is in the documentation. Unless it is documented and signed by an approving authority, usually QA, it is considered to be a rumor.

The most effective way of providing the necessary documentary evidence is to produce an instrument qualification document. This document gathers all relevant information and provides a single reference to assure validation.

It is important to define the requirements and the operational procedures to be used before producing the qualification documents. As a minimum the following procedures need to be in place:

- Calibration requirements.
- Production of instrument qualification documents.
- Method for preparing a calibration report.
- Calibration by work request.

All details of calibration are contained in the one document so that maintenance management systems can instigate a calibration campaign by referencing the document, rather than producing individual work requests for each element of the product critical instrumentation. If individual work requests are raised for each element of the product critical instrument, each one must have the required process accuracy and range when issued, and must record all raw data during the calibration.

Procedures must be produced for each activity, and a results sheet produced to record the results. Each result sheet must be countersigned by an authorized signatory, and space should be left for a formal audit.

At the end of each calibration campaign a calibration report must be produced which identifies any areas of concern, and gives authority for the process to be operated or prevents operation until specific actions have been completed.

A calibration report is prepared by the authorized technician responsible for carrying out the calibration work to highlight any concerns that have arisen following the completion of the calibration activity. This informs the production department of any instrument that might have failed, the degree of its failure, and allows production to discuss possible product implications with QA.

The calibration report is used to inform the production department of the instruments that have failed, and those replaced and adjusted. It is also used to assist the engineering teams to trend any instrument drift in order to justify its replacement on the grounds of reliability. This report must represent all the issues that arise from the calibration activity, even if action has already taken place to correct any concerns.

The calibration report should list all the instruments that have:

- Passed, as defined by the production department, but have required recalibration to return to the defined instrument accuracy.
- Failed the production defined limits, but were successfully recalibrated following an adjustment, also providing the exception report number and the reason.
- Failed the production defined limits and were replaced, providing the exception report number and the reason.

Test results summary must contain the following in tabular form:

- Type of instrument calibrated.
- Instrument tag number.
- Duty.
- Pass or fail.
- Date.
- Exception report number, if required.

Engineering observations should contain the following information.

- Any inaccuracies noted in loop drawings, user manual, P&ID drawings, and the calibration procedures.
- Any issues relating to access to plant and equipment requiring calibration.
- Any recommendations to assist future calibration activities.

Exception Report

The exception report must be raised when a "fail" occurs. It should be submitted at the end of the day's testing and not wait for the completion of the calibration campaign. The exception report must be sent to the process owner and the QA department. This is vital as a "fail" would mean that a product critical parameter is outside of its process accuracy. Hence all product produced since the last "pass" must be assessed to consider if a product recall is required. The consequences of this must be assessed by the process owner, and a formal response prepared and countersigned by QA. This report becomes part of the instrument qualification manual.

All of the response documents are added to the instrument qualification and form part of the validation of the process.

Calibration Results Sheets

It is important that a regime of auditing calibration results sheets should be in place. Errors can be easily made. Some of the errors commonly found are listed here.

- Incorrect results sheet for the device.
- Use of previous issue of the results document.
- Department, service, and location sections are incorrect.
- Tag number incorrectly entered.
- Incorrect device range.
- Critical device box has not been ticked.
- Results not entered in using blue ink.
- Process range is not within the calibrated range of the instrument? i.e.,
  Process range 20–80°C
  Calibrated range 0–100°C
- There is not a reasonable difference between the process accuracy and the device accuracy? i.e., a ratio of 10:1 is the norm for temperature but may be lower for RH!
- Entered information not in discrete units where possible.
- The test results do not cover the full process range, e.g., there must be as a minimum, a result above the upper limit of the process range, a result below the lower limit of the process range, and a result in the process range.
- Crossings out, that are not signed.
- Alterations made.
- Results sheets are not signed by the engineer or checked by someone independent.
- Not all sections have been filled in with the results information.
- If results are not within the device accuracy stated then the post adjustment calibration section must be completed. The comments section must contain a statement that the device is not within the stated device accuracy, and therefore had to be adjusted to meet the stated device accuracy and retested.
- If the results for the post adjustment calibration section are not within the device accuracy stated, then the comments section must contain comments that the device has been changed.
- Calculations are incorrect?
- If results within the process range band, are not within the stated process accuracy, the post adjustment calibration section must be completed. The comments section should also state that an exception report along with its reference number has been submitted, and that the instrument has been adjusted to meet the stated device accuracy and retested.
- If results outside process range band, are not within the stated process accuracy then, the post adjustment calibration section must be completed. The comments section must also contain a statement that the device was outside the process accuracy, but not within the process range band, and has therefore been adjusted to meet the stated device accuracy and retested.
- There has been no evaluation of the device accuracy.
- Incorrect rev number has been entered, i.e., the next consecutive number following on from the last results sheet.

Change Control

The essential element of change control is demonstrating that all changes are carried out in a controlled manner, from start to finish. The simpler the system, the better it works. The essence of making these statements is that if a company's existing change control system has been proven by audit, and fits the above statements, then the use of calibration certificates and document references within the change control document is all that is required. In some instances, companies may prefer separate change control for the calibration process, although this process should not be encouraged.

Change control should be used for changes in control or alarm settings as well as the removal of equipment.

As a minimum, any change control system needs to contain the data shown in Figure 11.2, which outlines the typical change control route.

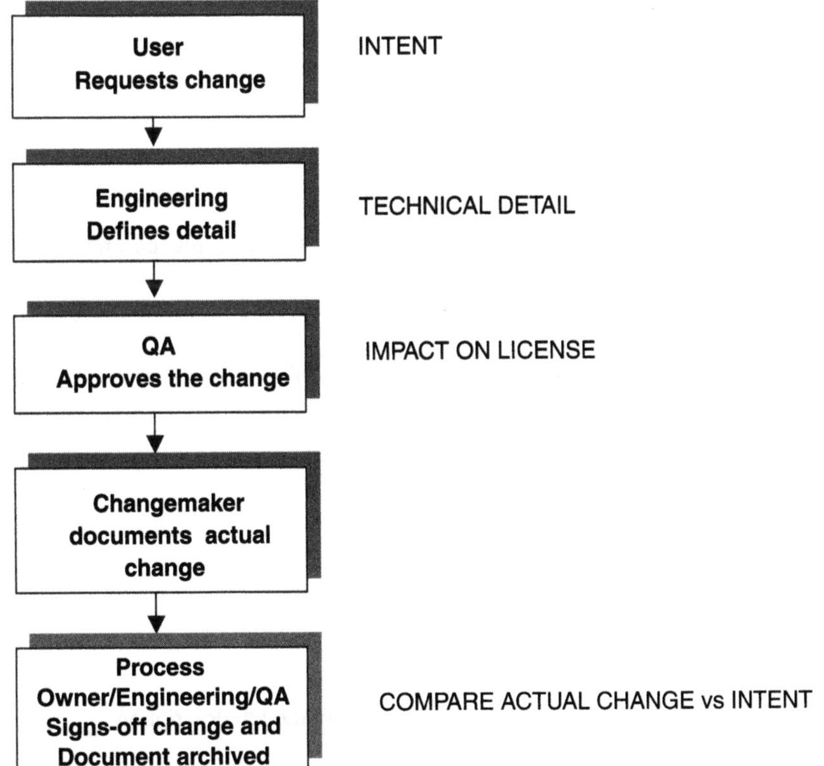

Figure 11.2 Typical change control route.

AUDITING

A formal process of regular auditing is necessary to ensure that the product critical calibration system is operating effectively. This should be performed by an independent standards or QA function as part of a self inspection program. Local audits by plant personnel are also useful in ensuring that standards are achieved and documentation is complete, signed, dated and where appropriate, scanned and registered.

Training

A person should be nominated for ownership of training and that person should ensure that all instrument calibrators are qualified as competent to carry out the required calibration to the required standard.

Training records should be maintained to demonstrate a robust system of training management.

Training Records

The training records should incorporate the following:

- Entry page:
  - To include full name; date record created; sample signature and initials; employers name and address; staff number.

- Role and responsibilities:
  - To include a copy of the "agreed" job description, giving responsibilities, key result areas, objectives, etc.

- Training record: (suggested sections):
  - Part (a) Future training need.
  - Part (b) Qualification record.
  - Part (c) Experience record.
  - Part (d) Competence record.
  - Part (e) Courses and presentations.

- Certificates:
  - To include certificates of training relevant to the job description.

- Competency:
  - To include copies of written assessments that demonstrate understanding of a procedure and "on the job" supervisor or workplace trainer assessments.

This style of record captures key elements of an individual's history, demonstrating the ability to carry out work competently.

SUMMARY

- Processes must be assessed to establish the criticality of all measurement and control parameters.
- Product critical instruments must be calibrated at sufficient frequency to maintain the processes in a validated state. This is a requirement of GMP, and hence a legal requirement.
- A system must exist, described by SOPs, to identify product, process and safety critical instruments, calibrate them to traceable standards at a specified frequency, label and document them, and to perform any calibration follow-up actions. This system must be audited at regularly defined intervals.
- There must also be an SOP to ensure that noncritical instruments are calibrated to ensure efficient and effective operation of the plant and equipment.
- Any system used is only as good as the documentation produced for regulatory approval.
- A consistent approach to validation across the pharmaceutical industry will improve understanding and efficiency, and give support to individuals in a regulatory audit situation as well as saving time and money.

GLOSSARY

NAMAS	National Measurement Accreditation Service
IPC	Industrial Personal Computer
DCS	Distributed Control System
UPS	Uninterruptible Power Supply
Smart	Intelligent transmitter
IQ	Installation Qualification
DQ	Design Qualification
OQ	Operational Qualification
ELD	Engineering line diagram
HAZOP	Hazard and Operability Study
RFI	Radio Frequency Interference
EMC	Electromagnetic Compatibility.
EMF	Electromagnetic Force

REFERENCES

Rules and Guidance for Pharmaceutical Manufacturers and Distributors 1997.

21 CFR Part 211 — Current Good Manufacturing Practice for Finished Pharmaceuticals.

21 CFR Part 11 — Electronic Records; Electronic Signatures.

Guidance on decontamination from the Microbiological Advisory Committee to Department of Health Medical Devices Directorate, dated June 1993.

1 European Union Directive 93/356/EEC and U.S. Code of Federal Regulations Title 21, Parts 210 and 211 detailing Good Manufacturing Practice for Pharmaceuticals.

2 Australian Code of GMP for Therapeutic Goods — Medicinal Products — Part 1.

3 U.S. Code of Federal Regulations Title 21, 211.65 Equipment construction.

4 U.S. Code of Federal Regulations Title 21, 58.61 Equipment design.

5 U.S. Code of Federal Regulations Title 21, 58.63 Maintenance and Calibration of Equipment.

6 U.S. Code of Federal Regulations Title 21, 211.63 Equipment design, size, and location.

7 U.S. Code of Federal Regulations Title 21, 820.61 Measuring Equipment.

8 U.S. Code of Federal Regulations Title 21, 820.80 Components.

9 U.S. Code of Federal Regulations Title 21, 820.60 Equipment.

10 U.S. Code of Federal Regulations Title 21, 21.34 Consultants.

11 *Instrumentation Reference Book*, 2nd ed., edited by Noltingk, B.E.: Butterworth-Heinemann, Oxford, 1996.

12 Ferenc, B.M., Kot, L., Thomas, R. *Equipment Validation in Pharmaceutical Process Validation*, 2nd ed., edited by Berry, I.R. and Nash, R.A.: Marcel Dekker, Inc., New York, 1993.

13 GAMP 4, GAMP Guide for Validation of Automated Systems in Pharmaceutical Manufacture, The GAMP Forum, International Society for Pharmaceutical Engineering, Tampa, Florida.

14 *Interpharm's Validating Automated Manufacturing and Laboratory Systems: Putting Principles into Practice*, Interpharm Press, Buffalo Grove, IL, 1997.

Chapter 12

Validating Legacy Systems

Siegfried Schmitt

CONTENTS

OVERVIEW

Automation is now part of everyone's life. Today's economy would cease to function without computers, and to blame this on the computers themselves is not entirely fair; they were after all, designed and put into use by man. We have only ourselves to blame when and if automated systems malfunction and we cannot understand why.

When we design and implement new systems, we are ideally placed to define them, test them, and approve their functionality. But most computer systems are existing installations and known as "legacy" systems, where we have a totally new situation. There may be no formal description of the system, the code may have been changed or replaced many times. Manuals will possibly have disappeared long ago.

Now we need to deal with the reality of such a situation, providing step-by-step guidance for those faced with assessment of legacy systems, for whatever reason that may be — perhaps to gain a better understanding of how a system operates, because of changed regulatory requirements, or simply to assess its performance and usefulness.

Much is written on new systems, with interest groups focussing on the "how to" element of system selection and installation. Little guidance can be found on legacy systems, guidance written in "plain English" rather than in technical terms. We try here to put that right, using a bullet point summary at the end of each section.

We refer frequently to the healthcare and pharmaceutical and allied industry sector, but we are not writing entirely for the life sciences professional. The principles discussed here, such as system assessment and evaluation, identification of remedial action and validation thereof, apply to all industries. Pharmaceutical, chemical, beverage, electronic, nuclear, cosmetic, animal health, and food personnel will all gain some benefit from the guidance, showing the steps which can lead to a fully-understood computer system, which does the job for which it was designed and intended — an eminently worthwhile result.

INTRODUCTION

Since this chapter was first drafted, a number of significant changes have occurred within the U.S. Food and Drug Administration (FDA), from both organizational and regulatory perspectives. The most significant change, introduced as part of FDA's initiative "cGMPs for the 21st Century," was the publication of the final guidance for industry document "Part 11, Electronic Records; Electronic Signatures — Scope and Application" in August 2003 [10]. In this document the FDA now makes significant concessions with regards to Part 11 compliance requirements for legacy systems; it does not, however, renege on the demand for fulfilling the requirements of the applicable predicate rules.

In the strictest sense of this guidance document, a legacy system is one that meets all the following criteria for a specific system [10].

- The system was operational before the effective date.
- The system met all applicable predicate rule requirements before the effective date.
- The system currently meets all applicable predicate rule requirements.
- You have documented evidence and justification that the system is fit for its intended use (including having an acceptable level of record security and integrity, if applicable).

If a system has been changed since August 20, 1997, and if the changes would prevent the system from meeting predicate rule requirements, Part 11 controls should be applied to Part 11 records and signatures pursuant to the enforcement policy expressed in this guidance.

There are indeed such systems still in use, although most applications will have had some upgrades or patches installed, not least to receive continued vendor support, or because upgrades became necessary with the migration to new or upgraded operating systems and changed hardware. There is a high risk of failure associated with such legacy systems; a dual risk, one of failing to work and one of no longer having a validated status. These "true" legacy systems are more of a curiosity than the norm.

Most users still consider any automated system already in operation as a legacy system, distinguished from new installations or upgrades to a new software version. As it is necessary to assess all existing systems for their validation status and whether the system has to comply with 21 CFR Part 11, it is only understandable to call them "legacy" systems. The scope of this chapter has thus not changed, and only minor amendments were made to ensure conformance with current guidance and regulations.

Despite FDA's initiative to reform the good manufacturing practices (GMPs) and with it 21 CFR Part 11, it is fair to assume that this guidance will be in place for the coming years, as it takes considerable effort to change the law, and to obtain buy-in from industry. Doing nothing or waiting for things to change soon is not an option if one wishes to stay in compliance. Where there are existing systems that have not yet been assessed and brought into compliance, this should be initiated and performed without delay. Following the advice and the processes outlined hereafter provides the reader with a pragmatic, proven and useful approach to achieving compliance for legacy systems.

It is hard to imagine finding a facility or a sector within the life science industry in this 21st century without some sort of automation and use of desktop computers. We are all involved in the deployment of information technology (IT) to complete our everyday activities satisfactorily. Automated and computer and IT systems improve business processes, ensure health and safety, and enable a company to function. The IT revolution has brought about an enormous change in both the way we work, and the way we document such work. This exponential evolution also means that today's computer or IT system is outdated tomorrow, whereupon it will become a "legacy system," or an inherited system.

Existing automated systems fulfil their role and run for many years, before replacement by new technology. Some of these systems fall under the regulations governing the healthcare (i.e., drug substance, drug product, and medical device manufacturers), food, cosmetics and nutraceuticals industries [1–7]. Legislation extends beyond manufacturing and associated laboratory activities; it encompasses all aspects of a product life cycle. Typical examples for IT applications which must comply are:

- A simple spreadsheet for yield calculations.
- An enterprise resource planning software package used as a worldwide manufacturing planning tool.
- A programable logic controller on a filling line.

This gives a flavor of the immense variety of systems with which a company must work successfully.

This chapter is aimed at the regulated life science industry, in order to assist management from all disciples in the assessment, qualification, and validation of their IT systems. It aims to provide a common understanding of the requirements for all parties involved, such as the IT, manufacturing, administration, quality control, and regulatory affairs.

Although most companies have implemented commissioning, qualification, and validation programs for their equipment and processes, some systems (such as servers, networks, or archiving systems) have often been excluded, particularly if not associated with processing or analytical equipment. The regulatory authorities no longer tolerate this negligence. This has resulted in many inspection report citings for deficiencies in this particular area in recent years.

Although industry started to look at ways in which automated systems should be commissioned, qualified and validated, it was only when the U.S. FDA published the "Blue Book" in 1983 [1], that the regulators provided rules and guidance. This was followed in 1997 by the requirements for electronic records and electronic signatures (ER/ES) in the U.S. Code of Federal Regulations [4], 21 CFR Part 11. This regulation, which was first published on March 20 1997 and came into force on August 20, 1997, provides the current impetus for industry to assess IT systems and take remedial action to attain this goal.

Because automated systems were not purchased and installed with this regulation in mind until recently, many companies have little or no knowledge of the compliance level of their automated systems. Companies not producing for or exporting to the U.S. market may think that they are excluded from these rules and regulations. This is a gross misconception. Regulatory authorities worldwide [5] are in the process of adopting the guidelines laid down in 21 CFR Part 11. The latest release of the European GMPs [14] mandates audit trails for electronic records, which goes beyond even the latest FDA requirements. The PIC/S inspection guideline [11] is now the *de facto* global inspection standard for automated systems, irrespective of the fact that the FDA will not be able to formally adopt the standard for legal reasons. All guidance and legislation have the same principles in common and by complying with the GMPs and 21 CFR 11 one will comply with most or all other applicable regulations. The focus of this chapter therefore is on Part 11 as the leading regulation.

Industries not directly impacted by 21 CFR Part 11 can also gain tremendously from understanding and implementing the principles of this rule. The pharmaceutical and medical devices industry should also look at other sectors, such as the food industry, for beneficial validation approaches.

While the authorities describe the *what* element of computer systems validation in their guidance documents, it is up to process owners and manufacturers to prove logically and consistently the *how* element. Consequently, sensible and affordable approaches are a *must*.

What are these approaches and how can they be implemented to comply with current regulatory requirements? This chapter provides answers to these questions.

THE ASSESSMENT PROCESS

Software is one of the most complex items man has ever created. Compared with other complex systems, developed software has the added disadvantage that one cannot see it, listen to it or feel it. Software can be defined as an assembly of a large number of elements interrelating in a multitude of ways. Therefore complex software cannot be understood in its entirety during development, testing, or use without the application of the assessment process, the primary tool for the appraisal and categorization of automated systems.

While for new systems, qualification and validation can be incorporated into the software development and implementation process, to ensure that the software can be fully understood and that quality is "programmed" into it [8,9], this is not always the case with *existing software*. The regulators would like to see the same level of documentation for existing and new automated systems [12,13], but in reality their expectations are rarely met. This is one of the main reasons why legacy systems need to be looked at from an entirely different angle.

Although it may sound trivial, the first thing you must remember is — *don't panic*!

Any attempt at problem-solving ahead without a strategy and sound planning is, at best, a waste of time and money. There is no "ready-made" legacy systems validation protocol, so it is quintessential to have a plan, i.e., *a strategy*.

This chapter is a cookbook with a variety of recipes to choose from; whichever recipe you select depends entirely on the particular circumstances for a given automated system.

The Strategy Document

Strategy should always be part of formal approved and controlled documentation, which can be changed and improved with the experience gained over time. The resulting strategy document is a vital component, and the team defining strategy and scope need to include members drawn from quality assurance, management, and IT departments.

The strategy document should define:

- The rationale for the assessment (reasons and expectations).
- Which parts of the enterprise shall be assessed (boundaries).
- Which regulatory rules and regulations must be referenced.
- Which internal guidance documents apply.
- The company's interpretation of the rules.
- Who will conduct the assessment.
- How the assessment will be conducted and documented.
- The required resources in monetary, time, and manpower terms.

The document should be written in a manner presentable to inspectorates, and also to the board of directors within the company, as it will outline the financial implications of the undertaking. Generally, the strategy is defined for an entire company or site. Careful consideration and planning at this stage is highly recommended, as the processes that follow generally take months or years to complete.

A uniform and consistent approach throughout the company is therefore advantageous from a project control and financial viewpoint. As a result of this policy, it becomes apparent that additional guidance documents such as clear standard operating procedures (SOPs), training procedures, or additional resources, are required. This approach will provide vital information on the length and breadth of the task in hand.

Recognizing the need to assess legacy systems and rectify any deficiencies may seem an obvious task to certain individuals within a company. All senior management must be made aware of the problem, must ultimately take responsibility for it, and act as sponsors for the legacy computer systems validation project. Quality assurance is a key component of automated systems validation and is the responsibility of senior management; although the task of assuring quality can be satisfactorily delegated, the responsibility for the end result may not.

It is strongly advised that a strategy document is written, approved, and ready for presentation in the event that it is required during a regulatory inspection. The strategy document provides evidence of a company's commitment and willingness to undertake the necessary steps. Without this documentary evidence, steps may be taken against the company by the regulators.

Recent citations by the FDA [1] were based on the fact that some companies had more than one approach to legacy systems validation within different parts of their enterprise. This resulted in contradictory protocols, interpretations, and results.

The favored approach must be having one approach and one interpretation within a company. The rationale for this is the adherence to existing laws and regulations, that require companies to apply qualification and validation to parts or all of their computer systems.

If this only applies to parts of the company then this must be clearly stated, reasons given, and the boundaries well defined. Although the number of regulations dealing directly with computerized systems is limited, others apply to systems supported by the automation in question. This interlink is crucial and again shows the need to ensure that the IT expert and the end user work together in a partnership.

The most inconspicuous entry in the list above deals with the company's interpretation of the rule. However, this is the one with the farthest-reaching consequences. This will become clearer when we have a look at the different assessment methods and the resulting consequences. The following example will illustrate just how far-reaching the consequences of the interpretation can be.

The FDA states in 21 CFR Part 11 [4] that:

> electronic signatures can be applied, and if they are then they must comply with the rule ... Clearly, the FDA does not require a company to apply electronic signatures, if they do not want to. A company may now decide that they interpret those cases where signatures are applied both electronically and by hand on a printout of a document, not to be electronic signatures. In the company's view this will eliminate compliance with the electronic signature rules for all cases where there still is a 'wet ink' signature. It is obvious that this will lessen the company's workload. Whether or not this interpretation is acceptable to the authorities is an entirely different matter.

Another major benefit immediately arising from a clear understanding of the requirements for automated legacy systems assessments is through the relationship between the suppliers and the users of automated systems. Suppliers need to understand their customers' specific requests, needs or wishes with respect to their approach and the contents of their automated legacy system compliance assessment. Often the customers, i.e., the users, have a much more in-depth understanding of the regulations, whereas the supplier may be selling mainly into a nonhealth care customer base, thus mainly unaware of the specific legal requirements. Texts in advertisements and product descriptions, claiming full 21 CFR 11 compliance or FDA approval for a product should be approached with care and apprehension. Only a few companies have so far proved to have the appropriate quality systems, inhouse expertise and build the right functionality for compliance into their products. As part of the assessment and remediation process, the users will regularly contact the vendors to obtain information to either fill gaps in the system assessment documents, or to discuss remedial actions, for example, migration to a compliant release version.

The decision as to who will conduct the assessment within the company should be based on staff availability, their training and understanding of the task, and particularly on the estimated time and cost expectations. Few companies have sufficient resources inhouse to conduct the assessment process with the necessary level of expertise and within the time constraints. The process is sometimes accelerated through involvement of the regulators.

Inspections may identify deficiencies or noncompliant practices, resulting in enforcement proceedings against the company, which require immediate action. In most cases external resources will be brought in to help with either part of, or the entire, process. If this is envisaged, it should be planned for in the strategy document.

In most cases, the overall validation process for both legacy and new systems stretches over months, or even years. It is therefore prudent to distinguish between immediate, i.e., short-term measures, and long-term activities.

Immediate activities are aimed at achieving compliance through measures implemented with limited effort, often resulting in "hybrid" systems. The term hybrid system [9,15] is generally used to describe a system that fails to fulfil all sections of the FDA ruling; those parts which fail are substituted by administrative or technical measures. The immediate aim is to secure the ongoing use of the system.

Long-term actions should always result in a fully compliant system, and this can ultimately mean replacing the system. There are a variety of good reasons why some tasks will take a long time, such as replacements not being available immediately, which then need to be handled as part of a long-term strategy.

Retrospective validation work is acknowledged to be considerably more expensive than prospective activities. The cost estimates included in the strategy document should also be included in the company's financial planning documents. Failure to do so may jeopardize the success of the project and could result in citations from the regulators. As mentioned many times before, the regulators only believe in documented evidence, not in "lip service."

Summary

- Create a rationale for assessing a large part of or the entire enterprise.
- Identify and interpret the applicable regulations.
- Define the assessment process.
- Establish the timetable for remedial action and plan the resources required.

The System Assessment Documents

The assessment process for legacy automation systems is comparable to the risk assessment process [9,16–18], something with which people from other departments may already be familiar with, such as manufacturing or production, health, safety, or the environment. As in these other areas, it is equally important to define the process, tools, deliverables, and associated documents. With regard to the computerized legacy systems assessment process, these activities are encompassed in the inventory and the assessment protocols. Without a complete, accurate, and constantly updated inventory no work should start; you will either find that you have to go back and do additional work (at inflated cost), or that an inspector will find those systems you have overlooked, and will challenge you. You do not want to be in either position. Thus the first step is the creation of the system inventory.

The System Inventory

IT infrastructure within a company comprises both software and hardware. For all existing legacy systems, a complete inventory is a prerequisite for any type of assessment. From experience this is an ideal opportunity to update or create the documentation for the IT infrastructure in a suitable manner for both internal and external presentation. Inventory tables should be complemented by graphical illustrations, where appropriate. The IT network configuration is a good example, where several layers of increasingly detailed maps provide a quick and efficient overview, both of the existing and the planned infrastructure.

Many companies in 1999 put much effort into creating comprehensive inventories in preparation for the Year 2000 (Y2K) problem; these inventories are today an excellent source of information for legacy systems. However, a word of caution is appropriate here. The Y2K assessment process focused on date fields and calculations based on (or for) yielding dates.

The legacy system assessment has a much wider focus and its consequences are more far-reaching. There is no easy fix for legacy systems, such as setting the clock back a number of years to fool the system. If we take an example such as Lotus Notes, the Y2K assessment would have been fine; but the legacy system assessment must pay attention to all applications created within Lotus Notes. The most striking difference between the Y2K problem and computer systems validation is simply this: there is no end date for computer systems validation.

Identifying those systems which fall under the GMP, good clinical practice (GCP), or good laboratory practice (GLP) regulations (generically known as GxPs), requires the assessment team to recognize whether a particular system can or will influence product quality. It is also prudent to simultaneously assess the impact of a system on business performance (e.g., a finance software package). Even if not GxP critical, it may still have a profound impact on business operations and the company may therefore decide to qualify it too. Knowing which of the product-quality critical systems is also business-critical will make it easy for the company to assign priorities. It is unlikely that the critical systems will be in compliance with regulations, so remedial work should start on systems assigned the highest priority. Those who do not have to comply with any of the GxP regulations may want to assess their systems with regards to the business impact only.

Information for the inventory is likely to be based on existing information, and is usually stored in either a spreadsheet or database form. Manufacturing, for example, is likely to maintain an up-to-date and complete inventory of all of its computerized systems. However, this may not be the case within administrative sections, although they are likely to handle quality-critical product data, such as customer shipment information. When deciding on the format for the inventory, it may be advantageous to make use of existing formats. Care should be taken to only use those formats that can be handled with ease, and are widely acceptable and suitable for all sites in all countries.

Even a "simple" paper document can cause endless problems. If for example, the original was designed in Europe in DIN A4 format, this can result in missing information on printouts on American standard format paper. When using electronic formats, care should be taken to allow for all alphabets and symbols in use in the company. Most modern software packages incorporate Unicode, which allows representation of any language, and by converting outputs to a generic format, such as PDF, shortcomings of other program outputs can be overcome.

Once the inventory is generated it will be subject to change as systems are added, modified and retired. As the inventory is a crucial document for continued compliance with regulations, as it provides an overview of all of the systems owned by the company, these changes should be managed under a formal *change management* procedure. It is not uncommon for companies to stop changes to the inventory immediately prior to the assessment process. If this were not done then, apart from the risk of missing certain changes, the inventory would itself become another legacy system, something that should be avoided if at all possible.

The authorities are very reluctant to accept noncompliant legacy systems and their patience is fast running out when they find new unqualified and unvalidated systems. For the authorities, it is no longer acceptable to find that companies are developing and implementing nonvalidated automated systems with quality critical components [1]. It is bad business practice to permit the uncontrolled development and use of any computerized system, irrespective of GxP criticality.

Whether the inventory is generated first, followed by the assessment, or whether the two tasks are carried out in parallel, is a decision based on practical considerations; most companies will attempt both tasks simultaneously. This is partially because the compilation of the inventory, and the assessment of the items it contains, requires the input of users and local support functions. As always, spare time is hard to find and it is often more economical to divert resources to this exercise once, if feasible. For examples of inventories see the sections on the assessment protocols.

Companies complying with GxP regulations and suppliers of software and hardware solutions regularly refer to and apply the guidance found in the Good Automated Manufacturing Practices (GAMP) [9] documents.

Summary

- Update the existing inventories.
- Classify entries.
- Reference legislation for additional guidance.

GAMP Categorization

The GAMP [9] documents have proven very popular with many companies for several reasons. In the absence of more detailed regulatory guidance, these guidelines provide the only international guidance documents. There are other guidance documents available [19, 20], but they are all limited either to particular countries or regions, or cover only one specific legacy computer system topic. The GAMP Guide provides guidance for users and suppliers, slotting all types of software into categories.* This simplicity makes this guide very attractive to industry.

The GAMP Guide† is currently in its fourth edition (published December 2001). Although GAMP is not an official guidance document it has been endorsed by all the major regulatory bodies, and is considered an international reference. The guide is not designed specifically for the retrospective assessment and validation of existing systems and is therefore limited in its usefulness for legacy systems.§

GAMP at present classes automated systems within five categories.

- *Category 1 Operating Systems*
  Established, commercially available operating systems, which are used in pharmaceutical manufacture.

- *Category 2 Firmware*
  Instrumentation and controllers often incorporate nonuser-programmable firmware. Examples include weigh scales, bar code scanners, three-term controllers. They are configurable.

- *Category 3 Standard Software Packages*
  These are commercially available, off-the-shelf standard software packages. Examples include statistical analysis packages and laboratory instrumentation software.

- *Category 4 Configurable Software Packages*
  These provide configurable standard software interfaces and functions. Examples include distributed control systems (DCS), supervisory control and

*See Vol. 4, Appendix M4.
†http://www.ispe.org.
§See Vol. 4, page 14.

Table 12.1 Assessment matrix

Company Name Department	Category	System	ID Number	GAMP category 5	GAMP category 4	GAMP category 3	GAMP category 2	GAMP category 1
IT								
	Network operating systems	Novell 4.11						
		Windows NT 4.0						
		Windows 2000 Server						
		Windows 2000 Advanced Server						
	Applications and systems	Microsoft Visio						
		Backup Exec						
		Adobe Acrobat Reader						
Quality Control Laboratory	HPLC							
		Waters						
		Agilent						
	GC							
		Varian						
		Spectra Physics						
etc.								

data acquisition packages (SCADA), manufacturing execution systems (MES) and some laboratory information management systems (LIMS) and management resource planning (MRP) packages. A typical feature of these systems is that they permit users to develop their own applications by configuring or amending predefined software modules and also developing new application software modules. Each application (of the standard product) is therefore specific to the user process.

- *Category 5 Custom (bespoke) Software*
  There are many instances of this type of system in the pharmaceutical industry that meet the specific needs of the user.

GAMP Category Application

It should be noted that complex systems often have layers of software, and one system could exhibit several or even all of the above categories. An off-the-shelf LIMS will require configuration, but links to existing applications are likely to call for customized solutions.

This classification strongly correlates with the suggested qualification, validation levels and efforts for each category. So this guide may seem to be the right thing to use. Before jumping to that conclusion, however, one should bear in mind that the above was written for new systems. Even the latest edition of GAMP [9] does not cover legacy (in the meaning of already existing) systems in detail; written for the pharmaceutical industry, it has a slight bias toward U.S. regulations. And last, but not least, it does not offer universal and easy-to-apply solutions to all legacy system problems. It is a valuable tool which should be used, as appropriate, in the qualification and validation of computer systems.

Table 12.1 is just one example of an assessment matrix categorizing automated systems according to GAMP.

The completion of this matrix will allow the grouping together of systems that require a particular level of validation. For legacy systems, this categorization is much too broad and simplistic to be of any significant value. The assessment protocols require a lot more refinement and the following chapters will detail how these assessment protocols can be developed and put to good use. Table 12.1 has already undergone a further categorization step by grouping the entries by department. Obviously, a breakdown of the automated systems inventory into segments such as LotusPage for your notes applications, process logic controllers associated with equipment in manufacturing, gas chromatographs in the laboratory, etc., can provide a much more manageable structure to the assessment process.

Summary

- Classify inventory entries according to system type.

- Gain guidance from GAMP.
- Feel free to refine and add information.

General and Detailed Assessment Protocols

The deliverable from the assessment process, initiated by the strategy document and based on the inventory, is a document providing details for all existing computerized systems, their level of compliance with the rules and regulations (in the understanding of the company), and any remediation work necessary. It should be noted that all inspectorates expect to find descriptions for all inspectable systems (their use, purpose and validation status, as a minimum). Often for existing systems this information has become outdated or is even missing.

The decision on whether the assessment process is divided into a general assessment and a detailed assessment, or whether only a detailed assessment will be carried out, is largely dependent on the size of the task, the available resources and is ultimately a management decision. As both approaches are successfully followed by industry, it would be difficult to make a recommendation on which to choose.

As a result, this chapter will present both ways in order to provide complete coverage. From a practical viewpoint the assessment protocols should be organized into categories, and grouped by department area, etc. For example, it is most likely that the automated analytical systems are assessed by qualified computer systems validation personnel, backed up by appropriate operators, scientists, and technicians from each area.

It is initially sensible to test more than one version of the assessment protocol to find the one most suitable for the company. It will become clear within a very short time which approach suits the business best, or is the most practical solution. This decision should then be recorded in the strategy document, and any deviations from this approach avoided, if that is possible. Any changes at a later stage in the process will have a knock-on effect, impacting on cost and efforts.

It must be reiterated at this point that the hardware is as much a part of the assessment process as the software. The hardware platform and its architecture has a profound impact on many regulatory aspects, such as security, access protocols, etc. Hardware is typically maintained by the IT department and may not have been assessed for compliance in the past.

To answer some questions, one has to look beyond the software and hardware aspects, and consider the system environment, such as facilities, company documentation procedures (including system manuals), or training programs.

The General Assessment Protocol

The assessment itself is often named a gap or risk analysis [9, 16–18]. The terminology is ambiguous and each company should define, either in the policy document or in the quality manual, the terms and acronyms used in connection with this task.

If it is desirable to gain a general overview or to collate a limited set of data for further refinement of the assessment process, then this general or high level assessment is the process of choice. As a minimum, it will identify and classify the systems into the following three categories:

- Computerized systems requiring qualification and validation because they impact on product quality.
- Computerized systems that do not impact on product quality but have a significant impact on business performance.
- Computerized systems that do not have an impact on either of the above.

These categories assume that systems affecting product quality implicitly also impact on business performance. From a regulatory standpoint, no further action is required for systems that impact neither of these areas. It may, however, become apparent that there are gaps in the documentation of these systems and the company may wish to correct this.

Systems not impacting product quality do not require qualification and validation. It is, however, prudent to determine if the existing procedures (e.g., backup, archiving, access control, etc.), and the life cycle documentation are of sufficient standard to enable system maintenance to be carried out under change control.

Often yes or no answers are replaced by more fine-tuned terms, such as: in full, to a greater part, partly, to a lesser part, not applicable. Another method is to assign numerical values to each term, thus providing a means for creating a "weighed" answer. Tables 12.2 and 12.3 are just typical examples.

Although this is a simple query matrix, completing it requires additional clarification and explanations. In this case such details should be found in the SOP referenced on the assessment protocol. The example document indicates that separate assessment protocols were created for each site and each building. In other cases it may be more sensible to break the documents down by department. A managed protocol numbering system is advisable for tracking and reconciliation purposes. System boundaries may not always be easy to identify. One may define physical boundaries or base the boundaries on system drawings. Printing system identification numbers may be helpful for grouping systems. We must remember that this protocol is mainly concerned with automated parts of the system.

So here inventory completeness refers to the inventory document, which must detail all automated system parts.

The questions on impact on product quality and business operations are usually straightforward. If either or both of these questions are answered with "yes" a detailed assessment will be required.

More detailed questions may be included in the general assessment, and while

Table 12.2 General assessment protocol for an existing computerized system

General assessment protocol for an existing computerized system

Manufacturing Site A
Building C

Document Number XXXYYYZZZ

Assessors (Name, Department):

Date of Assessment:

For help and advice consult SOP XYZ or contact the program manager at extension xxxx

system	inventory complete	impact on product quality	business operations	detailed assessment	electronic records	electronic signatures	system qualified	system validated	comments
	yes/no	yes/no	yes/no	yes/no	yes/no	yes/no	yes/no	yes/no	
shrink wrapper	no	no	no	no	yes	no	no	no	
FTIR	yes	yes	no	yes	yes	yes	yes	no	
etc.									

Table 12.3 General assessment protocol for an existing computerized system

General assessment protocol for an existing computerized system

Manufacturing Site A
Building C

Document Number XXXYYYZZZ

Assessors (Name, Department):

Date of Assessment:

For help and advice consult SOP XYZ or contact the program manager at extension xxxx

system	inventory complete	impact on product quality	business operations	detailed assessment	electronic records	electronic signatures	system qualified	system validated	comments
	%	3,2,1 (a)	3,2,1 (b)	yes/no (c)	5,4,3, 2,1,0 (d)	yes/no (e)	yes/no	yes/no	
shrink wrapper	no	1	1	no	–	–	–	–	
FTIR	yes	3	2	yes	3	1	1996	1997	
etc.									

(a) 3 = yes, 2 = indirect, 1 = no. (b) 3 = high, 2 = medium, 1 = low. (c) sum >3 = yes, sum ❑ 3 = no. (d) 5, 4, 3, 2, 1 = GAMP, 0 = no. (e) 3 = yes, 2 = not actively used, 1 = no.

providing a wealth of information, collating the answers may be too time-consuming. The assessments require a sound understanding of the issues, the company's interpretation of the rules and a certain amount of pragmatism. This may be beyond the requirements for the preceding questions.

The question of whether an electronic record is created may already be difficult to answer if the data is only stored transiently. The FDA guidance on "Scope and Application" [10] provides some pragmatic views, challenging the users to define whether the use of the automated system is purely incidental or whether an electronic record is created that the users rely upon. It may not always be easy to find an answer when carrying out the assessment and one should rather err on the safe side (consider it an electronic record), especially if the use of the record has not yet been defined in a written document.

Also, whether a legacy system is qualified or validated is never a trivial question. Even if archived validation protocols did not include testing for compliance with 21 CFR Part 11 (FDA's rule on electronic records, electronic signatures [4]) it is normal practice to consider the systems to be in a validated state. The shortcoming of not addressing the issue of e-records and e-signatures is the logical conclusion and result of the assessment process. Again, one should consult the FDA's "Scope and Application" guidance [10], which explicitly requires compliance with all rules and regulations in force at the time, i.e., compliance with the predicate rules, the current GMP.

As judgement and probably bias is unavoidable, it is good practice to provide comments with all entries to document the reasons for the choice of entry. One way to add more information to the entries is shown in the example in Table 12.3. It is the same as Table 12.2, but the answers are much more detailed and therefore fewer comments may be required.

More detail can, of course, be included in these tables and other aspects such as impact on safety, health, and environment (SHE) are also sometimes added. This all depends on the particular needs of each company, and no one example will suit everyone.

Where does a general assessment end and a detailed one start? The previous examples are suitable for high-level assessments. Although the systems are assessed and categorized, the high level assessment does not provide an answer to the question of what exactly is noncompliant with a particular system and what must be done about it!

An assessment without this information would be like a mechanic stating that there is something wrong with your car, but not what it is and how it can be fixed.

Summary

- Establish general assessment protocols.
- Include systems critical for regulatory compliance and business needs.

- Eliminate unimportant systems from further assessments.
- Provides a "feel" for the level of compliance of the systems.
- Use the information obtained to refine the project plan.

The Detailed Assessment Protocol

In-depth information on a system is obtained by conducting a detailed assessment. This allows the assessor to find deficiencies in compliance, identify recurring gaps and problems, and enables the analysis and design of remedial actions. It is clear that the completion of these protocols requires a thorough understanding of the assessment process and the automated systems concerned, including their use within the company. The topic of training becomes very important here and more information on this is given in the next section.

These detailed protocols can take different forms, e.g., spreadsheets, tables, and can be completed either manually or electronically. The following examples are suggestions and are by no means universal solutions.

The example shown in Table 12.4 and Table 12.5 was created using a flowsheet program. The selection criterion was the GAMP category 9 and for each separate category individual check sheets were created. The text of the applicable guidance document (21 CFR Part 11 [4]) is included and extended to provide additional guidance to the assessors, and to include the company's interpretation of the requirements.

Table 12.4 Title page

Site:	*U.S. East Coast* Document Reference Number: *2001/07-048*		
System name:	*Varian Gas Chromatograph*		
System reference:	*VCMG/A/1*		
System components:	*3300 Gas Chromatograph and 8200 Autosampler, Genesis Headspace*		
System category:	*GAMP Category 4*		
	print name	signature	date
Assessor:	*A. Senior*		
Asset owner:	*B. Junior*		
Quality assurance:	*C. Ontroller*		

Table 12.5 Assessment page

21 CFR Part 11 Assessment	Reference	**Specific requirements for compliance (bold)** *and recommended controls for compliance (italics)*	Complies Yes/No	Comments
Controls for closed systems				
Have the electronic records been defined?	11.1(b)	**All electronic records generated, held, manipulated or transmitted by the system have been identified and assessed if they fall under the part 11 rule, i.e., electronic data that are required under a predicated rule or are submitted to the FDA.**	Yes	Listed at end of table.
Has the "raw" data been defined?	11.1(b)	*Defining what is "raw" data helps in determining what electronic records apply to the system.*	Yes	Provide a reference to the document where the raw data definition or analysis can be found.
Can system be defined as "closed"?	11.3 (4)	*For closed systems §11.30 does not apply.*	N/A	
Is the system validated?	11.10(a)	**The system is validated to ensure accurate and reliable performance.**	Yes	Validation — IQ, OQ, and PQ completed.
	11.10(a)	*A current validation report covering the system is in place, demonstrating no significant deviations in system status from the regulatory requirements.*	Yes	Validation — IQ, OQ, and PQ completed — no validation report.
	11.10(a)	*Procedures specify periodic review of the validity of system configuration and performance.*	No	There is no periodic review, but if there is a change to the system this will fall under the current change control procedure.

The previous examples provide an insight into how detailed the assessment questionnaires should be.

Table 12.6 is typical of the variety of items found on a system inventory. It can be used as both a progress reporting tool and as a project-management tool.

The development of the questionnaires on which to base the necessary qualification and validation activities for compliance purposes or to satisfy internal business needs, is the most important step in the entire assessment process. Everything that follows is a direct consequence of these protocols. Now it is time to execute these protocols and it is vital that as much effort is put into their completion as was needed to initially create them. Only specially trained (internal and external) staff should be employed in the delivery of this task. Personnel training requirements are described in more detail hereafter.

Summary

- Write the detailed protocols for systems identified in the general assessment.
- Add detail as required by your industry and take into account relevant legislation.
- Include business requirements, such as document retention times.
- Provide guidance for the use of the detailed assessment protocols.

Training

With the strategy document and the general and detailed assessment questionnaires available, it is time to think about executing the assessment, collating the information, judging what actions may be necessary as a result of the assessment process and, most importantly, decide who will do it.

The system user generally has the best knowledge about the computerized system's use, but may lack knowledge or understanding of the underlying IT structures. Many staff will also have a deficit in understanding the requirements for regulatory compliance. In order to overcome these problems, it would seem sensible to adopt a team approach when executing the assessment.

There should be a core team of assessors who do understand the issues and have been trained in the applicable regulatory compliance guidelines. Depending on the size of the company or the specific task, it will be necessary to train additional staff from within the various departments.

Faced with such a task for the first time often seems daunting, and the question arises as to who will be suitably qualified to execute the assessment and how the chosen approach can be benchmarked against industry's best practice.

Many companies do not have sufficient or appropriate resources in-house to initiate the process and specialist consultants [20] will be hired to provide the necessary assistance. Although this is a sensible approach, care should be taken to

Table 12.6 Inventory

Department	ID	Description	Model, Vendor or Application	Category	Assessment
Formulation	58	Blender	Labmaster 2000	Equipment	complete
Formulation	77	Particle size analyzer	United	Equipment	complete
Information technology	60	Workstation	Agilent ChemStation	Equipment	to be done
Information technology	74	Server	Microsoft Windows NT	Equipment	complete
Information technology	76	Server	Oracle	Equipment	complete
Information technology	59	Software	Adobe Acrobat Reader	Software	to be done
Materials management	65	Batch status	MS Office Excel	Data file	to be done
Materials management	68	Inventories	MS Office Excel	Data file	to be done
Packaging	61	Bar code scanner	Allen Bradley	Equipment	to be done
Production	62	Check-weigher	Anritsu	Equipment	to be done
Production	64	Coater	GLATT	Equipment	to be done
Quality assurance	71	Rejection reports	MS Office Word	Data file	to be done
Quality assurance	72	Stability data	MS Office Excel	Data file	to be done
Quality assurance	73	Internal audits SOP	MS Office Word	Data file	to be done
Quality control	63	FT-IR spectrometer	Bruker	Equipment	to be done
Quality control	79	TOC analyzer	Sievers	Equipment	complete
Quality control	81	Workstation	Waters Millenium	Equipment	complete
Regulatory	69	Submissions	MS Office Word	Data file	to be done
Validation	70	Validation SOPs	MS Office Word	Data file	to be done
Validation	78	Portable calibrator	Gauss	Equipment	complete

ensure that the knowledge gained by the consultants is transferred to the team and becomes part of the knowledge pool of the company.

Simply purchasing the questionnaires should also be discouraged as only an understanding of the underlying principles and rationales can lead to a useful result. Thus front-end support and training using actual examples from within the company is a highly efficient way of getting started and getting it right first time.

An observation often made is the fact that quality assurance (QA) personnel have limited knowledge of IT systems and operations and IT staff have little appreciation for the regulatory environment and its implications. This is a primary area on which to focus training. In some cases it may be advisable to consider the appointment of an IT QA manager.

The training benefits are manifold. Staff training means that the workforce receives the qualifications required by the regulators. It also means that the understanding and awareness of the issues involved are improved. It is particularly interesting to see the considerable changes in the quality and numbers of entries in inventory lists once the contributors have received their training. What may have been a mere listing of hardware items will develop into a comprehensive systems inventory. The training should yield confident assessors, and users or system owners who have the knowledge to provide the right information.

Summary

- Establish training needs.
- Train the trainer or assessor.
- Bring in external resources and knowledge base if beneficial.

The Assessment

With everything in place, from the questionnaires to the training, the procedures and all of the support needed, the assessments should now get under way. Many entries on the inventory will not contain any electronic records or electronic signatures and will not be business critical.

Filling in the forms for these items will be an easy task, particularly if the inventory database and the forms are linked electronically to facilitate automatic data entry. It is an often voiced misconception that it is unnecessary to document and assess those systems that will not be inspected. Inspectors will want to see documented evidence of your decision process that leads you (the system owner) to believe that the system is out of inspection scope. Lack of such documentation can result in a deficiency citation.

Where the situation is not so obvious, and where the necessity for a detailed assessment can be assumed, the team needs to plan the time and location for it.

Sometimes the system owner or user is also the assessor; but more often than not the assessors will have to arrange for a meeting with the person familiar with the system. Time and progress estimates should be based on the latter scenario.

Depending on the complexity of the systems, the available documentation and information, experience shows that an assessor can complete between two and six detailed assessments per day. This will also include the time taken to formulate appropriate actions for those areas where deficiencies with the requirements have been identified. The limiting factor in most cases is the availability of the system user or owner, who is often occupied with meeting the daily needs of the business, which must be given first priority.

For a medium-sized establishment this assessment process will therefore take, on average, from several weeks to a few months. Multisite and multinational companies will probably need several months to complete the task. More likely, this will be an ongoing exercise, as there seem to be no relenting in the number of takeovers and mergers, which regularly create the need for additional assessments or reviews of those already completed. The time consumed by the assessment process will have significant financial implications, and these costs are often not included in the company's financial projects and budget forecasts.

Not all assessments will be as straightforward as was first thought, and the guidance documents may not give the answer, or at least not the detail, sought. In these instances it is advantageous to have a designated person (the project manager?) or a committee that will deal with any queries. In addition to providing guidance and answers to the assessors, there is also an opportunity to refine the internal guidance literature and to consolidate methods and solutions within the company.

The most efficient way to consider and decide on remedial actions for any type of deficiency identified is during the assessment itself. Often the system users or owners will already have deliberated on systems or procedures improvements and they should be aware of any limitations that would favor one solution over another.

The completed and signed-off assessment forms are collated and grouped, for example, by system type, department, deficiency profile, suggested remedial actions and any other sensible criteria. If there are more than just a handful of systems, such an approach is always preferable as it minimizes the workload resulting from the assessments.

The next section will provide more detail on the possible outcome of these assessments and potential corrective action measures.

Summary

- Prioritize the assessment exercise, e.g., by department, system, etc.
- Start with the most complex systems.
- Include the system user or owner in the assessment process.

- Decide on practicable short and long-term remediation work during the assessment.
- Group completed assessments by type of system or suggested corrective action.

Results and Options

With the exception of very specific systems or special circumstances, it is industry's experience that virtually no IT system is in complete compliance with the GxP regulations, and in particular with 21 CFR Part 11. This statement has several important implications.

- Pharmaceutical companies are using noncompliant IT systems and they are aware of it.
- So are the regulators, and they want industry to take action on this matter. That is what this chapter is about.

First we need to look at the options available to a company when the assessment comes up with a noncompliant system. There are five standard approaches:

- Redefine the use of the system — is it necessary for the application or is the use of the system purely incidental?
- Add procedural controls — this is often only a short-term solution.
- Upgrade the system — the preferred solution if cost and timescales are reasonable.
- Replace the system — a clean, but drastic solution.
- Retire the system — the medium- to long-term solution for systems that will never be compliant.

All options are open to a user but the implications vary widely. These are best explained using practical examples.

A laboratory is running an analytical test method and the result is calculated using an MS Excel spreadsheet which is stored on a networked PC with no particular access restrictions. All laboratory staff can use the spreadsheet when needed. The mathematical result is used in the release procedure for the product. There are clearly a number of deficiencies here that require immediate action.

Retiring the system would mean using paper again and using a second person to check the calculations. This may well be a suitable option in this case.

There is no obvious need to replace or upgrade the system as the spreadsheet itself is well suited for carrying out the calculations, and another system would probably require the same effort for bringing it into compliance.

Adding procedural controls may be a good option here. The spreadsheet could be password protected, it could be stored on a nonnetworked PC, and a standard operating procedure (SOP) could detail further control aspects.

Redefining the use of the system does not seem to be an option as the result would remain product quality critical.

A document management application is used for creating controlled documents, such as SOPs. The present program version does not have audit trail functionality.

One option would be to consider this system as purely incidental use of a computer system ("typewriter rule"). This will require the company to rely on the paper documents for daily use. In this case no further action is required.

If, however, the documents are distributed and accessed in their electronic format on a regular basis, then these will be electronic records and 21 CFR 11 applies. Retiring the system would mean reverting to paper again; not a likely solution. Implementing a paper-based audit trail is an enormous effort, particularly as a logbook alone cannot satisfy the requirements for complete contents and version control, including date and time stamps. As the system obviously satisfies most of the users' needs and the regulators' expectations, a good solution would be to approach the vendor for an updated version that provides the required functionality.

Clearly, each system must be analyzed for its merits and to determine the most appropriate way forward to achieve compliance or the users' requirements. This is a project in its own right and requires serious planning and the allocation of resources. This is discussed in detail in the following sections.

Summary

- All is fine? — Well done.
- There is a problem? — you have five options.

MANAGING LEGACY SYSTEMS (EXECUTION)

With few exceptions, there will be a short-term activity followed by a long-term strategy, that will bring the existing computerized systems into compliance with current legislation or users' requirements. These activities will have been defined and approved as detailed in the previous parts of this chapter. It is now time to execute these plans and we will look at the issues around the various options that may have been selected, and the associated project needs.

From the assessments, all of the information is now available: the number and particular types of systems, the associated deficiencies, necessary remedial actions, and the urgency with which these should be implemented. All of this information, when entered into a suitable planning tool, provides the company with an action plan, information on the project duration and milestones, plus associated cost and manpower estimates. This plan is exactly what the regulatory authorities are looking for. It is also the tool that management must have for the purposes of planning, budgeting, and project control. It does, however, make any weaknesses in the company's assets or procedures highly visible. To overcome or rectify these weaknesses, it is necessary to choose from one of the five options mentioned in the results and options section. Here we want to look at each option in detail to evaluate the pros and cons. Ultimately, the choice of action will determine the quality, cost, and time of the resulting solution.

Decommissioning (System Retirement)

When an IT system is obsolete, superfluous, inappropriate or unsuitable for validation, then decommissioning is the right choice. Again, this should be performed in a planned and documented manner. Depending on the type of computerized system and the volume of data, the archiving or migration of data should be considered. It is unlikely that none of the data are relevant to the business, which would be the only circumstance in which data deletion and system destruction is the straightforward option. If the use of the system is discontinued, the data will need archiving, using a suitable storage media and location. This procedure may either follow an SOP on data archiving or a specific protocol for the application concerned. In either case, data retrieval and the completeness and accuracy (trustworthiness) of the data should be tested on a representative sample. The verification process could employ check sums, file size figures, comparison of printouts, etc. The suitability of the archiving format should be assessed in advance. Following the data archiving the obsolete software application should be deleted from the system. Specialists from IT should ensure that the software application has been completely removed.

If the data are still required, then migration of the data to a new software application must be evaluated.

A typical example would be the replacement of workflow information stored as text and tables, which was created using standard text and spreadsheet software applications by an enterprise management system. Such a system can store information on batch sizes, status, location, etc. This information would have been held in numerous locations, on different systems, and in potentially incompatible formats by various people. Rather than having to address a large number of systems, these would be decommissioned and replaced by just one (new) system. The benefits are obvious and the applications would still be available, although in a different environment and format.

Systems that are especially prone to retirement are those that are only kept alive by the common notion that "We always do it this way." Where progress can provide improvement, progress should be made.

Redefining the System

Instead of retiring or decommissioning a system it may be possible, or desirable, to redefine its use or role. This would allow the continued use of the system without the need for potentially extensive remedial work.

In the context of 21 CFR Part 11, for example, the requirement to maintain records under predicate rules or submitted to FDA, and that are maintained in electronic format *in place of paper format*, are considered to fall under the rule [1, 10]. A laboratory may be used for the analysis of drug substances and for research purposes. If there are several systems serving this dual purpose, it may be possible to dedicate just some of these to analysis only. The regulators would not be concerned with any of the other systems. With this "simple" move the situation is simplified and savings are achieved. Clearly it is necessary to incorporate this procedure into the relevant SOPs and to train and audit staff working under these changed circumstances.

Where both electronic and paper records are created, it is now permissible to define (preferably in an SOP), which of these the master record is. This must reflect actual business practice. The system owner should be challenged if loss of the electronic record is acceptable. The answer should of course be yes. Where paper records can be defined as the master records, compliance with 21 CFR 11 is no longer a requirement.

Replacement or Upgrade?

This is probably the solution that first springs to mind when discrepancies are found with a system. However, unless the company using the system is producing its own hardware or programming its own software, obtaining a solution will be entirely dependent on vendor offerings. In most instances the latter will be the case. Few vendors will have a suitable upgrade or replacement available when needed. This is partly because many software packages or programs are written for clients from a wide range of industries, that typically are far less regulated than the pharmaceutical industry, and also because equipment or hardware vendors prefer to sell particular models in large numbers before they make available any new or substantially altered models.

It is not uncommon to encounter vendor claims of a "fully compliant" solution to whatever problem is most current in industry. These are often exaggerated and sometimes unsubstantiated or even false. Why should equipment and software producers have a better understanding of the regulatory requirements than the regulated industry itself? How can they know what the user really needs without having seen a user requirements specification? In conclusion, only the close cooperation of the vendor and the purchaser will allow a proper assessment to be conducted, whether a suitable upgrade or replacement is available.

No matter, whether a company chooses to replace or to upgrade a system, one is looking at new software or hardware, which will require formal qualification and probably validation [9]. All of the relevant documents like the user requirements specification (URS), functional specification (FS), design specification (DS), and the test protocols, must be established and executed. Code reviews and supplier audits must be conducted, change control procedures followed and other associated activities completed, as applicable, for the systems concerned. It is likely that the request for bid documents, together with the supplier selection process, will need to be redefined due to the experience gathered during the legacy computer systems assessment process. Such an action is not a "quick fix" and is rarely a short-term solution. In many instances replacements or upgrades are associated with substantial capital spending and will have to follow time-consuming internal procedures.

A number of factors may make it impossible for a company to obtain either an upgrade or a new system which fulfils all requirements, and not least the regulators' expectations. The reasons for this may be technical limitations, price, availability, unwillingness, and others. As always in such cases, a risk analysis should be performed, establishing the benefits compared with the risks of not upgrading or replacing the system. In any case, documenting this exercise will help to demonstrate to internal and external parties that everything humanly possible had been done to rectify the identified shortcomings of the existing system, even if only a partial solution or none at all can be found.

In some specific areas it is already apparent that client demand for certain features which are associated with demands from the regulatory bodies, has resulted in improved or compliant systems. At present, this applies mainly to sophisticated laboratory, enterprise resource planning, and materials or document management systems [20]. As demand grows, more solutions will become available, which should benefit all parties, not least the patients.

Hybrid Systems and Procedural Controls

Although "disliked" and discouraged by the regulators, hybrid systems are the short-term solution of choice in many instances. As discussed before, technical solutions may not be available currently, or too far into the future, too costly to implement, or unsuitable for a particular situation. The only way forward is to establish procedures for controlling the system until such time that appropriate solutions are made available. As this is the method used most often for immediate remediation, we will need to look at some of the solutions encountered more closely.

One of the most cited deviations [1] is the lack of, or insufficient, access control. The reasons for this are numerous, for example:

- The system has no, or limited, access control functionality (e.g., no password, one password only and no user ID, etc.).

- The functionality is not used or enabled (e.g., one password is used by all laboratory staff, etc.).
- The system is accessible from other applications (e.g., protected files can be modified and deleted using Windows Explorer, etc.).
- The physical location of the system is publicly accessible.
- There is no control over passwords and user IDs (e.g., expired user IDs are reused, etc.).
- The vendor or maintenance contractor has a "master" password or the administrator access codes are printed in the manuals.
- The passwords used for accessing the system never expire.

Where the system lacks access control it may be possible to physically secure the area, e.g., access by key or swipe card. In addition, it is necessary to establish a written procedure which details who has access and how this is recorded, managed, and controlled. Such controls must include any third party requiring system access.

Where access control functionality is available it should be used, and SOPs must detail the associated procedures to be followed. If correctly implemented and applied this will result in a compliant rather than a hybrid system.

Audit trails are another area of widespread concern. The regulatory expectations are such that an audit trail for electronic records should also be generated electronically and must be securely tied to that record. Few systems have this type of functionality and the audit trail information is not secure. As always, the authorities want to be able to detect fraud. For the company however, there is further interest in knowing when a particular event took place, and who was involved in it, because it may help to improve processes, avoid errors and faults, and therefore reduce system downtime.

Before the advent of electronic audit trails, paper based logbooks were used (and still are) to document sequences of events, and for providing the date and time, and the identity of the person who made the entry. In order to avoid fraud, two people had to be involved in this operation, the second person confirming the action or the observation made by the first. Automated systems were introduced to reduce the number of people involved in such operations. Modern processes are therefore no longer geared to cope with such procedures, which often prevents a company from reverting back to the old system. Clearly it is not acceptable to simply provide the operator with a logbook to fill in, as this would serve no purpose. It would be impossible to detect wrongdoing without an independent check.

In essence, where it is required, companies should attempt to bring in electronic audit trails because most other solutions are proving more complicated and costly. Exemption are locked-down databases, which do not allow record editing or deletion, only entry and export of new data entries, and automatically apply a date and time stamp. Data for export are additionally secured with a hash key to prevent (fraudulent) change before reimport. The absence of an electronic audit trail should always be described in a risk assessment document.

In this connection the issues of date and time must be addressed. Even companies with a single location should accurately date and time stamp on drug products, documentation, etc. Wristwatches and computer clocks are mostly out of synchronization with the national time standards. Providing accurate time on the system is not a big challenge and should be delegated to the IT department. Accurate atomic clock time signals can be either gathered from the Internet or a clock may be purchased and installed. (Improved accuracy can be obtained by coupling the system to a global positioning system (GPS)). The time signal can also be made available via the company's internal network.

What about companies with multiple sites and systems that are used globally? In the first case local time should always be used. Where one system is used on multiple sites in different time zones, it is often practical to use one time only. This may be the time at the location of the central processor unit, or it may be an arbitrarily set time for the system, such as Greenwich Mean Time (GMT). The FDA states in its guidance document: [10]

> "Although we withdrew the draft guidance on time stamps, our current thinking has not changed in that when using time stamps for systems that span different time zones, we do not expect you to record the signer's local time. When using time stamps, they should be implemented with a clear understanding of the time zone reference used. In such instances, system documentation should explain time zone references as well as zone acronyms or other naming conventions."

These few examples show that simple solutions can often be enough to improve the current situation and eliminate some of the computer system's deficiencies. Starting remedial action after the completion of the assessment process for all systems provides the opportunity to implement more far-reaching (site-wide or even global) solutions, with the obvious benefit of potential cost savings. It does not mean, however, that these procedural controls are always in full compliance with the regulators' expectations. It is likely that in many cases system upgrades or replacements must be considered as a long-term solution.

Summary

- Select the most appropriate solution for immediate action.
- If that is not sufficient, provide a plan for alternative long-term resolution.
- Remember: any solution must be practicable, sensible, and in accordance with regulations.

Practical Examples

The following examples are excerpts from actual assessments. They are meant to provide the reader with practical and pragmatic solutions to typical deficiencies and deviations from regulatory requirements. The examples were chosen as they represent typical and recurring deficiencies associated with legacy computerized systems.

Example 1 Remediation Planning and Risk Assessments

The completed detailed assessments for computerized systems with electronic records or electronic signatures contain the information where compliance with the regulatory requirements has already been achieved, and also any deficiencies identified. Industry's experience is that only some legacy systems are really fully compliant, and that for most systems some sort of remedial action is required. Where only a limited number of systems or deficiencies are identified, it may be possible to devise individual remediation plans for each automated system or application, without losing control over the task.

It is often advantageous to tabulate the findings from the detailed assessments, thus facilitating the information assessment process. Several advantages can be gained from this approach: similar or identical deficiencies or shortcomings can be grouped together, and a common solution can be potentially found. In addition, the deficiencies can be classified to form the basis for a risk assessment. The risk assessment process can also provide the information on the level of priority that should be given to a particular automated system or application. The plan for remedial action should take into account all of the information contained in the detailed assessments and gained from the risk assessments.

Excellent articles on the risk assessment process for computer software have been published in *Pharmaceutical Engineering.** These state that consideration should be given to the following:

- The risk that the system poses to product safety, efficacy, and quality.
- The risk that the system poses to data integrity, authenticity, and confidentiality.
- The system's complexity; a more complex system might warrant a more comprehensive validation effort.

The FDA guidance document, *Guidance for Industry, FDA Reviewers and Compliance on Off-The-Shelf Software Use in Medical Devices* [18], is much more specific about the particularities of the software risk assessment process:

> "Existing international standards indicate that the estimation of risk should be considered as the product of the severity of harm and the probability of occurrence of harm. On the

---

*Vol. 23, No 3 (May/June 2003) and No 6 (November/December 2003).

> software engineering side, probabilities of occurrence would normally be based on software failure rates. However, software failures are systematic in nature and therefore their probability of occurrence can not be determined using traditional statistical methods. Because the risk estimates for hazards related to software cannot easily be estimated based on software failure rates, CDRH has concluded that engineering risk management for medical device software should focus on the severity of the harm that could result from the software failure. Because risk analysis for software cannot be based on probability of occurrence, the actual function of risk analysis for software can then be reduced to a hazard analysis function."

Although this document specifically deals with medical devices, the FDA's conclusions are applicable to the software risk assessment process in general. It should be noted though, that there is no specific FDA guidance for computerized legacy systems.

Appendix M3, GAMP [9] details the risk assessment process for a given system function or system subfunction. Both the risks to GxP and the business are identified, and their respective likelihood and severity of impact assessed. The risk assessment process described is closely tied into the lifecycle and the validation process for a computerized system or application. It is therefore best suited to new systems.

The European GMP guidance document [5] has a section on retrospective validation for computerized legacy systems, which specifically requests a risk analysis for GxP impact.

Table 12.7 shows an example for a summary of the findings from the detailed assessments, with additional columns added for risk assessment information and the provision of priority levels. As all entries were identified to represent electronic records, they are therefore all GxP critical. Additional information on past performance and experience with the automated system or application can be provided in the history column. Additional information and guidance on how to describe or assess business risk and GxP risk can be found in Appendix M3 to the GAMP Guide [9].

In this example seventeen discrepancies from eleven systems or applications used by six departments are recorded. Closer analysis led to the following approach for remedial action.

Deficiency — No procedure for creating copies of electronic records for inspectors.

Solution — The existing SOP "Procedure for Regulatory Agency Inspections and/or Investigations" for this site was amended to include the submission of electronic records in electronic format. This ensures that the correct information is handed to the authority and by marking the data storage media label with the "Confidential Trade Secret Information" stamp, confidentiality is assured. This procedure will also cover the data format depending on the original application and the record contents.

Deficiency — Inadequate or no backup, archival, record retention, and data retrieval procedure.

Table 12.7 Risk Assessments

Inventory ID	Computerized System or Application	Short-term Remediation	Medium-term Remediation	Long-term Remediation	21 CFR Part 11 Detailed Assessment Entries	Deficiency Found	History	Business Risk	GxP Risk	Necessity or Need-to-Have	Priority
041	Department # 33 File Maker		Create procedure		11.10(b)	No procedure for creating copies for inspectors.	Not inspected	LA	H	N	2
051	Department #44 Easy Label 32 Software		Create procedure		11.10(b)	No procedure for creating copies for inspectors.	Software version release in 2001	H	H	E	1
090	Department #66 Calibration Manager Database		Create procedure		11.10(b)	No procedure for creating copies for inspectors. Export to readable format is possible.	Not inspected	LSP	H	Ni	2
012	Department #77 GLATT Coater	Provide retention of bespoke application with e-records.			11.10(b)	Requires bespoke application to view records. No procedure for creating copies for inspectors.	Reliable	H	H	E	1

Table 12.7 continued

Priority	Necessity or Need-to-Have	GxP Risk	Business Risk	History	Deficiency Found	21 CFR Part 11 Detailed Assessment Entries	Long-term Remediation	Medium-term Remediation	Short-term Remediation	Computerized System or Application	Inventory ID
1	E	H	L	E-records overwritten or deleted on purpose or by accident.	Document archival and access procedures inadequate, or missing. So far only documents were archived.	11.10(c)		Migrate to secure format (PDF or similar) or system (Lotus Notes, Documentum or similar). Create archival procedure.	All approved documents (i.e., electronic records or master paper documents) to be stored in one drive on one server only, ensures adequate access, maintenance identification and archival controls (SOP).	Department #77 NDA application in MS Word	016
1	E	H	H	Data retrieval successful in the past.	No backup and record retention procedure.	11.10(c)			Ensure adequate backup	Department #88 Analytical data server	072

Table 7.12 continued

Inventory ID	Computerized System or Application	Short-term Remediation	Medium-term Remediation	Long-term Remediation	21 CFR Part 11 Detailed Assessment Entries	Deficiency Found	History	Business Risk	GxP Risk	Necessity or Need-to-Have	Priority
016	Department #55 Approved suppliers list in MS Excel	All approved documents (i.e., electronic records of master paper documents) to be stored in one server only. Ensure adequate access, maintenance, identification and archival controls (SOP).	Migrate to secure format (PDF or similar) or system (Lotus Notes, Documentum or similar). Improve system.		11.10(c)	Document archival and access procedures inadequate or missing. So far only printed documents were archived.	Data loss in the past caused by accidental delection	LP	L	N	3
116	All data to be stored on CD, ensure adequate access, maintenance, identification, and archival controls (SOP).	All data to be stored on CD, ensure adequate maintenance, identification, and archival controls (SOP).	Create archival procedure.		11.10(c)	Document archival and procedures inadequate or missing.	Data available for past 3 years.	L	H	E	2

Table 7.12 continued

Priority	Necessity or Need-to-Have	GxP Risk	Business Risk	History	Deficiency Found	21 CFR Part 11 Detailed Assessment Entries	Long-term Remediation	Medium-term Remediation	Short-term Remediation	Computerized System or Application	Inventory ID
2	N	H	L	Spectrometer's hard disk filling up fast.	Document archival and access procedures inadequate or missing.	11.10(c)		Migrate to secure format (PDF or similar) or system (Lotus Notes, Documentum or similar). Improve system documentation controls.	Save data directly to server. Ensure adequate access, maintenance, identification, and archival controls (SOP).	Department #88 FT-IR spectrometer	066
1	E	H	M	Final/approved version always stored as read-only.	Document archival and access procedures inadequate or missing.	11.10(c)		Migrate to secure format (PDF or similar) or system (Lotus Notes, Documentum or similar). Improve system documentation controls.	All approved documents (i.e., electronic records of master paper documents) to be stored in one drive on one server only. Ensure adequate access, maintenance identification and archival controls (SOP).	Department #33 Departmental SOPs in MS Word	044

Table 12.7 continued

Inventory ID	Computerized System or Application	Short-term Remediation	Medium-term Remediation	Long-term Remediation	21 CFR Part 11 Detailed Assessment Entries	Deficiency Found	History	Business Risk	GxP Risk	Necessity or Need-to-Have	Priority
052	Department #44 Easy Label 32 Software	Define record retention policy.			11.10(c)	No record retention policy.	At present all records on hard disk.	H	H	E	1
091	Department #66 Calibration Manager Database	Define record retention policy.			11.10(c)	No record retention policy.	Not inspected.	LSP	H	Ni	2
100	Department #66 KAYE Validator	Define record retention policy. Implement appropriate backup procedure.			11.10(c)	No record retention policy. No backups.		LSP	H	Ni	2
013	Department #77 GLATT Coater	Store archive copies on more appropriate media. Clarify export of records in FDA readable format.			11.10(c)	Storage to Zip drive inadequate for long term retention. Current policy of monthly save to Zip drive not adequate for indefinite retention policy.	Zip files were never tested for data retrieval.	H	H	E	1

Table 12.7 continued

Priority	Necessity or Need-to-Have	GxP Risk	Business Risk	History	Deficiency Found	21 CFR Part 11 Detailed Assessment Entries	Long-term Remediation	Medium-term Remediation	Short-term Remediation	Computerized System or Application	Inventory ID
2	E	H	L	No problems in past.	Sequencing not validated.	11.10(f)		Validate system.		Department #66 KAYE Validator.	125
2	Ni	H	LS	No password or lock facility.	System left unattended during operation.	11.10(d) (Physical access).	Replace system.			Department #66 KAYE Validator.	101
2	E	H	L	Staff instructed verbally.	No procedure for physical access.	11.10(d) (Physical access).		Create procedure.		Department #55 MG2 Futura.	124

Abbreviations

H = High GxP risk
L = Low GxP risk
LP = Low/paper copy available
E = Essential
Ni = Nice to have
2 = 2nd Priority
RS = Replace system
M = Medium GxP risk
LA = Low/alternatives available
LSP = Low/services purchasable
N = Necessary
1 = 1st Priority
3 = 3rd Priority

Table 12.8 Table of Contents for the SOP "Procedure for Regulatory Agency Inspections and/or Investigations"

Table of contents

Purpose

Scope

Responsibility

Procedure

Overview

The archival requirements:
- Storage of electronic data.
- Storage of associated metadata, such as integration parameters or audit trail information, with the electronic records.
- Protection of the integrity of electronic records over the records retention period through appropriate policy and procedure.
- Detection of altered and deleted electronic records and their documentation in an audit trail.
- Accurate and timely retrieval of electronic records throughout the records retention period.
- Generation of accurate and complete copies of electronic records in both human readable and electronic form.

The archival process definitions:
- Definition of the record.
- Period or frequency of archiving.
- Integrity of the record.
- Maintenance of the record.

Deletion of records

Testing and qualification:
- Storage medium.
- Successful completion of the archival process.
- The accuracy of the records information.
- Data transfer method.
- Corruption (truncation, duplication, etc.).
- Record retrieval.

The archive:
- Access to the archive.
- The environment.

Maintenance:
- Reformatting and copying.
- Record integrity.
- Media performance and degradation..
- Migration.
- Disaster recovery.

References

Solution — A new site-wide SOP "Procedure for Data Archival" was drafted covering data storage, archival and retrieval, with the following table of contents as per Table 12.8.

Deficiency — No procedures for physical system access.

Solution — In one case the existing departmental system SOP is amended, following internal change control procedures. On one portal system physical access cannot be restricted, and there is no electronic access control facility. Replace the entire system.

Deficiency — Sequencing steps were not validated.

Solution — The existing validation protocol for the system is changed to incorporate the sequencing step tests. The protocol execution is therefore planned to coincide with the planned revalidation of the system.

This is an actual example showing that, by collating the information from the detailed assessments in a risk assessment type format, it is possible to limit the time and effort for deficiency rectification and to optimize the remediation effort. Five remedial actions covered all seventeen recorded deficiencies.

Example 2 Analytical System Deficiency Remediation

The results for the detailed assessment for a FT-IR spectrometer (electronic records yes, electronic signatures no, closed system) are given in Table 12.9. For reasons of clarity, only the comments for noncompliance are shown.

Deficiency — The ability to discern invalid or altered records was not validated.

Solution — The existing validation protocol for the FT-IR spectrometer is changed to incorporate the additional tests. The protocol will be executed during the annual system revalidation.

Deficiency — No backup or archival procedure.

Solution — Adaptation of the corporate SOP "Procedure for Data Storage, Archival and Retrieval."

Deficiency — There is no audit trail or audit trail functionality.

Solution — The system itself does not have the required functionality and a manual audit trail was not considered an acceptable solution. Furthermore, a system replacement or an application software upgrade, which would have rendered the system compliant, was unavailable. Therefore, it is necessary to acquire additional software that will make the system compliant. Various companies offer such software solutions, particularly for analytical laboratory systems. References to these can be found, *inter alia*, on the FDA website under Electronic Record — Electronic Signatures 21 CFR Part 11 Guidance Documents Dockets Established — Topics for Guidance Development [12]. Another popular source for solution provider information is the 21CFRPart11.com website [20].

Deficiency — The application developer has left and there is no qualification record for the developer or the maintainer. User training logs are complete.

Table 12.9 Detailed assessment form

21 CFR Part 11 Reference	Assessment results Compliant/Noncompliant/ Not applicable	Observation
Validation		
11.10.(a)	Noncompliant	The ability to discern invalid or altered records was not validated.
Inspectability		
11.10.(b)	Compliant	
11.10.(c)	Noncompliant	Data is on standalone PC with password protection. No backup or archival procedure.
11.10.(d)	Compliant	
11.10.(f)	Not applicable	
11.10.(g)	Compliant	
11.10.(h)	Not applicable	
Audit trails		
11.10.(e)	Noncompliant	There is no audit trail or audit trail functionality.
Personnel qualifications		
11.10.(i)	Noncompliant	The application developer has left and there is no qualification record for the developer or the maintainer. User training logs are complete.
11.10(j)	Not applicable	
Systems documentation ccontrols		
11.10.(k)(1)	Noncompliant	The number of copies and the location of the system documentation are unknown.
11.10.(k)(2)	Noncompliant	
Signature manifestations		
11.50 (a)(1)	Noncompliant	The printed names of the signatories are not on the document.
11.50 (a)(2)	Compliant	
11.50 (a)(3)	Compliant	
11.50 (b)	Compliant	
11.70	Compliant	

Solution — The history records for recent years show that the system and its application are very stable and operate reliably. The system vendor operates to internationally accepted software development standards and this was confirmed in writing. This information was considered sufficient, as it proved impossible to obtain the required records retrospectively. The existing SOP "Procurement and Invitation to Bid" was updated to require all qualification certificates for future purchases. The system maintainer's training logs were updated to include this particular system.

Deficiency — The number of copies and the location of the system documentation are unknown.

Solution — As this is a site-wide deficiency, a SOP "System Documentation" was established, describes the steps necessary for the review, approval, distribution, and use of system documentation for GxP critical systems. The documentation covered by this SOP comprises training manuals, applications manuals, operating systems manuals, configurable software manuals, SOPs, help files (online, on electronic media or on paper), security and access lists and drawings. In the case of the FT-IR instrument all documentation was collated and is now stored with the instrument in an access-controlled location.

Deficiency — The printed names of the signatories are not on the document.

Solution — It is possible to enter the printed name of the signatories on the document before the printout and the application of the wet signature. The existing SOP for the instrument was updated accordingly.

Validation

This chapter is not intended to provide in-depth guidance on the validation process for legacy systems, as this is dealt with in great detail in other publications [1,9,19]. However, the subject does warrant mention as one will come across the issue during the system assessment process. The question will be: Is the system validated?

We would like to assume that those companies obliged to validate systems would have done so. Nonetheless, having created this new awareness within a wide audience, it is very likely that gaps will be identified within the previous validation effort.

For example, many IT departments are prepared for a system crash and provide a backup service for that purpose. Few will have a system in place that allows for the archiving and retrieval of specific records for many years (often seven years or more), something that is required for electronic records, particularly under 21 CFR Part 11 [4].

Companies should assess if some or all of their existing computerized systems need to be reviewed, and the qualification or validation documents revisited in light of the newly-established requirements and needs. Excellent guidance for defining requirements and specifications, reviewing and testing systems against specifications, demonstrating that systems are being properly managed and performing ongoing evaluation is provided in the GAMP Guide Vol. 4. [9]

Summary

- Review validation procedures in the light of the newly gained information and awareness.

Ongoing Operations

Unfortunately time does not stand still and reviewing the automated legacy systems in a company does not stop day-to-day operations or changes to, or the purchase of, new systems. The process of introducing new items and administrative controls should always consider the impact these have on the legacy systems.

This may affect, for example, SOPs for:

- Data backup.
- Archiving.
- Disaster recovery.
- Data retrieval.
- QA audits.
- Purchasing procedures.
- Training.
- Error logging.
- Software and hardware maintenance.
- Change control.
- Organizational structures.
- Software and hardware distribution, etc.

SUMMARY

Assessing and understanding legacy computer systems not only helps to improve the operation and maintenance of the existing systems, it also has a profound impact on new systems or upgrades that are introduced into the company. The assessment effort and the associated training and awareness-building exercise motivates and empowers staff from all areas within the enterprise to understand the complex nature of computerized systems much better. It also helps to create a more common understanding of an issue that has been left to date, to a select group of computer system specialists, but which affects almost anyone in the business.

Furthermore, this retrospective assessment will only yield the expected results and benefits if there is thorough planning in the initial phases of the project, and if it is run as a team effort. For most companies this is an undertaking that will last for several months, if not years, and will incur substantial cost. For many of the regulated industries this exercise is definitely a must, as the inspectorates require them to be compliant. The mere fact that the regulators have not been enforcing the law to its full extent yet should not lull anyone into a false sense of security.

Understanding your legacy computer systems has enormous benefits, which outweigh the cost and effort of getting there.

Figure 12.1 provides an overview of the steps involved in the exercise.

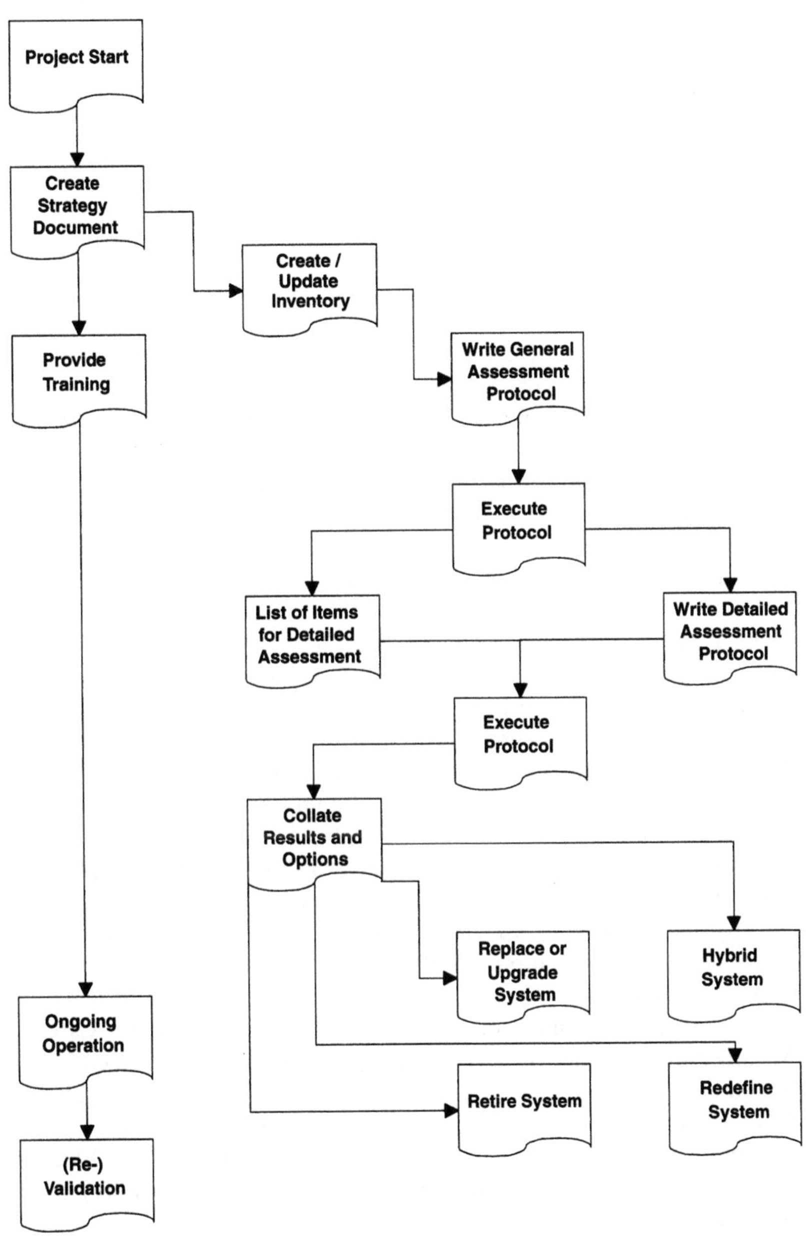

Fiigure 12.1 Project flowchart.

Much progress has been made in recent years, particularly in the wake of the year 2000 problem and following some high profile warning letters that resulted in multimillion dollar fines, to formally assess and document and, where applicable, to bring legacy computer systems into compliance with the rules and regulations. However, in our experience there are still many existing systems awaiting remediation; still a long way to go. Hopefully this chapter has helped the reader to get a few steps further down that road.

REFERENCES

1 U.S. Department of Health and Human Services, Food and Drug Administration. http://www.fda.gov/
2 U.S. Code of Federal Regulation. Title 21 Part 210 Current Good Manufacturing Practice in Manufacturing, Processing, Packing, or Holding of Drugs; General. http://www.access.gpo.gov/nara/cfr/waisidx_01/21cfr210_01.html
3 U.S. Code of Federal Regulation. Title 21 Part 211 Current Good Manufacturing Practice for Finished Pharmaceuticals. http://www.access.gpo.gov/nara/cfr/waisidx_01/21cfr211_01.html
4 U.S. Code of Federal Regulation. Title 21 Part 11 Electronic Records; Electronic Signatures. http://www.access.gpo.gov/nara/cfr/waisidx_01/21cfr11_01.html
5 The European Commission Directorate General 3. The Rules Governing Medicinal Products in the European Union, Vol. 4, Annex 11 Computerized Systems. http://dg3.eudra.org/F2/eudralex/vol-4/pdfs-en/anx11en.pdf
6 The Organization for Economic Co-operation and Development (OECD): OECD Series on Principles of GLP and Compliance Monitoring, Number 4 (Revised), Consensus Document Quality Assurance and GLP 1999. http://www.olis.oecd.org/olis/1999doc.nsf/LinkTo/env-jm-mono(99)20
7 The International Conference on Harmonization of Technical Requirements for Regiration of Pharmaceuticals for Human Use (ICH). http://www.ich.org
8 NAMUR, An Association of Users of Process Control Technology. http://www.namur.de/
9 Good Automated Manufacturing Practice Forum., The Good Automated Manufacturing Practice (GAMP) Guide for Validation of Automated Systems in Pharmaceutical Manufacture, Vol. 4, December 2001. http://www.ispe.org/
10 U.S. Department of Health and Human Services, Food and Drug Administration. Guidance for Industry, Part 11, Electronic Records; Electronic Signatures — Scope and Application, August 2003. http://www.fda.gov/cder/guidance/5667fnl.htm
11 Pharmaceutical Inspection Convention, Pharmaceutical Inspection Co-operation Scheme, Good Practices for Computerized Systems in Regulated "GxP" Environments, PI 011-1 20 August 2003. http://www.picscheme.org

12 U.S. Department of Health and Human Services, Food and Drug Administration. Electronic Record — Electronic Signatures 21 CFR Part 11 Guidance Documents Dockets Established — Topics for Guidance Development. http://www.fda.gov/ora/compliance_ref/part11/dockets_index.htm
13 U.S. Department of Health and Human Services, Food and Drug Administration. Title 21 Code of Federal Regulations (21 CFR Part 11), Electronic Records; Electronic Signatures. http://www.fda.gov/ora/compliance_ref/part11/Default.htm
14 European Union Commission Directive 2003/94/EC of 8 October 2003 laying down the principles and guidelines of good manufacturing practice in respect of medicinal products for human use and investigational medicinal products for human use — http://europa.eu.int/cgi-bin/eur-lex/udl.pl?REQUEST=Seek-Deliver&COLLECTION=oj&SERVICE=eurlex&LANGUAGE=en&DOCID=20031262p0022
15 The International Society for Pharmaceutical Engineering (ISPE). Good Practice and Compliance for Electronic Records Series. http://www.ispe.org/
16 U.S. Department of Health and Human Services, Food and Drug Administration. Guidance for Industry, E6 Good Clinical Practice: Consolidated Guidance, April 1996. http://www.fda.gov/cder/guidance/959fnl.pdf
17 U.S. Department of Health and Human Services, Food and Drug Administration. Guidance for Industry, Computerized Systems used in Clinical Trials, April 1999. http://www.fda.gov/ora/compliance_ref/bimo/ffinalcct.htm
18 U.S. Department of Health and Human Services, Food and Drug Administration. Guidance for Industry, FDA Reviewers and Compliance on Off-The-Shelf Software Use in Medical Devices, published September 1999. http://www.fda.gov/cdrh/ode/1252.html
19 The Parenteral Drug Association (PDA) — http://www.pda.org
Technical Report #31: Validation and Qualification of Computerized Laboratory Data Acquisition Systems.
Technical Report #32: Auditing of Suppliers Providing Computer Products and Services for Regulated Pharmaceutical Operations.
Technical Report #18: PDA Report on the Validation of Computer-Related Systems.
20 21 CFR PART 11 links — http://www.21cfrpart11.com/

SUGGESTIONS FOR FURTHER READING AND RELATED WEBSITES

Lopez, O. *21 CFR Part 11 Guide to International Compliance*. Sue Horwood Publishing Ltd., 2002.
Lopez, O. *21 CFR Special Edition Incorporating SCADA Systems*. Sue Horwood Publishing Ltd., 2001.

Wingate, G. *Audit Preparation for Suppliers*. Sue Horwood Publishing Ltd., 2002.

Lopez, O. *Retrospective Validation Plan for Computer-Related Systems*. Sue Horwood Publishing Ltd., 2001.

Clark, C. *Writing the Validation Report.* Sue Horwood Publishing Ltd., 2001.

Baker, Simmons, T. *Software Management Basics*. Sue Horwood Publishing Ltd., 2001.

Simmons, T. *Producing a Quality Plan*. Sue Horwood Publishing Ltd., 2001.

See also the web business card http://www.suehorwoodpubltd.com/ and websites for the following publishers.

http://www.dhibooks.com/ (Davis Horwood International Publishing)

http://www.pda.org/ (The Parenteral Drug Association)

http://www.crcpress.com/ (CRC Press)

http://www.ecec.co.uk/ (European Continuing Education College)

Chapter 13

Technology Transfer Keys

Stewart Green and Paul Warren

CONTENTS

INTRODUCTION

There can be few pharmaceutical companies over the last 15 years that have not undergone the maelstrom of takeovers, mergers, downsizing, centers of excellence or product rationalization. All these events can, and frequently do, result in product or products transfer between manufacturing sites. At best it will be a product or product type that the receiving site is familiar with, or at worst, one with which they are totally unfamiliar.

The challenges to effect technology transfer in a timely fashion, within budget and to achieve savings that have probably been precommitted, at the requisite quality, are approximately the same for each aspect.

This chapter provides a "ready reckoner" of the issues to consider to achieve these objectives, ensuring that the regulatory issues from both a licensing and inspection perspective are addressed, and maintaining the organization's integrity for its products and with its shareholders.

In considering the technology transfer process reference is made to the situation within the EU in the main; however, where useful guides or proposals are available from other regulatory authorities, notably the U.S. Food and Drug Administration (FDA), these have been included for completeness.

The purpose of this chapter is to present both an overview of the technology transfer process and to offer specific guidance concerning the key aspects of product transfer management, and how to document outcomes to completely satisfy both internal requirements and regulatory expectations. We provide suggestions on the personnel to be involved in the process, and a checklist to serve as an *aide memoire* to ensure that key steps have been covered.

This chapter discusses the principles behind the technology transfer process that can be applied in full or in part, dependent on the nature and complexity of the products involved in the transfer. The requirement to perform a formal technology transfer is prescribed — directly and indirectly — by the regulatory authorities within the EU For those markets regulated by the U.S. FDA, there are very specific requirements for transfer. While this guideline is focused on the EU, the principles, if applied in full, would also be expected to meet FDA requirements.

THE TECHNOLOGY TRANSFER TEAM

The decision to transfer products between manufacturing sites is frequently driven by economics. This may be the result of a global product or site rationalization program, or it may be driven by attempts to consolidate similar product types at a single site. It may result from a merger or takeover, which generates excess capacity in the supply chain leading to consolidation. Whichever the key driver for transfer, it is likely that due to the sensitive nature of the proposals, both in terms of affected sites and shareholders' confidence, this intention cannot be shared with the affected sites until timescales are already tight. It is against this background that the team responsible for the transfer process is required to operate. It must be accepted that although not ideal, this is an understandable consequence of operating in a highly competitive global business.

The structure of the validation team will depend on the degree of fit of the transferred product with the local site capabilities. For example, if the recipient site has a known expertise in solid dose formulations and the transferred product is a straightforward tablet formulation then the team members will be drawn from quality control (QC); quality assurance (QA) and production (or process support where this facility exists). If, however, the product represents a change in complexity (e.g., sustained release formulation) or a change in product type (e.g., capsule formulation where the site has previously only made tablets), then the core team may need to be enhanced for example, by the inclusion of engineering personnel.

Other disciplines, for example, the training function, also need to be considered. If there is a major impact on site quality systems or personnel knowledge base, then extensive training of site personnel throughout all disciplines, but particularly of operations personnel, needs to be considered. It is unlikely that the training can ever supplant the collective knowledge of the donor plant, but it should seek to identify key gaps in the process between donor and recipient plants and deliver a training program to close such gaps.

In many situations the timescales will preclude involving all team members full time on the process, unless an organization is specifically resourced to provide this service.

However, it is essential that at least one member is full time and has specific responsibility for the project. His role may be project management, co-ordinatory, or "hands on" in the process environment, but he must be focused and not distracted by the pressures of a "day job."

A regulatory interface is also essential. Despite a supposedly uniform regulatory environment in the EU, the reality for most companies is that even for a single product there may be divergent regulatory requirements; indeed the product registration may not be common to all markets and therefore the impact of change will also be variable.

The responsibilities for each team member need to be defined at the outset, so that all the bases are covered and all members understand what is expected of them.

Proposed Team Members and Responsibilities

Team member	Responsibilities
Process technologist	• Central focus for transfer activities. • Collates documentation from donor site (see the Documentation section). • Performs initial assessment of transferred project for – Feasibility.

- Compatibility with site capabilities.
- Establishes resource requirements.

QA representative

- Reviews documentation to determine compliance with marketing authorization (MA).
- Reviews analytical methods with QC to determine capability, equipment training requirements.
- Initiates conversion of donor site documentation into local systems or format.
- Initiates or confirms regulatory requirements, e.g., change to manufacturing license; variations to MA if process changes needed, etc.

Production representative

- Reviews process instructions (with process technologist) to confirm capacity and capability.
- Considers any safety implications, e.g., solvents; toxic; sanitizing materials.
- Considers impact on local standard operating procedures (SOPs).
- Considers training requirements of supervisors or operators.

Engineering representative

- Reviews (with production representative) equipment requirement.
- Initiates required engineering modifications, change or part purchase.
- Reviews preventative maintenance and calibration impact, e.g., use of more aggressive ingredients; more temperature sensitive process, and modifies accordingly.

TECHNOLOGY TRANSFER: KEY ACTIVITIES

Timelines

As previously indicated, the timelines for the transfer may well have been preordained by financial or marketing considerations. The first key activity of the team is therefore to do a "sanity check" to determine at the macro level whether those expectations can be met. If not, then senior management must be informed to ensure that the implications on the donor site (which may be closing), the recipient site (whose budget may have assumed the transferred volume) market supply, stock market confidence and so on, can be considered. The other time driver may well be the regulatory aspects (considered in the next section).

Initially the team will have to make a number of assumptions. For example, it will be assumed that process validation, analytical validation, and cleaning validation are trouble-free. It will also be assumed that actives, excipients, and packaging components are available on standard lead times. A complete time and event schedule at the macro level should be constructed on these assumptions, working backwards from the proposed transfer deadline. Key stages of the process such as:

- Data collection
- Data review
- Regulatory impact with particular emphasis on any change approvals
- Analytical validation
- Pilot or full-scale process batch
- Stability set down (if required)

should be mapped to determine whether the predetermined transfer timelines can be met.

Regulatory Issues

Changes to the approved MA can represent the greatest challenge to the transfer timelines. Most manufacturing units no longer supply a single market, and particularly where centers of excellence have been created, a single unit may supply on a global basis. For even a simple activity, such as registering a site change, the regulatory process can vary from 30 days to 12–14 months. This is why an initial regulatory assessment is so important in determining whether the overall timelines can be met.

Fundamental to the transfer process is the decision to implement little (if any) change in the transferred product or process. As the level of change increases, so does the regulatory complexity and the associated timelines. Guidance is available in assessing change in both of the major regulated markets, i.e., the U.S. FDA and the EU.

The FDA has published a series of proposals under the simplification process, for example SUPAC (scale up and post approval change) Guidance for Industry for Solid Dose Forms.

These provide guidance covering advice on so called “like for like” changes, i.e., the substitution of one granulator for another. A brief resume of some changes considered is given at the end of this section. By using this guidance it is possible to minimize the regulatory impact in those markets governed by the FDA.

Similarly, within the EU, at least for nationally registered products, guidance notes are provided for not only the type of change and its regulatory approval time, but also for the information required to support the change. Changes are divided into 30+ so-called Type 1 variations covering diverse changes ranging from change of site to changes in analytical methods, and other more complex variations, so-called Type 2 changes. In theory a Type 1 variation is approvable within 30 days and a Type 2 variation within 90 days. In practice only some member states of the EU achieve these approval timelines. As before a resume of the changes and their requirements is given at the end of this section.

EU Guideline on Variations to Marketing Authorization

(The full transcript can be found in *The Rules Governing Medicinal Products in the European Community, Volume 6A: Notice to Applicants, Chapter 5: Variations.*)

Nature of change	Documentation required
1 Change of manufacturing site	• No change in process, specifications, or test methods. • Proof that proposed site is authorized for the dose form production ("manufacturing licence"). • Declaration in writing of no changes in previously approved specification. • Batch analysis comparison; at least one full size batch, and two pilot batches compared with three full-scale from previous site.
4 Replacement of excipient with comparable excipient	• No change in dissolution profile for a solid solid dose form. • Justification for change including stability impact. • Commitment to provide ongoing stability and three months' data available up front. • Comparative dissolution profiles of "old" versus "new" product. • Declaration of no change in release or shelf life specifications.
8 Qualitative change in composition of packaging material	• Justification for change including comparative data, e.g., permeability. • For semisolids and liquids proof of no interaction between container and product. • Validation of any analytical methods used to control packaging material. • Ongoing stability and three months data available up front. • Declaration of no change in release or shelf life specifications.
11 Change in manufacturer of active substance	• The specifications, controls, and synthetic route should be the same as already approved (or minor changes justified).

	• Batch analysis of at least two lots from new source. • Declaration by the MA holder that there are no changes in finished product specifications.
15 Minor change in manufacturing process of product	• Product specifications not affected. • Dissolution profile for one "new" batch compared with three "old" batches (solid dose). • Justification for not submitting a new bioequivalence study.
25 Change in test procedures for product	• Appropriate validation data for analytical method and comparative data between "old" and "new" method. • Declaration that release and shelf life specifications remain unchanged.
30 Change in pack size for the product	• Declaration that specifications are unaffected. • Justification that new size is consistent with dose regime. • Declaration that container properties are unchanged. • Declaration that stability studies will be conducted.

NB. Only a selection of the 34 categories of change have been provided; the number is that used in the variations.

FDA Guidance for Industry: Changes to an Approved New Drug Application (NDA) or Abridged New Drug Application (ANDA)

Changes requiring prior approval:

- Move to a different manufacturing site when the new site has not been inspected by the FDA for the types of operation proposed.
- Move to a different manufacturing site when the new site does not have a satisfactory good manufacturing practice (GMP) inspection for the operation proposed.
- Changes that may affect the controlled release of the dose delivered to the patient.
- Changes in sterilization method for a sterile product.
- Changes in a viral removal step.
- Changes from dry to wet granulation or vice versa.
- Changes in synthetic route for drug substance.

- Addition of an ink code imprint to a solid dose form.
- Relaxing an acceptance criteria.
- Deleting a specification.
- Establishing a new analytical procedure.
- Changes in the immediate packaging material.

Changes which can be implemented in 30 days if no adverse comment:

- Moves other that those requiring prior approval.
- Moves of testing to another site.
- Changes in manufacturing process other than those requiring prior approval.
- Changes to aseptic filtration parameters.
- Changes from one sterilization autoclave or oven to another.
- Relaxing an acceptance criteria or deleting a test for a raw material.
- Change in an analytical method for a raw material.
- Change in size of a primary container.
- Addition or deletion of a desiccant.
- Reduction of an expiration date to provide increased assurance of identity, strength, or purity.

Changes which can be filed in annual report:

- Move to a different site for secondary packaging.
- Move to a different site for labeling.
- Changes to equipment of the same design (see SUPAC guidelines).
- Change in the order of addition of ingredients for a solution.
- Changes in specification to comply with *United States Pharmacopoeia* (*USP*).
- Tightening of specification.
- Change in container closure system for a solid dose form, e.g., adding a child-resistant closure; change from one plastic container to another of same type.

NB. Similar guidance for FDA regulated markets for making changes to NDA or ANDA. As for the EU guideline, only a selection of changes has been given.

SUPAC (Scale Up and Post Approval Changes) Guidance for Industry for Immediate and Modified Release Solid Oral Forms (FDA)

Operation	Equipment type	Examples considered essentially similar
Milling	Fluid mill	Tangential jet Loop Opposed jet Fluidized bed

Operation	Equipment type	Examples considered essentially similar
	Impact mill	Hammer air swept Hammer conventional pin or disk
Blending/mixing	Diffusion mixers	"V" blender Double cone blender Slant cone blender Cube blender Bin blender
	Convection mixers	Ribbon blenders Orbiting screw blenders Planetary blenders Vertical high intensity mixers
Granulation	Wet high-shear Granulator Wet low-shear Granulator	Horizontal Vertical Planetary Kneading Screw
	Extension granulator	Radical Axial Ram Roller or gear
	Fluid bed	All types
Drying	Direct heat, solid bed	Tray and truck Belt
Dosing	Tablet press	Gravity Power assisted Centrifugal Compression coating
	Encapsulator	Auger Vacuum Vibratory Dosing disk Dosator

NB. This guidance note provides guidance on what types of equipment can be considered essentially similar for each stage of the manufacturing process. Again only a selection has been given.

Determining the Process Scope

As previously stated, the ideal situation is to simply transfer the total process without change from the donor to recipient site. In practice this is seldom straightforward. During the initial feasibility assessment the comparability achievable is evaluated. Careful comparisons of processing equipment including the sophistication of the control mechanisms available, analytical capability, impact on other site processes, e.g., cleaning validation complexity, training and documentation requirements, all need to be factored into the process scope.

Excipients may not be available from the same source or the receiving site may have different preferred suppliers. Actives are normally sacrosanct, although in some cases even this change may have to be made because of other legislation, e.g., restrictions on crossborder trade in controlled drugs.

When all unavoidable changes have been identified then the scope of the transfer must be carefully formalized so that all involved parties are aware of the work involved.

Managing Change

Following the scope determination, the work needed to support any of the identified changes must be formalized. A single example will provide an illustration. Say, for example, it has been necessary to change the source of an excipient. The following list of questions, although not exhaustive, should be posed.

- Is the source of the excipient declared in the marketing authorization? If so, regulatory action may be required.
- Do the routine quality control tests provide sufficient control to characterize the practical use of the excipient? For example, is the particle size, shape, or distribution important?
- Are there any known interactions of the excipient in the formulation which may be enhanced with the proposed source?
- Are there any known interactions of the excipient with the container or closure system?
- Have any lots of donor site excipient been rejected and, if so, did this have any impact on the specification?
- Do both sources have European Certificates of Suitability, which would indicate that they are equally well characterized by the pharmacopoeial tests?
- Is the manufacturing process for the proposed excipient significantly different such that it may pose different problems (e.g., presence of solvents where previously none were used, aqueous based extraction which may lead to higher bacterial or fungal counts)?
- Is the proposed excipient available in manageable quantities (e.g., lifting restrictions may require availability in no more than 25 kg quantities)?

- Can it be assured that the proposed excipient will not interfere in the finished product analysis (particularly HPLC)? (A minor related substance may co-elute with the active product.)

As can be seen from the previous list, even what on the face of it may be a simple change, can, and does, involve complex issues.

Documentation

In order to maximize the chances of transfer success, as soon as dialog between donor and recipient site can take place, then the team should start to assemble available documentation. It is difficult to provide a definitive list of requirements as this will vary from product to product, process to process, and site capability to site capability. However, as a guide the following should be assembled.

- Production master formula:
  This should be compared to the formula actually dispensed and to that in the MA. It is not unheard of for differences to be seen.

- Manufacturing instructions:
  These should be compared to those in the MA. In our experience, for older products the detail is likely to be minimal (e.g., granulate the ingredients and tray dry to a predetermined moisture) and differences between actual and licensed can usually be accommodated. For recent products the detail may be substantial (e.g., granulate in a high-shear mixer using both granulator and chopper blades operating a high speed for 30 minutes) and changes require regulatory activity.

- Process validation studies or process development studies:
  These will provide valuable insight into process robustness, impact of variables on finished product quality, critical control points, etc.

- Rejects and deviations:
  Again these will indicate process robustness; determine whether manufacturing instructions contain the correct level of detail and whether the donor reacted appropriately to the failures.

- Analytical methods and validation:
  These should be compared against the MA with particular emphasis on the finished product specification. It is worth remembering at this point that the MA may vary in this and all other respects from market to market.

- Raw material specifications with particular emphasis on the active and key excipients:
  The latter may be of particular importance in modified release formulations. Care must be taken with any animal delivered products in the current climate of enhanced concern with transmissible spongiform encephalopathy (TSE). Certainly within Europe or where product is likely to be exported outside of the EU, most regulatory authorities will look for the absence of potentially compromising material. If it is recognized that product still contains material of bovine, ovine, or caprine origin (e.g., magnesium stearate), it would be as well during the transfer to substitute a vegetable equivalent. This is one case where like-for-like transfer should be avoided.

- Packaging components specifications:
  Again these should be compared against those in the MA and the specification should be as comprehensive as possible, particularly as the materials of construction of bottles, plastic tubes, laminates, etc., may well be commercial preparations for which equivalency is potentially difficult to establish.

- Safety data:
  Particularly where a material has specific safety issues (e.g., irritant or potent sensitizer, solvents, etc.) then all relevant data on handling requirements, disposal, environmental impact, safety data sheets, etc., should be collated.

- Other data which may provide a valuable insight into the robustness of the product and the production process:
  These include analytical deviation reports and customer complaints.

- Where a number of products are to be transferred:
  The collation of this repository of information may assist in the prioritization of the transferred products. Choices can be made on degree of difficulty, regulatory issues and the timelines involved, purchasing timelines or sourcing difficulties, and so on.

- It should be remembered that, where transfer results from the donor site closure, particular sensitivity is needed when dealing with the collation and evaluation of the information. Now is not a good time to be critical of the donor site practices and procedures!

Validation

This is one of the most critical issues in the technology transfer process because it frequently determines the complexity of the process and it is a focus for the regulatory agencies; not only from the licensing side but also during inspections.

The approach to validation for any transferred product must always be documented and science based. A number of regulatory guidelines are available: however, they are just that — guidelines. Of necessity they must deal in generalities. It is up to the receiving site team to evaluate each product and the information portfolio, and to determine the level of validation required. In the context of the transfer process we are usually referring to process qualification (PQ), unless of course equipment changes are also involved, in which case installation qualification (IQ) and operational qualification (OQ) may also be needed. Pragmatism also has a place in the decision making process. For example:

- If the product transferred is a simple liquid in which actives and excipients are dissolved by simple agitation
- If the equipment in donor and recipient plant is the same or essentially similar
- If no changes in source or type have been made to excipients and actives
- If the analytical methods are direct from a major pharmacopoeia

then it may be decided that no prospective validation is required and the transfer success will be measured by ongoing product monitoring.

There are usually three separate validation activities — namely process, cleaning, and analytical validation.

Serious consideration should be given to the merits of running a pilot scale (say 10% normal lot size) or even placebo product, if the evidence gathered during the transfer process suggests that the product may be complex or difficult to transfer or validate. This has three advantages. First, it allows all personnel involved to gain some familiarity with the production methods. Second, it may help to avoid costly "write-offs" and third, by working outside of the formal validation protocol, it provides an opportunity to address the issues without compromising the validation protocol or invoking a complex formalized investigation, in the event that something goes wrong.

Process Validation

Process validation has probably consumed almost as much time, energy, and money in the pharmaceutical industry over the last 10–15 years as manufacturing commercial products! Many companies also appear to have lost sight of the purpose of validation. In some circumstances, validation *appears* to be performed for the benefit of the validation department or, worse still, the regulatory agencies.

There is only one reason to validate a process. That is to *secure* the manufacture of a product, so that it can be *guaranteed*, with a high degree of probability, that the *patient* receives product of the requisite safety, quality, and efficacy each and every time. It also makes good business sense to be able to quickly and reproducibly release good quality products.

The approach to process validation will vary with product type and complexity. We will concentrate on the most common dosage forms, as discussion of the transfer of technologically sophisticated products such as inhalation aerosols, steriles, transdermal patches, etc., is best dealt with in a special treatise. As with most validation, three successive and successful repetitions of any of the validation processes given below are the norm.

Solutions

The key to validating solutions is to ensure that:

- Raw materials specifications for actives and excipients exercise control over critical parameters such as particle size and particle shape, partical size distribution and solubility.
- The manufacturing process parameters, be they temperature, order of addition, or agitation, are controlled and monitored to effect consistent dissolution of the ingredients.

Once such controls have been established then process validation can usually be effected by monitoring the active content of the individually filled containers produced throughout the filling period.

Creams

Creams may involve solubilization of the actives in either the water or oil phase, or dispersion without solubilization of the active in the water or oil phase. Where the actives are dissolved or dispersed during the cream formation, the energy involved to effect the formation of the oil and water micelle is such that homogenous distribution is almost assured. If the active is dissolved or dispersed after cream formation, this is likely to be a lower energy process and homogenous distribution through the viscous substrate may be more difficult.

In the former case, validation can be affected as for liquids by careful control of the physical attributes of the actives, in particular particle size distribution, and by careful control and monitoring of the homogenization conditions. The active distribution can then be monitored during the filling process by assay of individual filled units.

In the latter case, where distribution is effected after cream formation, then active ingredient distribution will normally be monitored at the bulk stage, taking samples throughout the blender as well as the filled units. The purpose of the blender samples is to determine whether the blending plateau is achieved under the prescribed conditions, i.e., the active has been evenly mixed.

Sampling of bulks can be technically very difficult: even the introduction of the sampling device may disrupt distribution of the active, although this is less likely in a viscous substrate than in a free-flowing powder (see section 2.5.1.4 on solid dose forms). The sampling regime is to some extent dependent on the blender type, but commonly a matrix of samples is taken by dividing the bulk into top, middle and bottom layers vertically and side — middle — side horizontally.

Ointments

Ointments pose similar, if potentially more challenging, problems than creams. Normally the active is distributed, not dissolved, unless it is reasonably heat stable when it can be dissolved at the molten "fats" stage. Ointments are generally relatively viscous, but due to the lack of water can be blended aggressively without fear of "cracking," i.e., separating phases, then the actives are usually incorporated using some form of high shear mixer. The degree of difficulty in doing this is to some extent dependent on whether the active can be incorporated either when the fats are molten or when they are cool. For the former, distribution should be relatively straightforward; for the latter, the viscosity may demand vigorous or prolonged mixing. Validation sampling is as for creams, i.e., bulk and filled units.

Solids

Validating solid dose forms after transfer has generated significant debate with the industry and its regulators as to the complexity of the validation process. There are probably several reasons for this.

- The multistage nature of the typical solid dose process, e.g., sieving, mixing, granulating, milling, drying, compression, and coating.
- The low level of active in the typical tablet.
- The impact changes or variations in the manufacturing process have on disintegration or dissolution and hence possibly bioavailability.
- As in most cases the active is not dissolved in the substrate, distribution is accomplished by physical dispersion only.

The U.S. FDA has insisted on blend uniformity studies, even to the extent of requiring them as routine. Within the EU the regulators do not have a declared policy and are driven by good science; normally this requires blend uniformity studies on validation only. A number of companies have taken such studies to extremes and have performed blend studies at every stage of the solid dose process.

This is probably reasonable at the development stage of a product to demonstrate exactly when and under what conditions the mixing plateau, i.e., the point at which the active is homogenously distributed occurs, and to ensure that subsequent demixing does not happen. However, for a previously manufactured product, particularly one for which a large number of lots have been manufactured, consistency of the finished product results should provide a reasonable indication that the process is under control; hence blend homogeneity and finished product homogeneity studies only are required.

Sampling at the final blend stage poses particular problems when powder sampling; the introduction of a so-called sample "thief" has been shown to disrupt mixing. Multipoint sampling throughout a blender is normally used, sampling wherever possible a sample size equivalent to the final dose form weight. The regulatory authorities (predominantly the FDA) will accept sample sizes up to three times the dose weight, but even this size is difficult to sample consistently.

Most granulates consist of granules or powders of different flow indices, which upon the introduction of a multipoint sampling device can differentially flow into the sample cavity, leading to apparently heterogenous samples. Even the angle of introduction of the "thief" can impact on the sample characteristics.

Final product sampling is usually performed by taking compressed tablets throughout the compression run. Variables that need to be considered are:

- Interchangeability of compression machines to provide production flexibility.
- The impact of the change of overhead feed drums and whether segregation occurs as the drum or hopper empties.
- The impact of compression machine speed on dose reproducibility.
- The impact of vacuum transfer parameters such as velocity, fluidization air volumes.

Direct compression formulations can be more problematic than wet granulation formulations as the incorporation of active in the former is physical only.

Each formulation transferred should be considered on a case-by-case basis to determine the most appropriate validation approach. It may be appropriate, if time and economics permit, to manufacture a 10% scale pilot batch with additional sampling to gain an understanding of the manufacturing dynamics before resource is committed to a full-scale batch.

Acceptance Criteria

It is difficult to set general acceptance criteria for each dose form as it is dependent on so many different factors. However, as a guide the following criteria have gained acceptance within the industry and with the regulatory authorities.

For a *tablet product* the criteria outlined in the *USP* for uniformity of dose should be applied, but the relative standard deviation (RSD) should not be greater than 5.0%. If it is wished to control content uniformity by weight during routine manufacture, it will be necessary to demonstrate a closer relationship of weight to content. It is unlikely that this may be assured with an RSD greater than 3.0%.

For *liquids, creams, ointments and gels* it is normal to take samples at several stages during the production process. The sampling points are dependent on the complexity of the manufacturing process and the mechanics of incorporation of the active. For example, if there are several aggressive mixing stages in the process it may be possible to only sample at the end of the process; for a more gentle process it may be necessary to demonstrate homogeneity at several steps.

For *intermediate* stages acceptance criteria using a 95% two-sided confidence interval about the mean could be used which would ensure that the true batch mean is contained within the data with 95% confidence.

The calculation:

$$X \pm t_{df,0.025} S\sqrt{n},$$

where

X = mean of n values
S = standard deviation of n values
n = number of unit samples
df = n–1
$t_{0.025}$ = 97.5 percentile of the t distribution with df degrees of freedom.

For *final* product it is normal to expect all finished product samples taken throughout the filling run to meet in full the finished product specification.

Cleaning Validation

This is another area in which careful risk assessment is required when transferring products.

As a practical example, the receiving site is used to dealing with fairly innocuous solid dose forms and then has to manufacture a tablet containing highly potent active. It is quite possible that local cleaning methods will prove inadequate based on the normal criteria used to assess cleaning efficacy (less than 0.1% of the standard daily dose of the "contaminant" present in the daily dose of the recipient product).

Consideration would need to be given to either:

- Reevaluating the cleaning methods, which might be an onerous task requiring extensive revalidation.
- Assessing whether a change in detergent might be sufficient to effect removal.
- Or whether a facility would need to be dedicated to the new product.

Similarly, if the receiving site was used to handling creams and then had to deal with a fatty ointment, once again current cleaning methods may prove inadequate.

Depending on the status of the donor plant, analytical methods may be available which are sufficiently sensitive to detect around the parts per million rate, and this method development will need to be factored into the timelines.

Finally, a new product may bring with it additional microbiological demands, e.g., products containing natural ingredients, high sugar concentrations, poorly preserved, and so on. This will probably need the services of a competent microbiologist to assist in the risk assessment.

Analytical Validation

The technology transfer of analytical methods can almost be considered as a project within a project, in that the ideas and thinking behind the overall product transfer apply equally to the analytical area.

All relevant documentation, method validation reports, out-of-specification reports, laboratory investigations and typical analytical results, should be reviewed by a transfer team. This transfer team should consist of all parties who will be using the methodology, and should include a minimum representation from all those involved in routine testing, stability, and process validation support, plus at least one knowledgeable individual from the donor site, when possible.

Each test should be reviewed against its history in the hands of trained analysts, the skill set of the receiving site, and the sophistication of the methodology.

In addition, emphasis should be placed on site-specific operating procedures, to highlight ways in which differences could impact the way the test is implemented at the respective sites.

A record of the rationale used to decide on the level of technology transfer necessary for each test should be made at this stage. The preparation of a validation master plan (VMP) may prove a useful vehicle in which to record these decisions.

Guidance on the level of technology transfer necessary for specific test procedures is given in the IPSE guidance on technology transfer. However, recommendations on some of the more common test requirements as applied to common pharmaceutical formulations are detailed below.

Assay

Assays should always be transferred although matrixing can be used on similar formulations. Typically this will be carried out by two analysts at each site, in triplicate, on three batches, on three different days. The analysis should consist of independent preparation of reagents, standards, etc., and should use different batches of analytical columns if appropriate. During the analysis any standard system suitability tests must be met and the acceptance criteria are usually based on the mean assay and variability obtained together with a visual comparison of the chromatography. Typically limits of plus or minus 5% of the mean assay between donor and receiving site are considered acceptable.

Impurities and Degradants

These should always be transferred. The samples analyzed and the analysts used are the same as for the assay. Transfer should also include confirmation of the limit of quantitation and response factors for those substances where quantitation is calculated from the relative response to that of the drug peak. Old samples are often useful in these transfers, especially for products that typically have low levels of impurities.

Acceptance criteria are usually based on mean and variation values (variation may be expressed in absolute rather than relative terms) and a visual comparison of the chromatography.

Dissolution

Typically transferred but often limited to one analyst, one batch and a dissolution profile on 12 units at each site. Acceptance criteria are typically mean meets specification with an absolute difference of not greater than plus or minus 5% and profiles are comparable.

Identity

Identity varies widely in techniques and complexity but is typically carried out on one batch only with acceptance criteria based on showing equivalence.

Microbiological Testing (including Sterility and LAL)

Transfers are not normally carried out on these test procedures as these are usually subjected to "in house" validation before use. Validation is usually completed in triplicate on three different batches.

Compendial Methods

Transfers are not normally considered necessary. However, care should be taken. These methods are not always described in sufficient detail to ensure comparable results are obtained (e.g., column packing details, extraction times, etc.). If the receiving site has had no experience of the formulation, a limited transfer may be prudent.

As with all such guidance different approaches are equally valid, and provided a sound rationale is recorded then this should be acceptable to the regulators.

The conclusions reached should be acceptable to all parties involved but, in general, and in the experience of the authors, this is not always the case. There are a number of pressures present at this time: some subconscious, others more direct. The vast majority are to reduce the workload and speed up the whole process, but it is our experience that more time has been lost through foreshortening of the process, than in carrying out unnecessary additional work.

It is important to remember: this is a *knowledge transfer* process as much as a *technology transfer* process.

Protocol

For those methods where a formal technology transfer has been deemed necessary, it is important for the whole process to be recorded in a protocol, prior to any completion of testing. This protocol should ideally be generated by the donor site, since it is considered expert in the methodology. However, alternative arrangements can be made if necessary, but it is preferable that any such protocol be generated by individuals who will not participate in the subsequent analysis.

This protocol should include the following sections:

- *Objective* — a clear statement of the objective of the transfer, from which laboratory the method is transferred and which of the receiving sites' laboratories are included in the transfer.
- *Scope* — a clear statement of the methods transferred and what is involved in the transfer.
- *Definition of responsibilities* — who is responsible for what and when, e.g., who writes the report, who signs the report, when does responsibility for the method transfer from the donor site to the receiving site.
- *Definition of terminology* — do not make assumptions that everyone has the same understanding of terms used (this is especially important in transfers between different countries).
- *Materials, methods, equipment to be used* — should include details on how the transfer analysis will be transferred, define the samples to be used, the number of replicate sample preparations, different analysts, days on which the analysis is to be completed, replicate injections of samples and standards and how they should be treated (individually, meaned, etc.).
- *Prequalification activities* — what training, if any, is required to be carried out by staff at the receiving site before the main part of the protocol is executed. What if any trial runs will be completed and what will happen to the results.
- *Experimental design used* — if a number of similar formulations are transferred at the same time it may be prudent to investigate the potential for reducing the workload by the use of experimental design. If this course is followed the design and the rationale for its use should be included.
- *Acceptance criteria* — detail what acceptance criteria will be applied to which results, include any statistical assessments to be made.
- *Remediation process* — if all goes well this section should not be needed, but including it at this stage enables subsequent actions to be more easily justified. It should include details of those involved in any investigations undertaken and any additional training requirements.
- *Documentation* — should make reference as to whether the transfer will be completed using the donor site's documentation or whether this is to be converted to the receiving site's format ahead of the transfer work. It should also

include how documentation generated during the transfer is identified, handled, reviewed, and stored.

- *Raw data* — how the raw data is to be identified, handled, reviewed, and stored.
- *References* — references to any external documentation used during the assessment prior to generating the protocol and any site SOPs used during the transfer.
- *Approval signatures* — who will approve the protocol and subsequent report. Should include name, job function, date and where working across time zones, the time and time zone.

For older products, where validation data to modern standards is not necessarily available, consideration should also be given to revalidating the methodology to International Committee for Harmonization (ICH) requirements as the movement of the product may open up discussions with the regulators on these aspects of the license.

Only when this protocol has been agreed should analytical work commence.

When the analytical work is complete there are, in common with other qualification-type work, a number of possible outcomes. Hopefully these and the necessary remediation were included in the original protocols. However for those that were not, the normal processes of investigation and further work should be followed.

Do not forget that the underlying reason for the transfer is to ensure that the method is robust, compliant, and can be used reliably at the new site.

The outcome of the protocol should be recorded in a formal report, any deviations discussed and justified and the report duly approved by the same signatories.

Depending on the sophistication of the test and the general skill set of the receiving site, consideration should be given to how additional staff will be trained in these new methodologies.

Packaging Issues

This section will concentrate on primary, i.e., product contact packaging, although the regulatory issues involved in declaring a change of site on label, leaflet, or carton can be considerable!

Issues to be considered are availability and comparability.

Most sites will have a purchasing strategy of preferred suppliers to secure economies of scale. Major items will be purchased from a single supplier, bottles and laminates often fall into this category. Wherever possible, supply chains will also be kept short, purchasing from as close to the manufacturing unit as possible.

Where product is transferred across countries or continents this may cause conflict between the needs of purchasing and the regulatory position in a product transfer. Significant changes in primary packaging are likely to require at least 3 months upfront stability and for sensitive products possibly 6 months at 25°C and 60% relative humidity (RH) and 3 months at 30°C and 75%RH.

Compatibility may also be an issue on a number of fronts.

First, as the plastic compounds used in both bottles and blister pack laminates are often commercially sensitive, it is sometimes difficult to directly compare them except by resorting to IR trace comparison. While this may provide a chemical compatibility, the bottles or laminates may still have different barrier properties and it may be necessary to compare minimum vapor transmission rates (MVTR) as well.

Second, although not normally considered a problem with solid dose forms, liquids, creams or ointments may need data generated on extractables and there is a potential for migration of the printing inks into the product. Similarly, some products may interact with the container causing discolouration or even cracking.

Stability Requirements

In the previous sections the need to consider stability for transferred products has been mentioned several times. As before, the best avoidance tactic is to make no changes in either process or packaging components. Practically this can be a difficult position to sustain, and in most cases sufficient changes will need to be made which precipitate a stability requirement.

By the time a 10% pilot scale batch has been produced, samples taken (and presuming stability indicating assays are available and validated), 3 months may have elapsed until the first stability time point; a further 1 month for results generation and reporting; then a total of at least 6 months can elapse. Clearly, this has an important impact on the transfer timelines.

If changes appear unavoidable then an early dialogue with the regulatory authority is recommended, to ascertain whether upfront or concurrent stability is required. Provision of previous data coupled with MVTR data, product compatibility studies or declarations from the container manufacturer of its suitability (conformance to FDA or DIN standards) for pharmaceutical use may be sufficient to allow stability data to be produced post-commercialization.

If there are a number of different strengths of the same formulation, it may be possible to use matrixing, i.e., provide data on the lowest and highest strength to negate the need for data on products in between.

For older products another complication may be the stability conditions themselves. Older products may only have had stability data generated at room temperature (18–25°C) and ambient humidity. Upon transfer, stability data meeting ICH conditions will be expected, i.e., 25°C and 60%RH. This may be too severe a challenge for either the formulation or the packaging system.

The latter may be correctable by increasing the barrier properties of the bottle or blister film (although not forgetting that this may have an economic impact) while the former may stop the transfer at worst, or require a reduction in the shelf life. Depending on the market competition, even this option may be unpalatable to the sales and marketing group.

Training

Regulatory agencies are paying increasing attention to training of operational staff, as do most companies. This assumes even more importance during technology transfer for a variety of reasons.

First, time constraints are normal and cutting training may be considered a soft option to save time. Second, the formulation, its manufacturing process, and the handling characteristics of the ingredients, may all be unfamiliar to operational staff. Third, the transfers will be under scrutiny, both inside and outside the operational unit, thereby increasing pressure on the staff.

Spending time on involving all relevant personnel in the process, providing appropriate and timely training, and encouraging staff to contribute to the process itself, will all help to minimize the likelihood of failure at what can be a stressful time for the organization. It perhaps goes without saying that all training must be documented and increasingly "validated."

THE TECHNOLOGY TRANSFER REPORT

Regulatory inspectors and sometimes assessors will ask for evidence of successful transfer. This is more likely when the technology transferred, be it the process or analytical method, is new to the site or poses particular challenges, e.g., the introduction of bioassays. The report should also serve a similar function to the original development pharmaceutics report in that it provides a "ready reckoner" of key aspects of the product and a reference point in the future if problems are encountered.

Contents

Generally the process consists of two stages:

- The generation of a protocol (a proposed structure for which is given below).
- A final technology transfer report, which includes all the raw data, or reference to where it can be found, together with a critical evaluation of the results.

Protocol structure

- *Scope* — a clear statement of the transferred product and of what is involved in its transfer, i.e., process validation, analytical validation, cleaning validation, etc.
- *Change management* — a statement of any changes being made as a result of the transfer, e.g., changes in source of actives, excipients, components, analytical methods and equipment, together with justification.

- *References* — cross-references to the original donor site documentation, e.g., manufacturing formula, manufacturing and analytical methods, specifications for actives, excipients and components. Copies of these documents may usefully be attached to the report as appendices.
- *Acceptance criteria* — a statement as to how the success of the transfer will be measured (see the Acceptance Criteria section) for each of the processes involved.
- *Sampling regime* — a statement of the number, size, and source of all samples and at what stage they will be taken.
- *Recipient site documentation* — reference to any source documents used in determining the transfer approach, e.g., pharmaceutical development reports, analytical validation or process validation reports from the donor site.
- *Additional requirements* — for example, if it has been determined that stability is needed then a copy of the protocol or reference to where the report may be found.

It may also be worth considering adding a section regarding the level of training considered necessary if the production, cleaning, or analytical methods are complex or new to the site.

The completed protocol will be supplemented with all the raw data (or references to workbooks, data files, etc.), to form the final report and a clear critical evaluation of the data and conclusion. If all acceptance criteria have not been met then a number of options need to be explored.

The transfer team, together with regulatory support, need to consider the nature of the failure and its impact on the robustness of the transfer. For example, if the cleaning validation fails, it can be considered that the manufacturing process is uncompromised, but a report addendum will have to be prepared clearly stating what corrective action has been taken and what results were achieved after implementation of the action.

Failure of the analytical validation clearly disrupts the program as process validation cannot be initiated with a flawed analytical technique; or indeed any stability testing initiated.

Failure of the process validation is clearly very significant and it may be very difficult to pinpoint what actions are required to correct the process. The normal causes of failure are inadequate distribution of the active and change in the dissolution profile.

Causes for the former may be:

- Inadequate mixing, over mixing (leading to demixing).
- Disparate particle sizes of active and excipients.
- Physical segregation caused by vacuum transfer systems.
- Different bulk density leading to higher or lower loading in the granulator and subsequent changes in swept volume.

For the latter, over-mixing leading to "slicking" of the lubricant is a common source of failure.

Normally an extensive sampling regime is required to determine the root cause, taking samples potentially at every stage of the process. This additional testing should be defined by a new protocol which once more sets out the purpose of the additional work, the acceptance criteria, etc., and the work carried out. It may be helpful to include the corrective action report as an addendum to the original report. It may be wise to maintain an increased sampling regime following any corrective action, to provide additional confidence that the source of variability has indeed been identified.

It should be noted that the technology transfer report may be requested by the licensing authority in approving the site transfer, or by the inspectorate, as part of a preapproval or normal GMP inspection.

Approval Process

The normal signatories of the technology transfer protocol are the team involved, regulatory affairs personnel, with a final approval to start from quality assurance. If the process involved is technically very complex it may be worthwhile, at the protocol initiation stage, to seek sign-off from experts at the donor site to ensure that (based on their better understanding of the process) all key criteria have been covered.

Once the work required to enact the protocol has been completed, and where timescales are very tight, it may be worth considering if commercial production can be effected against a review of the raw data, rather than waiting for the completion and signoff on the finally completed report. This decision should be formalized prior to the initiation of the transfer process, not subsequent to it.

POST-TRANSFER EVALUATION

During the period of the transfer, close scrutiny of the process involved is maintained by the transfer team and hence it can be considered that the validations are somewhat "artificial." It is therefore worth considering putting in place a post-transfer evaluation process where, say, the first 6 or 10 lots produced under standard production conditions are reviewed. Additional final product samples may be analyzed and the results plotted using Shewarts charts or similar to establish process robustness.

Dissolution profiles rather than simply drug availability after a set time period may be considered. These results can be collated and added as an addendum to the original technology transfer report to provide powerful evidence of the success of the transfer validation. In those countries where annual product reviews are mandated, then any recently transferred product should be given priority review status.

TECHNOLOGY TRANSFER CHECKLIST

Below is a checklist that summarizes the details that should be collated during the process, the majority of which have already been referenced.

- Copy of Part 2 of marketing authorization.
- Production master formula.
- Manufacturing instructions.
- Dispensing instructions.
- Analytical methods.
- Previous process validation.
- Previous analytical validation.
- Cleaning instructions and previous cleaning validation.
- Stability reports.
- Excipient specifications and source.
- Active specifications and source.
- Primary packaging material specifications and source.
- Packaging instructions.
- Customer complaints.
- Process deviations file.
- Analytical deviations file.
- Reject and rework file.
- Specimen manufacturing batch record.
- Specimen cartons, labels, leaflets.

SOURCES OF INFORMATION

Analytical Procedures Technology Transfer. ISPE Draft Guidelines. International Society of Pharmaceutical Engineers, ISPE European Office, 7 Avenue des Gaulois, 1040 Brussels, Belgium.

Cleaning Validation. Pharmaceutical Quality Group Monograph No. 10. Institute of Quality Assurance, 12 Grosvenor Crescent, London SW1X 7EE, U.K.

Comments on the European Commission Guideline on Dossier Requirements for Type 1 Variations. MCA Eurodirect Publications.

Draft Guidelines for Validation of Analytical Procedures. International Committee for Harmonization (ICH).

Guidance for Industry Changes to an Approved NDA or ANDA. Center for Drug Evaluation and Research (CDER), Food and Drug Administration (FDA).

Guidance for Industry SUPAC Manufacturing Equipment Addendum. Center for Drug Evaluation and Research (CDER), Food and Drug Administration (FDA).

Guidance for Industry Variations in Drug Products that may be included in a Single ANDA. Center for Drug Evaluation and Research (CDER), Food and Drug Administration (FDA).

Guideline on Dossier Requirements for Type 1 Variations. European Commission Enterprise Directorate-General.

Reviewer Guidance, Validation of Chromatographic Methods. Center for Drug Evaluation and Research (CDER), Food and Drug Administration (FDA).

EU documents are available on the website: www.eudra.org
FDA documents are available on the website: www.fda.gov

Chapter 14

Qualifying SCADA Systems in Practice Acquisition*

Orlando Lopez

CONTENTS

BACKGROUND

The introduction in 1997 of 21 CFR Part 11 (hereafter referred to as Part 11), established the exact regulatory requirements applicable to the Supervisory Control and Data Acquisition (SCADA) systems.

---

*Originally presented in the International Validation Week '98 Conference, Mahwak, New Jersey, November 1998, this paper was originally published in 2000 by Sue Horwood Publishing Ltd. This article updates the original published article and incorporates the most recent (February 2003) Food and Drug Administration's Part 11 draft guidance.

The main function of the SCADA system is to collect product-related manufacturing data linked to programmer logic controllers (PLC). PLCs are used to control and monitor data acquisition of manufacturing equipment (e.g., fluid bed granulator).

Computer systems used to create, modify, and maintain electronic records must be validated to ensure accuracy, reliability, consistent intended performance, and the ability to discern invalid or altered records.

In addition to the implications of Part 11 to the SCADA systems, this chapter addresses the importance of the factory acceptance test (FAT) and commissioning to expedite implementation of such systems.

The scope of the following discussion covers SCADA systems supporting cGMP-related electronic records in which Part 11 is applicable.

INTRODUCTION

Cell controllers are used for manufacturing control and data acquisition. In their most basic form, these systems process inputs and direct outputs. Everything else is simply an activity supporting inputs and outputs (I/Os) [2]. The primary concern for cell controllers is working accurately in the intended process. This is dynamically verified during the qualification [3] of the cell controller. The qualification of automated cell controllers is "essential to ensure proper functioning of the process and product quality" [4].

Cell controllers fall into a specific category, such as a distributed control system (DCS), PLC or SCADA. Historically a DCS was meant for analog loop control, a PLC for replacement of relay logic, and a SCADA system was used when data collection was needed. Currently a DCS can replace relay logic, a PLC can implement analog loop control, and SCADA can do both. In addition to the above-mentioned categories, cell control can be implemented using personal computers. This category is called "soft PLC."

As depicted in Figure 14.1, PLCs are always used linked to a process plant via a real-time link. PLCs cannot exist in isolation to electronically record data. The PLC must be linked to a SCADA system. The combination of a PLC plus a SCADA system gives functionality close to a DCS.

In addition to the integration issues associated with the implementation of SCADA systems in a GMP [5] environment, this chapter addresses issues on these systems concerning Part 11.

Part 11 allows the regulated industries to electronically maintain records required to be kept by the predicate regulation [6]. Records that are electronically maintained following the provisions of the Part 11, can be used to satisfy a predicate rule.are recognized as equivalent to paper-based records.

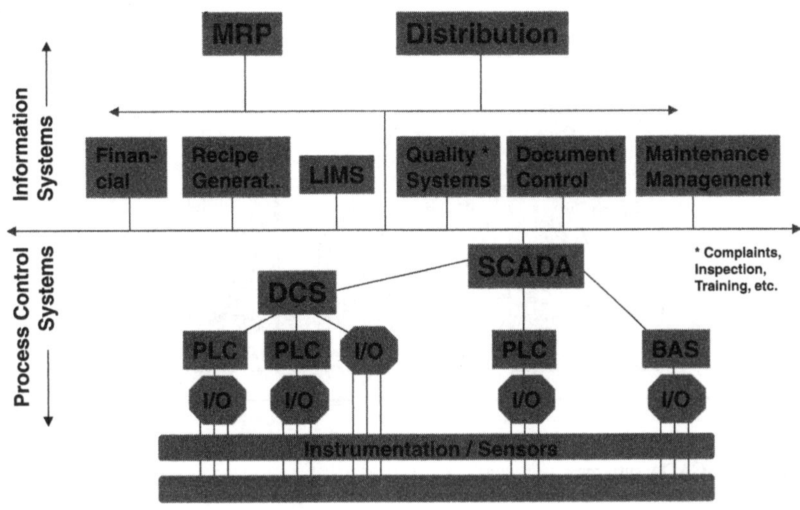

Figure 14.1 Integration.

SCADA SYSTEMS

SCADA software monitors and collects data from remote functions and processes by using serial communication links between master and remote locations. It is primarily concerned with I/O monitoring and the passing of setpoints or open loop commands to remote controllers.

SCADA application software, which is normally implemented by the SCADA system supplier, performs such functions as database management, scan I/O data from the remote terminal units (RTUs), log and report scheduling, display drivers, perform on-line calculations, call mathematical subroutines, and protocol conversion.

These systems are responsible for the control of electronic records and their display, but usually not their final storage. SCADA systems, as illustrated in Figure 14.2, are supervisory in nature because they are not responsible for the primary control functions. They gather and send information to remote locations, interface with the primary controllers by sending set points or calculated values, and are capable of communicating over telephone lines, UHF or VHF radios, microwave systems, satellite systems, and fiber optic cables.

SCADA systems comprise master control stations, equipment installed at the remote sites, and the human machine interfaces (HMI). The computer-based system at the control center is referred to as the master control station (MCS). The MCS may be a single computer with display and logging peripherals. For more demanding requirements, the MCS may be composed of multiple computers

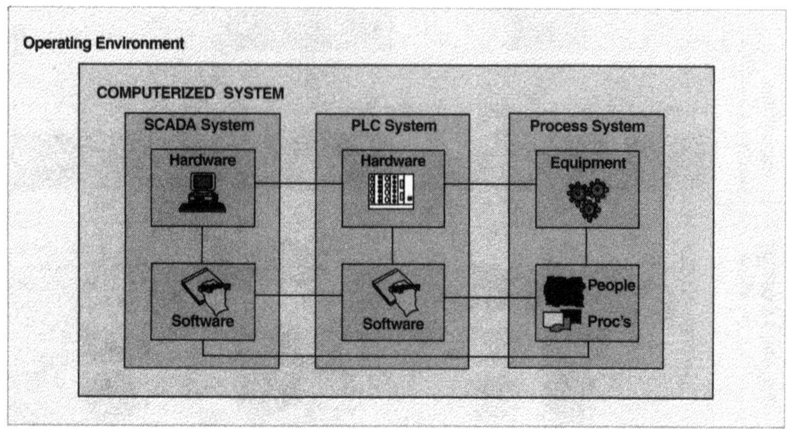

Figure 14.2 SCADA systems.

networked together. The multiple computer system configuration provides both added workstations and redundancy protection against computer failure. Small- to medium-sized MCS requirements are met with the application of a high performance PC running SCADA software under a real-time operating system. For a very large SCADA system MCS, with measurement databases exceeding 50,000 points, mainframe computers are needed.

The MCS might also be a hardware module that functions as a data concentrator for yet another digital system (such as DCS). Usually any PLC linked to a SCADA system acts as the central controller.

At the control center, computers acquire the data measurements from all of the stations and present a complete dynamic profile of the entire process. The readings are displayed and recorded in graphic and text formats, and control commands to effect changes in the process are transmitted back to the remote sites. The transmission to the remote sites is performed either automatically or is initiated by the operators.

The equipment installed at the remote sites is called an RTU. An RTU is a box positioned in substations and it will never disrupt the system's process. Instead, PLC/controllers do control the process based on set points. RTU units measure voltages, currents, pressures, temperatures, device positions, equipment alarms and they compute flow rates and volumes. The measurements and calculations are performed at very high rates of speed with high degrees of accuracy under all conditions of the rugged environment in which they are installed. The RTUs are intelligent, normally containing multiple microprocessors with sophisticated real-time software programs. They are configured to fit the specific needs of each individual station and they are designed to be applicable to a variety of differing station requirements.

HMI and the data collection systems provide the operators with a central interface into the operation of the remote stations. They also provide the ability to make changes in the operational parameters. The HMI application is used as the reporting mechanism for the system and it maintains the historical database for the system.

In general, the communication between workstations, master, and remote stations is performed by:

- Multiple workstations accessing the master station and sharing system and process data.
- The master station polls blocks of data to and from remote stations.
- Remote stations collect data. They have blocks of data waiting to send when the master polls them.

In summary, SCADA systems:

- Collect and store historical data.
- Monitor the process and provide information to make decisions on products and processes.
- Provide supervisory control such as: analysis, yield reports, and product information.
- Provide a mechanism to access real-time data in the PLCs.
- Detect system alarms.
- Report problems: displays, summaries, and acknowledgments.

PART 11 [7]

The scope of Part 11 was updated as the result of the February 2003 draft guidance. This guidance has a significant practical effect on enforcement decisions by adopting a more reasonable and risk-based approach. The draft guidance clearly states, "fewer records will be considered subject to Part 11." There is a predominant focus on predicate rules. The U.S. FDA emphasized that records must still be maintained or submitted in accordance with the underlying predicate rules. FDA will enforce predicate rule requirements for records that remain subject to Part 11, and intend to enforce all provisions of Part 11 other than legacy systems, [8] audit trails, record retention, and record copying requirements.

The regulated industry will continue to have responsibility for maintaining and submitting secure and reliable records under predicate rules, and for meeting all other predicate rule requirements.

Under the new scope, Part 11 applies to:

- Records that require maintenance by predicate rules and that are maintained in electronic format in place of paper format.

- Records that are required to be maintained by predicate rules, are maintained in electronic format in addition to paper format, and are relied on to perform regulated activities.
- Records submitted to the FDA, under the predicate rules (even if such records are not specifically identified in Agency regulations), in electronic format (assuming the records have been identified in the docket as the types of submissions the Agency accepts in electronic format).
- Electronic records required to be maintained by a predicate rule and represented on a printout, but the electronic records are relied on to perform regulated activities.
- Electronic records required to be maintained by a predicate rule, not submitted, but are used in generating a submission.
- Electronic signatures that are intended to be the equivalent of handwritten signatures, initials, and other general signings required by predicate rules.

Part 11 regulations does not apply to electronic records that are not submitted to the Agency, not used to generate a submission, and not required to be maintained by a predicate rule.

In addition the U.S. FDA will not impose Part 11 requirements on legacy computer systems, as long as the records that these systems generate meet Part 11 requirements.

Records, in which Part 11 is applicable and maintained following its provisions, are to be recognized as equivalent to traditional paper-based records.

The Part 11 requirements applicable to a typical SCADA system are discussed in the next section.

PART 11 AND SCADA

As already stated the SCADA system is typically a hybrid [9] computer system that saves on magnetic media manufacturing data required by the cGMP regulations. One possible example consists of a SCADA system in which historical data collection is archived and production batch reports are printed directly from the SCADA station. These reports are usually signed manually. These records are relied on to perform regulated activities.

On hybrid systems, the subpart B in Part 11 is the relevant regulation applicable to these electronic records. These records, in which Part 11 applies, must be maintained and retained in electronic format for the period established by the cGMPs. The retention requirements of cGMP records can be found in 211.180(a).

Based on the new FDA approach, the areas in Part 11 impacting the SCADA hybrid systems are:

1 Audit trails and metadata.

2 System security.
   a. Codes and passwords security.
   b. Codes and passwords maintenance.
   c. Passwords assignment.
   d. Records protection.
   e. Authority checks.
3 Operational checks.
4 Location checks.
5 Document controls.
6 Open or closed systems.

The discussion of the above items can be found elsewhere [10]. Readers may differ the inclusion of the audit trails in the above list. The decision to apply audit trails [11] is based on the need to comply with the predicate rule requirements. The inclusion of audit trails is considered "as a check of accuracy" [12] of computer outputs in a cGMP environment.

The SCADA systems are responsible for the management of manufacturing-related electronic records (e-recs) but usually not its final storage. As part of the cGMP requirements on data integrity, it is important to describe the entire path that the data follows and where manipulations to that data take place. This description could start from the sensor in the field and go as far as the electronic batch record system (EBRS).

The SCADA application software managing electronic records must conform to the following requirements:

- The changes to the e-recs do not obscure earlier modifications.
- There is no possibility to alter in any way the audit trail of changes made to electronic records.

Security can be viewed in many ways. Preventing access to data or records is one view. It may also pertain to accidental or intentional data manipulation, corruption or destruction that may occur through environmental factors such as a power failure that causes data to be lost. The SCADA application should be designed, verified, and tested so that these accidental, intentional, or environmental data losses do not occur.

Authorized parties may also view security as allowing access to the records. These are called authority checks.

Security is very important for the integrity of the cell controller's data and will be discussed later as part of the discussion on validation.

QUALIFICATION PROJECT LIFE CYCLE

Figure 14.3 depicts a sample cell controller development life cycle in a regulated

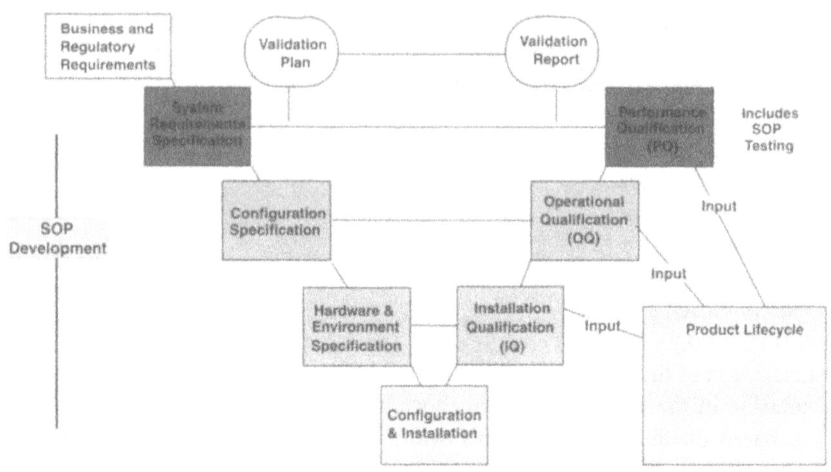

Figure 14.3 Typical project development and testing framework.

environment. When evidencing cGMP compliance, in each of the phases identified in the project life cycle, certain deliverables are expected.

It is very important to define all deliverables, to perform rigorous review cycles, and to establish a multidisciplinary project team to analyze the design in an orderly and consistent fashion. These activities are defined in the computer systems' validation procedure or in the validation plan.

The qualification of SCADA systems introduces particular issues that must be addressed and verified during the project development life cycle. Some of these issues are:

- SCADA systems integrate components from several vendors, each emulating the host protocol. Integration of all of these components can be challenged.
- The security of the system parameters is an issue in any cell controller. This concern is simplified in recipe-based systems where values are overwritten with each production run.
- PLC and SCADA systems often have critical timing and environmental requirements.

As shown in Figure 14.3, the project can be arranged as follows:

- Business and regulatory requirements.
- Software configuration and hardware specifications.
- Configuration and installation.

- Qualification testing.

In this chapter the maintenance and system retirement are out of the scope.

BUSINESS AND REGULATORY REQUIREMENTS

During this phase the evaluation of the business needs and modeling of the technology operation take place. The end-users analyze and confirm the proposed scope of the project, including the SCADA requirements. The term "requirement" defines a bounded characterization of the scope of the system. Some of these requirements include:

- Functional capacity.
- Execution capability.
- Operational checks.
- Installation.
- Documentation.
- The user's manual.
- Training.
- The maintenance manual.
- System maintenance.
- The system test plan.
- Acceptance criteria.
- GMP compliance.

The requirements contain the information essential to support the process, operators, regulatory, safety, and many more.

The system requirements document includes a review of the process to familiarize the software supplier or integrator with the user, process and data acquisition requirements, and special considerations of the project. Specifically for SCADA systems, the requirements document must include a definition of the data to be collected, how the data will be used, how it will be stored, what the retention requirements are, what the data requirements are, and where each function is to be executed (e.g., MCS, remote location).

This process view is essential when software must interface with other elements such as hardware, people, and databases. It incorporates requirements from the system level with a small amount of top-level design. Each SCADA element must be well defined at the outset in order to provide prospective suppliers with enough information to provide a detailed and meaningful quotation.

The requirements document addresses:

- Control philosophy: project description, references, objectives of cell controller, definitions, conceptual automation system architecture, level of automation required, and area-specific philosophies.

- Functional requirements: batch control, operator interface, timing, security, data archiving, audit trails, logging, reporting, alarming, recipe management, interfacing to other systems, and production scheduling.
- Performance requirements: expandability, responsiveness, and redundancy.
- Hardware requirements: system hardware requirements and third party cell controllers hardware requirements.
- Required standards: software development SOPs, design/programming, and other standards.
- Plans: execution, testing, and staging.
- Redundancy and error-detection protocol.
- The role of the SCADA in the communication interface to field devices, data acquisition, reports, and HMI.
- Input gained from operators and supervisors into the system design to influence how the system is operated.
- Type of control and process to be performed.
- Level of automation (e.g., fully automatic batch execution).
- Timing, safety, and regulatory requirements.
- The central processor, memory, bulk storage equipment, peripheral devices such as printers, video display units, operator consoles, and system support devices.
- Scan cycle and the response time required to accomplish the users' needs.

Adverse environmental conditions may affect the operation of the process control system, including the SCADA. It is necessary to specify key environmental parameters and operational limits of the system components. The facility and supporting utilities must be designed to maintain control within the specified operational limits.

Each requirement in the requirements document must be "testable." This means each requirement must have an objective criterion and must be nonambiguous. All of these requirements are tested during the performance qualification (PQ).

The requirements document also includes a risk assessment that pays attention to the system operation and the impact of the implementation to the product for which the process was designed.

The requirements contained in the system requirements document can be used to select the standard software, the developer of the SCADA configurable elements, and to put together the design documents.

Software Configuration and Hardware Specifications

After the process, operators, regulatory, and safety requirements are established, the vendor-supplied standard software and the system integrator can be selected. The system is delineated based on the selected standard software.

The software configurable specification and the hardware specification represent the adaptation of the system integrator's project bid and the owner's proposal to a final design of the system.

Before purchasing the SCADA vendor-supplied standard software, an audit is performed to assess the developer's software quality assurance (SQA) program. A proper SQA program assures software correctness, reliability, testability, maintainability and compliance with standards, procedures, instruction codes, and contractual and licensing requirements. In addition this audit is used to evaluate the vendor's personnel and the hardware quality assurance procedures. The personnel involved in developing, approving, and implementing the hardware and software can have a dramatic impact on the project success.

The software configuration specification includes the capability of the SCADA application to implement the data acquisition functions as required in the system requirements document, such as:

- Batch processing sequence.
- Graphics standards and displays (detailed schematics, primary control, monitoring data, overview graphics display maintenance screen, help screens).
- Operator interface requirements (display performance) and display formats.
- Logical security options and capacity (21 CFR 11).
- Data storage and communication capabilities, including error-detection protocol.
- I/O list, protocol, and data link requirements.
- Database (I/O) listing, log and reports specifications, alarm handling, history and trending and documentation standards.
- Potential expansion of services requirements.
- Format and content of reports.
- Method of communication.
- Subsystems' components and interfaces, data structure, design constraints, algorithms, and system decomposition.

This document is also maintained under a configuration management to always reflect the current project scope.

The software configuration specification is tested during the operational qualification (OQ).

The hardware specification describes the hardware design used to maintain the implementation of the cell controller and the collection of batch records. This includes signal, power, redundancy, quantity, and complexity of the data acquisition required of the cell controller.

The hardware specification includes a description of the design of the central processor, memory, peripheral devices such as printers, video display units, operator consoles, and system support devices. It includes the detailed design of the scan cycle and the response time required to accomplish the users' needs.

The hardware specification contains hardware architecture block diagrams. These show the conceptual hardware architecture including interfaces between levels, operator interface terminal locations, vendor-supplied controls and interfaces, printers, highway connections, and so on. This is specific to the vendor-supplied hardware.

The hardware specification may include cell controller specification including I/O estimates by area and the application software needed to support each cell.

The risk analysis is revisited and updated based on the software configuration and hardware specifications. The revisited risk analysis document contains how the risks inherent to the system are to be mitigated.

The hardware specification is tested during the installation qualification (IQ).

The software configuration specification and the hardware specification define the equipment or system in sufficient detail to enable the integration of the hardware and the code to be developed.

SCADA systems' application software and hardware are configurable. These systems comprise a number of modular blocks or packages providing the system functionality. The configuration of the predefined modular blocks or packages is therefore specific to the user process. For these configurable elements the full development model must be followed. The software architecture consists of: database, human–machine interface (HMI), statistical process control (SPC), alarm processing, trending, batch data reports, and batch data storage.

The configurable elements developed by the integrator are specific in accordance to the user requirements. Quality audits to the software supplier and the integrator can be performed to evaluate the level of quality and testing built into the standard and configurable products components.

The in-process audits verifies the consistency of the product as it evolves through the configuration by determining that the system requirements are fully tested and the design of the product satisfies the requirements depicted in the software configuration and hardware specifications. The integrator's quality assurance group can perform this audit.

Factory Acceptance Test (FAT)

A FAT is a mutually agreed detailed test performed by the vendor or integrator at the vendor's or integrator's site. It is an integration test executed in an environment very similar to the hardware and software interfaces encountered in the operational environment. In replacing the process equipment the system can be subjected to a real-world environment by using emulators [15]. The user's representative evaluates the supporting documents, the operation, the functionality, and the reliability of the cell controller.

One of the main functional tests during the FAT is the implementation of the error-detection protocol to the SCADA systems. The error-detection protocol provides information about data corruption and can be used as an ongoing monitoring tool. Part 11 requires that the integrity of data must be safeguarded. Batch records can be built based on production data collected electronically.

Another issue regarding electronic recipe-based systems and the associated security is the audit trails and the process parameters. Recipe values can be overwritten with each production run. Using the single loop controller's approach, control of the process parameters must be proven in two places: within the PC which contains the recipe set points to be downloaded, and at the controllers themselves, which may be configured through their own operator panels. In the PLC approach, the program can be written so only a programing terminal can change the data memory for either the stored recipe blocks or the active block. An advantage, then, of the PLC-based cell controller is that the operator may choose only those values that exist in the PLC and have been validated. In case of overwriting a recipe value there must be a time-stamped audit trail to document who did what, wrote what, and when.

By necessity, SCADA systems will be required to interface with a broad spectrum of electronic equipment. Many techniques have been developed over the years to accommodate most of the requirements.

Interfaces to information technology (IT) systems are normally handled by providing a direct network interface from the SCADA system equipment to the information technology systems.

Some SCADA system suppliers have developed protocol converter products that allow interfacing RTUs and other remote equipment into the SCADA system. Interfacing is a major concern in the application of SCADA systems.

Proper integration of the SCADA hardware for its designed operation is demonstrated through suitable tests. Many times SCADA systems are built utilizing components from several vendors, each emulating the host communication protocol. In order to support this varied architecture, an alternative is testing using communication protocol simulators. These simulators monitor network traffic, log network and station errors, and provide real-time master and remote simulation. Control over pretransmission mark time, squelch time, data framing, and error checking is provided. In addition, a hardware trigger output is available that can be used to trigger an external device such as an oscilloscope or a logic analyzer. These capabilities allow you to verify the operation of each subsystem before it is put into service. These simulators have proved to be invaluable for commissioning new equipment, troubleshooting network problems, and routine maintenance.

In addition the FAT includes verification of (as applicable):

- Database structure, files, tables, dictionaries, and data archiving.
- Selected configuration or control file parameters.
- Proper communications between the computer system and the peripherals.
- Startup and shutdown of the computer system.
- Startup and shutdown of the software.

- Restart and recovery functions and procedures.
- Application availability to an authorized account.
- Application primary menu availability.
- Application major component and function availability.
- System-wide "function key" processing.
- Any vendor-supplied diagnostics.
- Data acquisition (e.g., scan I/O data from RTUs).
- Loop tests and operational checks.
- Batch control.
- Recipe management.
- Alarming.
- Timing.

During the FAT a functional audit and a physical audit may be performed. A functional audit compares the configurable code with the documented software configuration specification. Also, the review of the in-process audit results may be coordinated.

A physical audit compares the configurable code with its supporting documentation. Its purpose is to assure that the documentation to be delivered correctly describes the code. Inputs to the physical audit consist of all design documentation.

If the FAT results and audits conform to the contractual agreements, especially to the software configuration specification, the system will be accepted for shipment and installation. All identified critical problems found during the execution of the FAT must be corrected before shipment.

Configuration and Installation

The configuration and installation of the system comprises the deployment of the automated cell controller, including the SCADA at the operational environment. It includes the controlled equipment, the process control hardware, and the application or configurable software.

For cell controller hardware, this deployment involves the integration of PLC, SCADA, and associated hardware components based on the system configuration documents.

The implementation of SCADA software involves configuration of the custom configurable package, debugging, and formal configuration inspections by the developer. The major elements to be configured in a SCADA system are:

- Data channels, including ports and the number of messages that can be buffered. Device equipment connected to the serial and parallel ports (e.g., modems), including communication settings.

- Master configuration, including master station address, error detection protocol, and response time.
- Node definition: PLC, DCA, BAS bridge or sensor device connected to the data channels.
- Master pool list.
- Scan classes: scan period, i.e. of how often the address is scanned.
- Database: tag type and associated data structure.

Items that may be checked during the configurable testing include the following:

- Functionality as per design document.
- Results of subjecting the unit to maximum or minimum limits.
- Reaction to incorrect inputs.
- Exception handling.
- Algorithm checking.
- Adherence to documented standards.

Commissioning

The commissioning or site acceptance testing (SAT) is performed after the configuration and installation of the system in the operational environment.

During the commissioning many of the FAT verifications are reproduced. The commissioning is the set of activities comprised of the system installation, start-up, operational verification, and turnover performed by the cell controller supplier in the operational environment [16–18]. As in the FAT, the user's representative evaluates the results of the commissioning.

The most important test is the hardware configuration and qualification. This is probably the first time that the complete system hardware is available. The hardware configuration provides an equipment installation and configuration, and an inventory list for each device or piece of equipment associated with the SCADA system. Vendor manuals for each piece of hardware are required.

The hardware commissioning includes:

- System description and schematic drawings.
- Piping and instrument drawing.
- Instruments list.
- I/Os list.
- Wiring checks.
- Loop diagrams.
- Calibration.
- Hardware configuration.
- Interface verification and integration.

- Verification of hardware integration.
- Security verification.
- Control equipment configuration verification.
- Control equipment interface verification.
- Hardware redundancy verification.

The software commissioning includes:

- Man–machine–interface installation verification.
- Security verification.
- SCADA database and configuration verification.
- SCADA interface verification.
- Catastrophic recovery verification.
- Man–machine–interface functional verification.
  - Boundary values.
  - Invalid values.
  - Special values.
  - Decision point and branch conditions.
- Reports generation tests.
- Data acquisition and database access controls.
- Loop tests and operational checks.
- Network connection (as applicable).
- Trending and alarms processing.
- Interface with other applications (e.g., SPC).
- Timing (as applicable).
- Sequencing and operation.

Qualification Testing [19]

In process control systems, qualification testing is necessary on the levels where the physical process is carried out, where manufacturing procedures, control, instructions, and specifications are loaded to the PLC, and where quality data related to the product or process is manipulated and recorded. Qualification testing is necessary at the sensor or data collection devices, process control, supervisory or line control, plant integration, and control levels. These levels affect how the physical process is carried out. Qualification testing is also necessary for the retention and manipulation of data relevant to the quality of the product or process.

The computer system qualification testing incorporates the typical IQs, OQs, and PQs.

The IQ establishes confidence that computer hardware and ancillary systems are compliant-approved design intentions and that manufacturer's recommendations are suitably considered.

The OQ establishes confidence that computer system is capable of consistently operating within established limits and tolerances described in the software configuration specification.

The PQ provides documented evidence that provides a high degree of assurance that the computer system and the operating environment perform as established by the requirements specification deliverable.

A comprehensive commissioning testing following approved qualification protocols incorporates the typical qualification testing found in an IQ and OQ. Much of the documentation may be used to support the qualification activities. Based on a comprehensive commissioning, the qualification testing may include only a performance qualification (PQ).

Figure 14.4 depicts typical qualification activities and the associated time line.

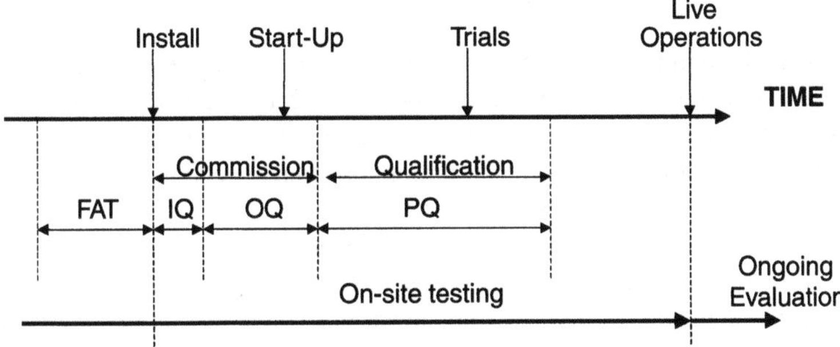

Figure 14.4 Qualification timeline.

The PQ is an exhaustive system performance test designed to determine the degree of accuracy with which the system correlates to the SRS. The PQ should not be confused with the process performance qualification and the product qualification as defined in the FDA Guideline on Principles of Process Validation. The PQ occurs under operational conditions but not as part of the actual operational process.

The specific test objectives for SCADA systems include:

- Determination that the system is accuracate in receiving, recording, storing, and processing electronically manufacturing information.
- Determination that the system is accuracate in arriving at the appropriate disposition decision based upon the data received through the SCADA system.
- Determination of the integration between all SCADA components.
- Platform security.
- Audit trail reporting.

- System backup.
- System restoration.
- Database recovery.
- If SCADA database conversion, migration, or preloading with data is to occur prior to PQ testing, the verification of these activities and their associated data may be addressed in the PQ.
- Test that SCADA databases files, or tables are appropriately scaled versions of the production datasets. Test data must contain a well-designed representation of production data that allows all conditions to be tested and all defects uncovered so that they can be corrected. Test data must be clearly identified and retained.

Summary Report

Once the qualification testing has been completed, the test results and data need to be formally evaluated. The written evaluation needs to be presented clearly and in a manner that can be readily understood. The report should also address any nonconformance or deviations to the validation plan that are encountered during the qualification and their resolutions.

The summary report addresses the results of each qualification protocol. In addition, all inspections and technical review results must be summarized.

A summary of nonconformances and deviations, their resolution, and impact must also be included.

The summary report is linked with the validation plan.

System Use and Performance Evaluation

During the operational phase, the procedures and systems needed to insure the acceptability of the system over time are inspected at system start-up.

Operating Manuals and Procedures

Operating manuals should be available to the users of the system at all necessary locations. These manuals must be written at a level such that the actual operator can utilize them.

SOPs required for manual steps must be completed. These procedures should include operations performed on a routine basis, as well as procedures needed for occasional use. Some of these procedures are:

- Configurable code management.

- Preventative maintenance.
- Environmental control.
- Backup.
- Recovery (data).
- Specific training.
- GxP training.
- Security.
- Disaster contingencies.
- Changes to validated systems.
- Supplier audit.
- System management.
- Periodic review.

Change Control

Maintenance in SCADA systems becomes a key issue, particularly when a new version of the vendor-supplied standard software is updated. A change control procedure must be developed whereby changes in the software and computer hardware may be evaluated, approved, and documented.

As necessary, additional qualification may be needed to evaluate changes (e.g., impact analysis) on SCADA systems. The procedure should allow for both planned and emergency changes to the system.

The procedure must include a provision for the updating of pertinent documentation on the system. Records of changes to the system must be kept for the same period as any other regular production document.

Environmental control

A procedure should be in place for the ongoing monitoring and documentation of key environmental parameters. Environmental parameters may include:

- Temperature.
- Relative humidity.
- Power levels and conditioning.
- Static electricity.
- Dusty conditions.
- Electromagnetic interference affecting system components or communications lines.

Backup

Procedures should be in place to assure that data backups are performed on a regular basis and are stored in a secure location.

System Recovery Plan

This plan focuses on the procedures for returning the system to full and proper performance after a catastrophic condition. It includes data recovery, system restart procedures, and addresses all aspects of recovery from loss of a hard drive, corruption of a file or database, or loss of power to the system. The evaluation of these procedures as part of the OQ or PQ is recommended.

Training of Personnel

Each user of the system must be trained on the various functions he/she will be performing. All such training should be documented.

System Security

The documentation should describe the physical (hardware) security employed to protect the system, as well as software security.

Support Personnel

A listing of support personnel and their responsibilities and qualifications should be included as part of the documentation.

System Performance Evaluation

In the operational environment the automated cell controller shall be monitored. System outputs should be periodically examined for accuracy and discrepancies.

Many I/O systems provide capabilities in terms of self-diagnostics. Events such as a broken wire or a shorted contact can be quickly diagnosed to the I/O point level through built-in fault tables. The verification of these diagnostics is an essential element in system evaluation.

Another element that should be verified periodically is the configurable data. Import and export utilities at all levels allow consolidation of configurable data from PLC and supervisory software. All data is fully documented and can be verified on a continuing basis.

As in any CGMP environment, the performance monitoring activity is guided by a standard operating procedure and the results must be documented.

REFERENCES

1 The process of determining whether a system or component is suitable for operational use (IEEE).

2 Snyder, D., "Take Advantage of Control Options," *A-B Journal*, March, 1997.

3 The process of determining whether a system or component is suitable for operational use (IEEE).

4 Motise, P. J., "Human Drug CGMP Notes," Volume 6, Number 2, June, 1998.

5 GMP is an abbreviation that encompass the current U.S. FDA current Good Manufacturing Practices (cGMP).

6 Predicate regulations are the Federal Food, Drug, and Cosmetic Act, the Public Health Service Act or any FDA Regulation, with the exception of 21 CFR Part 11. Predicate regulations address the research, production, and control of FDA regulated articles.

7 Guidance for industry, *21 CFR Part 11; Electronic Records; Electronic Signatures, Scope and Application*.

8 A system which is in place and is used and which is deemed to have aged with respect to the application of the regulations (ISPE).

9 In the context of Part 11, hybrid computer systems save required data from a regulated operation to magnetic media. However, the electronic records are not electronically signed. In summary in hybrid systems, some portions of a record are paper and some are electronic.

10 Lopez, O., FDA Regulations of Computer Systems in Drug Manufacturing — 13 Years Later, *Pharmaceutical Engineering*, May/June, 2001.

11 Comment paragraph 186, 1978 CGMP revision.

12 FDA, CPG 7132a.07, "Computerized Drug Processing, I/O Checking," 9/4/87.

13 Tetszlaff, R., "GMP Documentation Requirements for Automated Systems: Part I," *Pharmaceutical Technology*, March 1992.

14 Motise, P.J., U.S. FDA, e-mail: motise@cder.fda.gov

15 Emulation: the imitation of all or part of one computer system by another, primarily by hardware, so that the imitating computer system accepts the same data and executes the same results as the imitated system (ISO).

Simulation: the representation of selected characteristics of the behavior of one physical or abstract system by another system. In a digital computer system, simulation is done by software (ISO).

16 Wheeler, W.P. Commissioning: A Vital Precursor to Validation, *Pharmaceutical Engineering*, July/August, 1994.

17 Angelucci, L.A., Validation and Commissioning, *Pharmaceutical Engineering*, January/February, 1998.

18 ISPE, *Pharmaceutical Engineering Guide: Oral Solid Dosage Forms*, February, 1998.

19 Testing conducted to determine whether a system or component is suitable for operational use (IEEE).

Chapter 15

The Application of GAMP 4 Guidelines to Computer Systems Found in GLP-Regulated Areas

Paul Coombes

CONTENTS

PART 1 THE ACADEMIC SIDE OF THE SUBJECT

To explore the question given to the author of this chapter "how can GAMP 4 be applied to GLP?" we must first confirm our definition of GLP (Good Laboratory Practice) and quickly eliminate some common misunderstandings. The term GLP refers explicitly to laws concerning the area of investigation where toxicology and safety studies on chemicals are carried out — which may include animal and other *in vivo* and *in vitro* testing. This work is performed in the so-called preclinical (or nonclinical) phase of drug product development in the pharmaceutical industry — but toxicology testing is also carried out in the industrial chemicals and defence and military sectors. The key defining aspects of this type of regulated work are chemical and biochemical analysis. This sometimes involves animal testing carried out in laboratories and other controlled areas, performed on chemicals and new molecular entities (which may become medicinal, therapeutic, cosmetic, or industrial products) to determine toxicity and safety data using explicit and implicit scientific and ethical approaches named the "Principles of GLP" [1]. Often, but not always, the work in GLP areas of the pharmaceutical sector is on new compounds not yet approved for use in humans or animals.

GLP regulations do not apply to most analytical development laboratories or quality control (QC) laboratories in drug manufacturing — GMP is the applicable regulatory framework in these cases. GLP is therefore *not* a general guide on how to do good work in all types of laboratory. However, the term "good laboratory practice" is used as a self explanatory term in many laboratories whether they are GMP, GLP, GCP regulated, or regulated by other bodies, or not regulated at all. (Please see the end of this chapter for more detailed definitions and references about GLP.)

GAMP (good automated manufacturing practice), as the name indicates, originates from the world of automated manufacturing. It provides its audience with comprehensive and authoritative guidance on the validation and control of process automation and other automated and computerized systems. Process automation systems used for drug product manufacture are clearly absent in the world of GLP — but other types of computerized systems mentioned in GAMP 4 certainly abound. A huge variety of computer controlled scientific instrumentation, electronic data processing systems and electronic information systems are employed in GLP laboratories. There is an explicit requirement to validate those computer systems used in GLP studies if one follows the OECD GLP and U.K. GLP regulations and guidance:

> "The computerized systems used within the study need to be reliable, accurate, and have been validated". [U.K. GLP Schedule 2 Part 1, 11. (2)]. [2]

Or

> "All computerized systems used for the generation, measurement or assessment of data intended for regulatory submission should be developed, validated, operated and maintained in ways which are compliant with the GLP Principles". [3]

Perhaps surprisingly the FDA GLP regulation (21 CFR Part 58) does not include the word "validation," and the words "automated" or "computer" are only meaningfully mentioned in the definitions section for "raw data":

> (k) "Raw data" ... Raw data may include photographs, microfilm or microfiche copies, computer printouts, magnetic media, including dictated observations, and recorded data from automated instruments. [Section 58.3 21 CFR Part 58]

We can continue the same "word search" approach looking in a different direction, namely, checking how many of the key words associated with GLP are found in GAMP 4. This exercise provides an initial feel for the level of correlation between GAMP 4 guidelines and GLP principles.

Cross-checking in the text of GAMP 4 for some of these key GLP words, we find:

- No reference to "chemical or biochemical analysis," "scientific," "animal testing," "study director," "study protocol," "toxicity," or "test facility" in GAMP 4 .
- References to "laboratory" and "laboratory equipment or instruments" are all in sections concerning QC laboratories or included as GMP equipment.
- "Raw data" only appears as an excerpt from the OECD GLP Consensus Document [3] and is not elaborated upon in GAMP 4 itself.

We therefore can conclude that GAMP 4 does not explicitly speak to the defining purposes of GLP, or the defining management roles and responsibilities and processes of GLP (for example: study director, study protocols, raw data, test facility), nor specifically the specialist computer-controlled laboratory and scientific equipment used in GLP studies. This is hardly surprising given the provenance of and the main audience for the GAMP initiative — namely the GMP regulated manufacturing world. However, because many of the typical IT and laboratory systems found in GMP are similar to those in GLP environments, there is still some common ground on which GAMP 4 guidelines can operate and be of value to computer validation workers in GLP areas.

Is there guidance on computer validation that is specifically targeted to the GLP environment? Yes, the OECD document [3] deals directly with computers used in GLP and provides an authoritative source of guidance. This is the primary reference document for computer validation in GLP. However, this document does not detail how to achieve the prescribed activities or give any examples. What are needed are further specific interpretation documents with appropriate examples.

It is at this level of guidance where GAMP 4 could prove valuable to practitioners of computer validation in GLP. GAMP 4 provides very practical example standard operating procedures (SOPs) and guidelines for each specific aspect of current computer validation practice. The minimum required procedures for computer systems used in GLP are conveniently listed in the OECD document [3].

Table 15.1 matches the minimum required computer validation procedures for GLP systems as stated by OECD to those provided in GAMP 4 and comments on their applicability.

It is clear that much of GAMP 4 is useful for computer systems validation and control in the GLP world. Most of the required procedures for GLP computer systems have an analogous guideline procedure and example provided by GAMP 4. This is potentially very useful for those who perform validation and those who act as QA in GLP studies. It is unsurprising, given the "generic" applicability of many aspects of computer validation and control, that although the starting point principles of GAMP are dissimilar to the "Principles of GLP," there is large overlap when it comes to computer validation methodology.

Table 15.1 GLP vs. GAMP 4 review

Minimum GLP procedures list for computer validation and control as stated in OECD document [3]	Nearest GAMP 4 SOP or guideline title	Comments
Procedures for the operation of computerized systems (hardware or software), and the responsibilities of personnel involved.	Operational SOPs — none	Naturally each system operational SOP is specific so no guidance document can provide operational procedures.
	A "Roles and Responsibilities" heading section is included in many GAMP 4 SOPs and guidelines reminding readers of the need to determine and record the responsibilities of personnel involved in a computer validation project.	The roles and responsibilities in the world of GLP are prescribed in the OECD document — these should be followed. GAMP titles and roles do not exactly map to GLP principles so they are of only general interest to workers in GLP computer validation.
Procedures for security measures used to detect and prevent unauthorized access and program changes.	O3 Guideline for Automated System Security	GAMP 4 security guidelines are equally appropriate to GLP systems and can be applied.
Procedures and authorization for program changes and the recording of changes.	O4 Guideline for Operational Change Control	GAMP 4 change control guidelines are generally appropriate to GLP computer systems and could be applied but the examples in GAMP are PLCs (unlikely to be relevant), reference is made to "experimental work," which is not same as the sense used in GLP. Avoid the full exact implementation of this GAMP 4 guideline and the example forms except for the major IT systems. Lab systems change routinely and need a different Change Control approach to GMP process automation.
Procedures and authorization for changes to equipment (hardware or software) including testing before use if appropriate.	O4 Guideline for Operational Change Control	
Procedures for the periodic testing for correct functioning of the complete system or its component parts and the recording of these tests.	O1 Guideline for Periodic Review	GAMP 4 periodic review guidelines are equally appropriate to GLP systems and can be readily applied.

Procedures for the maintenance of computerized systems and any associated equipment.	No specific SOP or guideline for maintenance	
Procedures for software development and acceptance testing, and the recording of all acceptance testing.	All of the development appendices D1 to D6	GAMP4 development guidelines are equally appropriate to GLP computer systems and can be readily applied with the addition of scientific based testing approaches for the lab science systems (absent from GAMP4).
Backup procedures for all stored data and contingency plans in the event of a breakdown.	O7 Guideline for Back Up and Recovery of Software & Data O8 Guideline for Business Continuity Planning	GAMP4 back up guidelines are appropriate to GLP systems and can be applied with the additional knowledge of "raw data" (such guidance is absent in GAMP4).
Procedures for the archiving and retrieval of all documents, software and computer data.	O6 Guideline for Record Retention, Archiving, and Retrieval	GAMP4 archiving guidelines are appropriate to GLP systems and can be readily applied. GLP record retention periods are typically "indefinite" or 10–50 years, which is much longer than GMP batch records. GLP electronic records are typically much more diverse in format and type compared to GMP e-records. The technology challenge for e-record archiving is therefore greater in GLP than GMP.
Procedures for the monitoring and auditing of computerized systems.	O5 Guideline for Performance Monitoring	GAMP4 performance monitoring guidelines are equally appropriate to GLP IT systems and can be readily applied.

However, GAMP 4 for GLP is not a perfect marriage. Some of the GAMP 4 guidance does not quite fit GLP and some key aspects of GLP are absent in GAMP 4, largely due to the differences between the starting principles and practices of GMP and GLP. For GAMP guidelines to more precisely map to GLP requirements a new revision would be required, written to specifically and deliberately incorporate the principles and practices of GLP.

One very good guideline document that does give a precise interpretation of the OECD GLP consensus document [3] has been prepared by a Swiss working group AGIT (Arbeitsgruppe Informations-technologie). Entitled "Good Laboratory Practice (GLP) Guidelines for the Validation of Computerized Systems," it is currently in draft form. [4] This document provides excellent computer validation guidance appropriate to the GLP environment. It is recommended reading for those involved in computer and laboratory systems validation in GLP regulated organizations. The document provides detailed guidance on developing the validation plan and report for a range of systems commonly used in preclinical laboratories. However it lacks the detail that GAMP 4 provides for the preparation of procedures and SOPs. It also lacks guidance on the preparation of suitable requirements specifications and any best practice testing approaches to verify the system requirements statements. In the meantime, GAMP 4 can therefore provide guidance in preparing the requirements documents and testing strategies for computer validation and is applicable to GLP systems for those specific procedures highlighted in Table 15.1.

A crosscheck mapping of the key points in the AGIT document versus the GAMP 4 contents and philosophy is provided in Table 15.2. This is provided to facilitate the use of both GAMP 4 and AGIT guidelines in GLP computer systems validation.

The schematic in Figure 15.1 attempts to show that GAMP 4 and the various other guidelines can assist with computer systems validation in GLP, but all activities must fit within the principles of GLP.

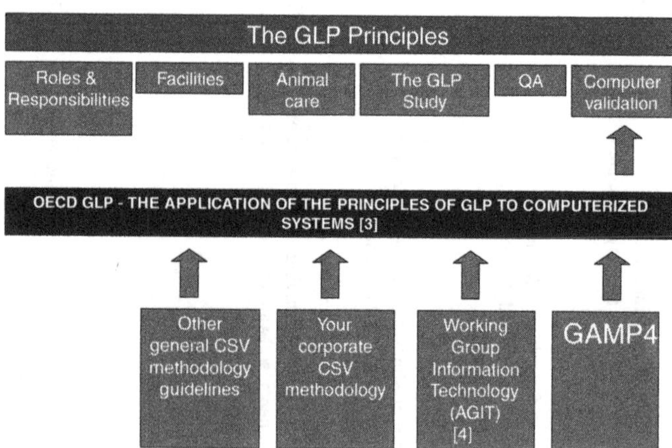

Figure 15.1 The GLP principles and computer systems validation.

PART 2 THE PRACTICAL SIDE OF THE SUBJECT

Part 1 of this chapter discussed some possible answers to the questions "what are the regulations?" and "what guidance is available for the validation of computer systems used in GLP?" We found that it is a requirement that GLP studies need to follow the principles of GLP. Where computerized systems are used in the conduct of these studies (which is inevitable nowadays) they should be validated. Another point worth mentioning here concerns the increasingly strict requirements in the case of patent applications in U.K., Europe, and the U.S.A. A trustworthy and detailed record of the development of a new medical product with reliable dates, times, and attribution of the people involved, is required. To achieve this the trustworthiness of the computer systems used and the electronic records produced during the development of the drugs for patent application must be demonstrated. This is one of the main goals of proper computer system validation (CSV). It could be in the future, that the research and development departments of pharmaceutical companies will view the need for fast and successful patent applications as an equally important driver for validation of computer systems and laboratory systems as the GLP regulations themselves.

This part of the chapter briefly discusses the considerable practical problems associated with the application of computer validation guidelines in preclinical areas of the pharmaceutical industry. These findings are based on extensive first-hand experience in a number of international pharmaceutical companies over a couple of decades. For convenience, the discussion is presented from the point of view of a QA person charged with the task of ensuring compliance to GLP on a particular site within a company.

The first problem you will encounter is convincing many of the top management and study directors that CSV is a required part of GLP and the validation activity itself needs to meet certain standards of depth and quality. (These are additional to the traditional instrument checks found in laboratories and more than just accepting standard commercial software and computer products as OK and therefore "validated.")

Reference to Part 1 of this chapter might help clarify the need for computer validation in GLP to senior management.

Since computer validation requires people, time, and money, then the winning of adequate budget and resources predicates all other considerations in computer validation. The biggest problem found in "real-life" is first calculating then gaining "adequate" budget and resources for computer validation.

It is vital to know what:

- Existing computer systems are in scope.
- New systems will be introduced within the budget timescale (usually a year).
- New preclinical studies are coming up. How do they affect prioritization?
- CSV methodology is intended to be used.
- Training (of users, management, QA, validation workers) is required.

Table 15.2 Comparison of key points of AGIT and GAMP 4

AGIT Document [4] section or reference	Analogous GAMP 4 section or reference	Comments
GLP principles	None	Already established difference in starting point between the two guidance documents, GAMP 4 primarily addresses the GMP environment.
Inventory	Main body 11, M1, M9, O1	Both agree on requirement for inventory of computer systems.
Source code	D5	GAMP 4 devotes a whole section to source code maintenance and review. Code review is absent in AGIT the only advice is: "The source code of application software should be accessible for at least 10 years after the first use of the software at a test facility. It is not necessary that it is available at the test facility, but the test facility has to ensure that the vendor of the software keeps the source code at a save place so that it is available to GLP authorities if necessary." This rather large philosophical gap arises again from starting point differences. GAMP 4 concerns primarily process automation and the FDA interpretation that the "code" controling process automation (often bespoke designed) can be considered equivalent to the other records making up a GMP master batch record. In GLP there is, naturally, no such analogue. In addition the OECD and AGIT documents are written with the presumption that the vast majority of computer systems are vendor-supplied standard systems with little or no bespoke design. This presumption holds true for most automated control systems found in GLP. Robotic lab testing systems are examples of automation systems with a high level of bespoke design employed in GLP studies.
"Commitments" (to quality standards)	M2	The AGIT document speaks of need for a quality system during system development (usually by a system vendor). GAMP 4 has a section on this subject. Also see guidance for computer system vendor and supplier audit by Wingate (Chapter 5 of this book).
Software and hardware categories	M4	GAMP software and hardware categories are probably the most well-known aspects of the GAMP guidelines. The AGIT document also attempts its own categorization. It provides three software categories and three "tentative" equipment categories. GAMP categories are essentially based on "the increasing risk of failure with the progression from standard... to bespoke..." (with "a GxP risk assessment" as an additional consideration). Whereas the AGIT document distinguishes systems and software based only on their complexity, and assumes *a priori* that each system is equally GLP critical (otherwise it would not be in scope). AGIT also admits that systems (even in the same

Table 15.2 continued

AGIT Document [4] section or reference	Analogous GAMP 4 section or reference	Comments
		complexity category) may have different “functional risks.” Both GAMP 4 and AGIT see the purpose of their categorization to assist in the determination of a suitable scale of validation effort. An intelligent consideration and application of both categorization schemas would assist workers in GLP computer validation.
Validation plan	M1 (and M3)	Both AGIT and GAMP 4 agree on the need for a validation plan (VP), and many of the proposed contents of the VP document overlap. Functional risk assessment is mentioned in AGIT as a VP deliverable. The risk assessment process itself is covered in greater detail by GAMP 4 (in the M3 guideline), and could be usefully applied for GLP validation projects. (GLP workers can ignore the purely manufacturing examples given in GAMP 4, and concentrate on risks to the scientific validity of GLP data associated with the functional and performance characteristics of the computer system validated.) Both AGIT and GAMP 4 provide a skeleton template VP document for their readers’ convenience.
User requirements (URS)	D1	AGIT only briefly mentions URS and does not consider functional and design specifications guidance. (The only reference is in the standard “V” model diagram provided as an appendix.) Conversely, GAMP 4 has devoted individual sections on user, functional, hardware design and software design specifications (D1, D2, D3, and D4 respectively).
Testing	D6	AGIT includes only cursory advice on testing in the VP section. GAMP 4 section D6 provides expanded generic guidance.
Validation report (VR)	M7	AGIT and GAMP 4 are in broad agreement on the purpose and contents of the VR.
Archiving	O6	GLP archives are well established and most large organizations have a GLP archive department with a GLP archivist whose instructions are paramount.
Retrospective validation	O9 — APV interpretation of EU guideline	AGIT seems to allow retrospective validation of computer systems. Although GAMP 4 presumes prospective validation and explicitly states that it is not written for retrospective validation purposes (main body section 3), guidance is provided in section O9 by the APV. An intelligent consideration and application of both GAMP 4 and AGIT guidance on retrospective validation would assist workers in determining how to perform retrospective GLP computer validation.

Finding the optimum balance between the benefits and the business risks is the continual challenge in this field. Benefits are gaining compliance and improving scientific data quality. Risks are doing too much CSV in the overall sense and for each individual system, doing it too slowly in general and causing delays in particular for each individual system, doing it too expensively.

I have witnessed many CSV and QA professionals spend too much time on:

- Gathering inventories and making complex prioritization methodologies without starting real validation.
- Making overly detailed and complex project plans not based on experience of typical metrics.
- Spending years defining and then constantly refining (or radically changing) CSV methodology.

All these mistakes tip the cost/benefit balance way past the optimum before any meaningful CSV work has even started.

One of the key differences in the preclinical compared to the manufacturing area is the speed of change and turnover of computer systems (especially those involved in scientific measurement and analysis, and knowledge management). This is driven by three main factors:

- The turnover of new investigational compounds. Therefore the need for new preclinical studies. New GLP studies often need new or different types of lab instrument and computing to be introduced and validated.
- The constant introduction of new scientific technology (almost invariably computerized systems) and new software promising better scientific analysis.
- The introduction of enterprise-wide computer systems for knowledge management, gathering and sharing, and changes to IT infrastructure and platforms.

The types of computer system and software found in GLP areas that have been included in CSV projects in my experience are:

1 Information databases, such as LIMS and EDMS.
2 Statistics software packages, such as SAS, Minitab, WinNonLin, GraphPad and Excel.
3 Scientific research and information systems often web based with Internet search engines.
4 Computer controlled science based instrument systems, such as mass spectrometers, HPLC, NMR, imaging systems, biometric data collection and processing systems, bioanalytical systems, DNA sequencing, etc.
5 Electronic laboratory notebook and electronic data archive systems.

Type (1) systems use essentially the same technology and require the same level of development and validation in GLP as in GMP environments. So there is no reason why the application of GAMP 4 guidelines should be any less successful in GLP, than the proven benefits of using the GAMP approach found in many CSV projects in manufacturing on such systems.

The same logic applies to the statistics software applications (type (2)) except that in GLP there will probably be many more statistics software packages in use than in manufacturing. The depth of functionality required and complexity of statistical problems encountered is higher in GLP than GMP. This means specialist expertise in performing CSV on statistics packages is more important in GLP areas because there are more software products to validate, more bespoke configurations the applications, and the validation usually needs to include a greater depth and breadth of testing.

The knowledge management systems (type (3)) are rarely found in GMP, and not explicitly mentioned in GAMP 4. These system types are as likely to be excluded from a company's CSV projects (on grounds of not being directly GLP critical systems) as they are to be included, and then subsequently found to be the most difficult to validate! The difficulties in validating such systems arise from their open nature, the rate of change in design and usage, and the inability to effect meaningful change control. All these aspects effectively preclude use of GAMP 4 guidelines because these guidelines are only designed for closed and readily controlled systems, entirely under the governance of the company owning the computer systems. I suggest, therefore, GAMP 4 guidelines are not applicable to these kinds of computer system.

The bulk of the systems requiring CSV in GLP areas is always the laboratory instruments (type (4)). GAMP 4 is not especially focused on this type of system, so if guidance is needed this should come from other publications and experts in the field. The variety of systems found in this category is much greater in GLP than that found in QC labs in GMP areas. In addition, this variety is ever increasing as new scientific analysis technology is introduced and taken on by scientists in preclinical areas. Experience has shown that workers with a background in instrumental science and analytical chemistry are essential in this particular field of CSV of scientific computerized systems. I have never yet seen a high quality validation of a computerized laboratory instrument performed by CSV professionals who come from a pure IT or engineering background. Even those CSV professionals with proven skills in laboratory systems validation in GMP environments need some time to adjust to the different culture, workflows, and requirements of the scientists and their systems in the GLP environment.

In GMP (and the new 21 CRF Part 11 scope) the "risk analysis" approach to CSV decisions involves estimating the effect of a computer system on patient safety and drug product quality. In the GLP environment this is meaningless as there is no need to consider drug product or patient. This is one of the more obvious differences between the two fields. In GLP the "product" of the scientists' endeavors is data. The customers of the data are the corporate panel charged with deciding whether to advance a compound to the next stage of development. Eventually the relevant regulatory reviewers may become customers of the data. Computer systems must be validated in GLP, therefore, with the goal of ensuring the quality, confidentiality, integrity and lifetime availability of the electronic data they collect, process, share and store. The validation of type (5) systems and maintenance of their data is more relevant and challenging in the GLP than the manufacturing environment. The retention periods for toxicity data enforced by GLP are much longer than GMP records. In this instance again, GAMP 4 provides no explicit guidance.

Finally in this chapter, the subject of grid computing is raised. This is where multiple networked and shared PCs are connected and used to perform number crunching tasks not possible on single PCs. This concept, if adopted in the pharmaceutical industry, will surely be found only in the discovery and pre-clinical areas.

The challenge grid computing poses to current concepts of computer validation as outlined in GAMP 4 and other similar guidance is enormous, and not yet met by any authoritative guidance on the subject.

DEFINITIONS OF THE MAIN ACRONYMS IN THIS CHAPTER

AGIT Arbeitsgruppe Informations-technologie. A Swiss Working Group in GLP matters URL: http://www.glp.admin.ch/

EDMS Electronic Document Management System.

GLP Rules and guidelines concerning testing of compounds for safety and efficacy but not to do with manufacture of drug products — that is GMP. There are many GLPs, but they all have the same overall purpose. The main U.S., U.K., and European GLPs are noted here.

FDA GLP In response to criminal behavior exhibited by a few members of the toxicology testing industry in the mid 1970s, the U.S. Food and Drug Administration (FDA) published regulations governing the conduct of safety tests on regulated products (21 CFR Part 58). The purpose of the regulations is to assure the quality and integrity of the data used by the government to arrive at sound regulatory decisions (i.e., to grant approval for marketing a new drug or pesticide). The regulations are process oriented and address such matters as organization and personnel, facilities, equipment, facility operations, test and control articles, and study protocol and conduct. In all, the regulations contain 144 requirements controlling the procedures and operations of toxicology laboratories.

OECD GLP The primary objective of the OECD Principles of GLP is to ensure the generation of high quality and reliable test data, related to the safety of industrial chemical substances and preparations in the framework of harmonizing testing procedures for the Mutual Acceptance of Data (MAD). They set out managerial concepts covering the organization of test facilities as well as those under which preclinical safety studies are planned, performed, monitored, recorded, and reported. The OECD Principles of GLP, an integral part of the 1981 Council Decision on the Mutual Acceptance of Data in the Assessment of Chemicals, were revised in 1997.

U.K. GLP and E.U. GLP Good laboratory practice (GLP) embodies a set of principles providing a framework within which laboratory studies are planned, performed, monitored, recorded, reported, and archived. These studies are undertaken to generate data by which the hazards and risks to users, consumers and third parties, including the environment, can be assessed for pharmaceuticals, agrochemicals, cosmetics, food and feed additives and contaminants, novel foods, and biocides. GLP helps assure regulatory authorities that the data submitted are a true reflection of the results obtained during the study and can therefore be relied upon when making risk and safety assessments. GLP is concerned with the organizational processes and the conditions under which laboratory studies are planned, performed, monitored, recorded, and reported. Adherence by laboratories to GLP principles ensures the proper planning of studies, and the provision of adequate means to carry them out. It facilitates the proper conduct of studies, promotes their full and accurate reporting, and provides a means whereby the integrity of the studies can be verified. The application of GLP to studies assures the quality and integrity of the data generated, and allows its use by U.K. and EU government regulatory authorities in hazard and risk assessments of chemicals.

The U.K. GLPMA will enforce compliance with the Good Laboratory Practice Regulations 1997 (the "GLP Regulations"), which contain all the legislative measures necessary for the implementation in the U.K. of the three EC Directives on GLP: Council Directive 87/18/EEC, Council Directive 88/320/EEC and Commission Directive 90/18/EEC. The GLP principles originally adopted by the European Community (article 1.1 of Council Directive 87/18/EEC) were those published by the OECD in 1982 in Chapter 2 of "Good Laboratory Practice in the Testing of Chemicals — Final Report of the OECD Expert Group on Good Laboratory Practice." A modified version of this chapter (modified to take into account legislative drafting requirements) is contained in Schedule 1 to the GLP Regulations. Commission Directive 90/18/EEC also endorses some OECD recommended adaptations of the original principles published in OECD Environment Monograph No. 47 set out in the annexes to that Directive. The sections of Annex B of Commission Directive 90/18/EEC which are directly relevant to an understanding of GLP principles are contained in Schedule 2 to the GLP regulations.

HPLC High performance liquid chromatography.

LIMS Laboratory information management system.

NMR Nuclear magnetic resonance.

OECD Organization for Economic Cooperation and Development. URL: http://www.oecd.org

REFERENCES

1 OECD Series on Principles of Good Laboratory Practice and Compliance Monitoring No. 1: OECD Principles of Good Laboratory Practice (as revised in 1997). Environment Directorate, OECD, Paris, 1998.

2 U.K. GLP — Statutory Instrument 1999 No. 3106 The Good Laboratory Practice Regulations 1999. URL: http://www.hmso.gov.uk/si/si1999/19993106.htm

3 OECD Series on Principles of Good Laboratory Practice and Compliance Monitoring No. 10: GLP Consensus Document. The Application of the Principles of GLP to Computerized Systems. Environment Monograph No. 116; Environment Directorate, OECD, Paris, 1995.

4 Good Laboratory Practice (GLP) Guidelines for the Validation of Computerized Systems [draft] Working Group Information Technology (AGIT) Release Date: 22 June 2000 Version: 01. URL: http://www.glp.admin.ch/legis/val1_0.pdf

Chapter 16

The Validation of a LIMS System — A Case Study

David Hogg and Fernando Pedeconi

CONTENTS

OVERVIEW

This chapter discusses the validation of a LIMS system from the end-user perspective. The first sections deal with the general technical aspects of the validation of such systems, while the later sections deal with the project management approach adopted for one such validation project.

LIMS IN THE PHARMACEUTICAL INDUSTRY — INTRODUCTION

LIMS systems are computerized information management systems. These have been increasingly widespread since the 1980s onwards not only in the pharmaceutical world, but also in the forensic, food, medical devices, clinical trials, academic and research and development arenas; and in general in all sectors of industry that have, as a common characteristic, a need for a source of laboratory information organized in a such a manner that it allows easy handling. A minimum workflow for a typical laboratory can be the following:

- Creation of a sample.
- Analysis.
- Calculations of physical or chemical parameters.
- Analysis report.

To reproduce these minimum tasks electronically, the main reasons for which a company or institution has LIMS are:

- Organized storage and retrieval of information generated in the laboratory, either across a site or a corporation.

- Dedicated chain of custody of information.
- Reporting.

The above-mentioned features may be performed either automatically or manually, but other secondary desirable features are now increasingly becoming more important.

- Automated data collection.
- Automatic reporting.
- Interfacing with other business systems.

That means that the industry is adopting the available technology very quickly, particularly as the cost–benefit ratio is more attractive now than previously. For example, the features available today for servers, workstations, storage devices, and network hardware make the systems more and more complex in structure not only in terms of the hardware involved but also in terms of the software features available, while the costs have not increased at the same rate.

Regarding the software, LIMS can be seen as a client–server application that stores data in a centralized database, composed of many tables. There are several database models available, but nowadays the most important, from the LIMS perspective, is the relational model, which allows for easier design and use of customized databases.

There are, though, some points in which the use of these systems differ between industries. In particular, and because of the regulations affecting the pharmaceutical and medical devices industries, the design, use, and features of any LIMS system will be different from those in other industries where there are fewer regulatory restrictions.

LIMS SOFTWARE DEVELOPMENT LIFECYCLE AND VALIDATION

Validation in a software context means "confirmation by examination and provision of objective evidence that software specifications conform to user needs and intended uses, and that the particular requirements implemented through software can be consistently fulfilled."

In the case of a LIMS system, validation starts from the same moment of gathering the business and regulatory requirements for such a system.

Whatever the requirements may be, there are a number of basic areas to consider in a LIMS application, whether bespoke or standard-off-the-shelf software. These are the database and its tables. If the system is a standard commercial one, it will be supplied with a set of minimum database tables in order to run as supplied. That can be enough for some laboratory needs, although it is almost always necessary to customize the number and layout of the tables composing the database. In the case of full-bespoke systems, that task will be carried out from scratch, designing the whole set of tables (and their corresponding relations).

There are two important types of tables composing a database. One group is formed by the so-called *dictionaries*, which store "static" or support data composed of product specifications, tests, calculations, users, in short, all the information not directly associated with a sample. The other group of tables is related to information associated with sample results, which means values entered either manually or automatically as a result of performing tests on samples using laboratory instruments. The most important of all the tables in a typical sample-oriented LIMS is the samples table, which stores all the sample-related information by means of indices. The key index is normally the sample number, which is automatically generated by the application.

There are two scenarios for the development and customization of the LIMS database and its tables (also called the "back end" of the LIMS). The LIMS might rely on its own proprietary-developed database or on a widely available, non-proprietary database management environment. Use of open or well-known models such as SQL, My-SQL is recommended, otherwise a very well-tested and documented model, instead of starting with a new model for databases. This is for reliability, support, and maintainability of the system itself.

The LIMS team must decide to which model the database will adhere. Normally LIMS supplier companies also provide database support for their products for both design and maintenance. Where the LIMS design will rely on an open database, there are several tools available to accomplish those tasks.

The front-end of any LIMS system is composed of the user interface and its elements (macros, scripts, routines, etc.), and outputs (data tables, reports, exported files, etc.). Again, a commercial-off-the-shelf application will be supplied with a minimum set of screens and elements to facilitate the interaction with both the end-user and the database, while in a custom-built application all the screens must be built from the ground up. It will be very unlikely that two laboratories, even as part of the same company, could ever use the same front-end application layout, since the screens and their associated elements are related to each particular laboratory's needs, tasks, and products or materials for analysis.

In the case of a commercial application, it will come supplied with developer tools for screen customization, report creation, script editing, and whatever is necessary to set up a system from the front-end side. If the system is going to be built from scratch it is advisable to use well-known, supported, and documented applications for its development. In particular, it is good engineering practice to use code writers, compilers, and profilers that have been broadly tested and are well-known in the industry.

The remaining area that requires detailed attention is the interfacing of the LIMS with instruments for automatic data collection, and with other systems for data exchange. This is a relatively new area in industry but due to the availability of cheaper, more reliable and higher capability hardware is growing steadily. Interfacing to instruments is a business decision that may require very different levels of work, depending on the nature of the instruments to be connected. In general, the LIMS can be interfaced either directly or indirectly to the instruments: in the first case this is done by means of a commercially available or company developed interface. Such a bespoke interface requires detailed knowledge of both the instrument electronics and software and the LIMS end, but nonetheless it is not normally a huge task. Indirect interfacing is found when an instrument (or a series of them) is connected to the LIMS application by another software system acting as signal collector and digitizer, which then parses the data into LIMS. This is normally the case found in chromatography equipment, for instance, when specialized software such as chromatography data systems act as instrument data controllers, sending the sample-related data onto the LIMS application afterwards. The amount of work done by the LIMS team is, therefore, variable.

Interface with other business systems comes from the need of two or more business users to share of the same piece of information. This concept should be borne in mind when buying a LIMS or when starting to develop a new one, regardless of the timescale. Every LIMS design should keep open the options of exchanging data with other business systems (statistical packages, enterprise resources planning, etc.).

It is clear now that the amount of work necessary on development, customization and validation, once the LIMS project and its philosophy have been agreed by the user company or institution, will depend upon the end-users, business and regulatory needs, and on the decision to develop a fully bespoke system or to customize an existing commercial one.

The Validation Roadmap — Requirements for a New or Existing System

The main "user" of the LIMS will be the quality assurance department. It will use the LIMS to organize its laboratory duties and to store and report the information for the analyses generated. That information will be represented in several ways, and decisions will be made using this information that will impact on the business itself. Also, inputs and outputs to and from the system might have an impact on other departments' operations. Hence, whether the need is for a new application or an existing one is judged to be insufficient for the business, at the outset, the LIMS team must gather all the requirements from the different departments and affected users of the system. Typical requirements specify:

- All inputs the system will receive.
- All outputs the system will produce.
- All functions the system will perform.
- All performance requirements the system will meet (data throughput, reliability, timing, etc.).
- Definition of all internal, external, and user interfaces.
- Operating environment for the software (hardware and operating system).
- All ranges, limits, defaults, and specific values the system will accept.

There are many techniques available to actually gather the requirements for a solution. In the pharmaceutical industry the best way to effectively carry out this exercise successfully is to determine the requirements for each concerned area separately. This is based on the nature of the different areas present within the typical pharmaceutical manufacturing company, but it should also allow for the different backgrounds, education, and experience of the individuals involved in different tasks. The better and the clearer the requirements, the more chances for success in any project.

The LIMS team should categorize the requirements into at least two categories, depending on the current and prospective needs for the system.

- Mandatory requirements: ones that the system needs to meet, otherwise it will not be fit for its intended purpose.
- "Nice to have" requirements: Those ones that it would be desirable for the system, but not of immediate need. In a LIMS these might include barcode readers and label printers, or a module for interfacing with certain types of instruments, for instance.

These requirements are gathered in a document which states the expectations for that system at a high level. That document will be the "guideline" for the analysis of the different options available to the LIMS team — can all the requirements be satisfied with a commercially available system, or it is necessary to develop a tailored one?

The team will then go a step further in this process. Once the user requirements for this application have been gathered, the LIMS team will need to produce a high level document called software requirements specification. This describes, at high level, the requirements for the software application as a whole, a system or subsystem, or simply a "bolt on" to the existing system, depending on the case.

With all these requirements on the new or existing system, the LIMS team will start to survey the different options. Typically, the team will translate the user requirements into a request for proposal (RFP) document, that will set the basic criteria to be met by either the software developer contractor, the internal software developer group, or the off-the-shelf software supplier. The solution for any particular need will be agreed and then analyzed; it might be either for a entirely new system or subsystem. The extent of the documentation produced will depend on how bespoke or standard the solution is, and its technical complexity.

Risk Management and Traceability Matrix

Risk management is a necessary activity not only in a regulated environment, but in all the activities related to software conceptualization, design, implementation, and ongoing operation. In this context a business and regulatory risks analysis must be made, with flexibility to be adapted to changes. As with any other activity related to software there is a high probability that the risks will change during the software development life cycle process due to redefinitions of requirements, changes of the design philosophy, or other parallel changes not originally taken into account. There are many published frameworks for risk management, one of the most widespread is that proposed in GAMP 4, which provides a good methodology for identification and measurement of risks associated with the system under analysis.

The complexity of project management of this nature, regardless of whether a new or existing application, grows along with the progress of the project itself. It is good business and engineering practice to keep tracking the requirements to the specifications and then to the design and build of the software, as well as taking the same approach with the associated risks and their mitigating actions. Some risks may be mitigated by putting written procedures in place, in other cases the developer or whoever configures the system should be aware of the risks that require remediation or mitigation in the system itself. Whatever the case, the evaluation of risks throughout the entire lifecycle of the project should be traceable.

21 CFR Part 11 — Considerations within a LIMS Environment

The U.S. 21 CFR Part 11 rule is related to the use of electronic records and electronic signatures in a regulated environment. This U.S. FDA rule, as well as other equivalents worldwide, means to promote technology to reduce the amount of paperwork typically generated within a quality assurance structure, and therefore to speed up and streamline the process of batch approval.

The rule sets the minimum criteria that any system* should meet to consider the electronic records generated by it as equivalent to paper records, and the electronic signatures applied to these electronic records as equivalent to the handwritten signatures. Broadly speaking, the system must ensure:

- "Data accuracy, reliability, consistent intended performance and the ability to discern between invalid or altered records." Requirement met by design and validation of the system.
- "The ability to generate accurate and complete copies of records in both human readable and electronic form suitable for inspection, review, and copying by the agency." Requirement met by the design of the system.
- "Protection of records to enable their accurate and ready retrieval throughout the records retention period." Requirements regarding data backup, disaster recovery, and archiving.

---

*It is important to make clear that for "system" it is understood as the computerized components plus the people, the procedures, and the environment.

- "Limiting system access to authorized individuals." Requirement met by design and configuration of the system. Most (probably all) of the commercial LIMS applications allow different access levels, and the configuration of different privileges for each chosen access level. That means in practice that a particular individual within the organization should have access to perform actions and to read or write data, according to that individual's job description and responsibility.
- "Use of secure, computer-generated, time-stamped audit trails to independently record the date and time of operator entries and actions that create, modify, or delete electronic records...." Requirement met by the design and configuration of the system. The fact that the LIMS systems core is the database tables does facilitate compliance with this aspect of the rule. Special care, however, has to be taken during the configuration of the audit trail before going live since the data generated by the use of this feature adds data to the data tables and therefore the whole system's performance may decay as a result of too much data added to the database. Also, this data is necessary for review and auditing purposes; it is not data that will normally be used externally. Therefore, special effort should be made at the time of configuring other tools or interfaces needed within the system to avoid creating this information if the process does not require it.

  It is also expected that static or support data will be at least version-controlled. The system must allow the storage of previously entered information for specifications, calculations, test specifications, and other support data that could be required for auditing or regulatory purposes.
- "Use of operational system checks to enforce permitted sequencing of steps and events, as appropriate." Requirement met by design and configuration of the system.
- "Use of device checks to determine, as appropriate, the validity of source data input or operational instructions." Requirement met by design of the system.

Another part of the rule requires that the users of the system shall be made aware of their accountability in using electronic signatures. In fact, this aspect relies on the procedures and practices across the company or division actually using the system, according to the FDA's applicable predicate rules. In this context, the LIMS team should map the actual paper process and establish when the paper signatures are required, and translate the conclusions of this exercise to the developer or eventually the system administrator, who will actually implement the electronic signatures as required. This ensures that the quality assurance department will provide a rationale whenever a signature is required. All the decisions made by the LIMS team should be documented and archived, since they are subject to future changes, as any other aspect of the LIMS system itself.

The developer or customizer of the LIMS application should be aware also of the fact that the definition for electronic signature is "... a computer data compilation of any symbol or series of symbols executed, adopted or authorized by an individual to be legally binding equivalent to the individual's handwritten signature," and that even biometric methods can be applied for the identification of any individual executing an action on a record contained in the LIMS system. The manifestation of an electronic or biometric signature, nonetheless, has to adhere to the following.

- It must have the name of the individual executing the signature.
- It must have the date and time when that signature has been applied.
- It must also contain the meaning of the signature (approval, reviewing, for instance).

It is important to take this into account when configuring reporting tools, or for review purposes when creating a screen showing the workflow on a given sample.

Building or Customizing the System — Giving Shape to the Application

Once all the requirements have been gathered, the supplier's ability to deliver a quality and reliable product assessed (or assembled by the developer team), the risks determined and all regulatory requirements have been taken into account, the next step is to build the system or to buy the most appropriate off-the-shelf option offered to the company's LIMS team. Requests for proposal are matched against the different solutions offered. The cost–benefit analysis is made, a potential provider (or more than one in the case of very complex systems) is selected and audited for compliance with the company's own quality systems, all concerns about business continuity are resolved (availability of technical support, local helpdesk, and other related issues), and then the developer's group within the LIMS team will embark on customizing the application and making it suitable for the business, according to the requirements set previously.

The customization of an entire LIMS application comprises several related tasks, which can be divided in layers:

- User interface.
- Interfaces with "external" systems.
- Database tables and core program settings.

The System Database

The most extensive work to be done in the whole LIMS system is on the database, in customizing the system tables. This in turn will determine how the system and user data will be stored. The behavior and features of that set of tables depends greatly on the available technology. In the past most systems used commercial proprietary databases, whereas today the model and technology supplied by

Oracle™ has been more broadly accepted. This is becoming the *de facto* industry standard for many reasons:

- Ability to handle data transactions very effectively.
- Ability to easily interact with other commercial systems (or bespoke ones) for reporting.
- Use of well-known database languages such as SQL in a user-friendly environment, among other reasons such as worldwide customer post-sales support.

The LIMS system will be supplied with a minimum set of tables and a configuration that will make the application operate once installed, but nonetheless the company must adapt the system to its needs. To achieve this, the database developer must "map" all the data that will need to be stored and their inter-relationships, define data types, define all the attributes for every single piece of information to be handled by the database's tables. Then the prerelease test plan must be developed, which can constitute the basis of the operational qualification testing phase during the validation exercise.

Interfacing with Other Business Systems

Very rarely will a LIMS system operate without interacting with other business or laboratory systems. In most cases it will be necessary to develop or configure either bespoke or commercial interfaces. For extensive and complex interfaces, the LIMS team may well define the need to treat this aspect as part of another separate project, since some interfaces at instrument level might involve extensive programing tasks, as in the case of software used to control hardware such as chromatography or spectroscopy equipment, for instance. In other cases, the interfaces may consist of a simple series of scripts using some features of the operating system underlying the application. The LIMS team will decide and prioritize according to the business needs of the systems to interface initially, and dedicate more effort to those. In any case, extensive testing must be planned for these interfaces, which can also be used as part of the operational qualification for the whole application.

When choosing commercial off-the-shelf interfaces for laboratory instrumentation or other business system interfacing, part of the problem has been already defined. It is already known that the interface has been designed to operate with both systems to be interfaced, and therefore the LIMS team should only be concerned with the interface settings and other constraints, such as network hardware and overall performance. The LIMS team must make sure that the interfaces have been thoroughly challenged and tested to ensure that they will perform as desired; again, these tests can be part of the operational qualification of the entire application.

The User Interface

The layout of the user interface will begin to be defined within the software requirements specifications and the functional specifications as provided by the system supplier or the developer's team. At this stage the system will consist, in a minimum configuration, of screens at user level, which need to be adapted to the business needs. The developer must "map" the end user needs and define:

- The type of screens needed.
- The sub screens.
- All the elements required to successfully make the system operate in a clear and safe manner.
- How the screen elements will interact with the database fields.
- What the general behaviour will be, paying particular care of the regulatory requirements.

The more the constraints on the data analyst, the less the possibilities of making errors afterwards, so whenever possible the developer should base its strategy on limiting the choices of making decisions or entering information by the end user. The use of pull-down or option lists instead of free text input fields will make the data more consistent across the system and minimize the probability of error. The design of queries is an activity to which special care should be given. The entire functionality of a screen may depend on the use of such queries, therefore the developer must ensure that the information retrieved matches exactly with the intent of each individual query. A slight difference in the criteria applied to sort the information out from the database may deliver undesirable results.

The allocation of privileges and permissions to different levels of authorized personnel is sensitive to the configuration of the access levels, so the developer must pay particular attention to the configuration of the requirements in this area.

Another special requirement is introduced by electronic signatures. The developer must base the implementation of e-signatures based on the rationale provided by the quality assurance department.

At this stage, the planning of the testing of the whole should commence. This will constitute another element for the basis of operational and installation qualification.

Pre- "Cut Over" Testing and "Go or No Go" Decision

Exhaustive testing must be carried out on all the components that will form the system to be delivered to the business. Modules will be tested by using normal cases, boundary limits and worse case scenarios, the code will be inspected, and integration tests done. When the final release is ready, the developer's team should have already planned the necessary installation qualification tests, which will verify that the application is installed according to its design specifications. All the tables, modules, scripts, routines, user interface elements, scripts, and other files for both the server application and the terminal clients must meet these specifications for naming, versioning, length, location, operating system, and the hardware should be qualified so that it meets the application's needs.

The system as a whole must be challenged against the operational situations it was designed for. Operational qualification must include both functional testing (the functionality meets the requirements) as well as boundary and worse case scenarios (the functionality is still performing without showing failure outside its normal value range). The team may decide which functions are more important and prioritize them (producing a rationale), and test these more important functions more thoroughly than the others, saving time and effort.

The test plan should be created during the software development phase. The methodologies used to identify test cases should be independent of programming personnel, but they should take account of the technology of the application and the software and programming concerns related to testing. The methodology for testing typically will consist of:

- Module testing. This focuses on the examination of subprogram functionality and ensures that functionality not visible at system level is examined. This should be done before the integration of the entire system.
- Functional testing. Tests to expose program behavior in response to the normal case and in response to worst-case conditions. The application will be challenged against the domains of input and output, responses to invalid, unexpected and special inputs. This type of testing should be applied at the module, integration, and system levels of testing.
- Integration-level testing focuses on the transfer of data and control across a program's internal and external interfaces. If the LIMS contains a large number of modules this type of testing should be conducted to demonstrate that the added modules do not affect the behavior of the existing ones.

These activities must be carefully documented, test scripts must be followed in full, and any rationale for not doing so must be documented. Deviations (internal to the project) will be raised if a test does not match with its expected outcome. At the end of this exercise the team must review the results of this activity and if errors are found they should be categorized, in order to make the "go or no go" decision of implementing the system in the "live" environment.

- Irrelevant errors, such as typographical errors at the time of writing the test scripts.
- Minor errors, such as the use of upper- or lowercase letter in fields not constructed for them.
- Tolerable errors that must be communicated to the supplier.

- Severe errors, such as algorithms performing wrongly, that must be communicated to the QA department, which lead to the failure of the validation exercise until resolution.
- Disastrous errors, such as database integrity. Impossible to go any further with the validation effort.

Test scripts should be written in such a manner that do not allow ambiguity of interpretation. This aims to achieve two objectives:

- The scripts will be executed without leaving the tester to follow paths other than stated.
- The review process will be aligned with the same level of criticality as when the test has executed them.

The minimum content of test scripts are as follows:

- Test script identifier — unique identifier of the test script.
- Purpose — description of the feature to be tested.
- Special requirements and prerequisites (other subsystem running and providing data input, for instance).
- Test procedure steps.
- Cross-reference with documents, such as the user manual, whenever applicable.
- Test log — expected outcomes and observed results.
- Unexpected events.
- Resolution of unexpected events.
- Pass or fail criteria: State the criteria to successfully pass the test. Does the test pass or fail?
- Sign off by tester and peer reviewer.

Post "Cut Over" Testing — Performance Qualification

Once it has been decided to release the final candidate version of the system, it will be installed in the live environment. At that stage, some of the errors found in the previous tests may have been already resolved, and the system will be tested to assess that it meets the user requirements specifications. The system will be tested as to how it will operate in "live" business conditions, therefore the ability of the system to transport data among the other different systems by means of the interfaces will also be tested.

Standard operating procedures for all the instances of operation of the system must have been produced or updated, whichever is applicable.

SPECIAL CONSIDERATIONS

Data Archiving and Migration

Whenever the quality assurance department has previously had a LIMS system, existing data will need to be migrated between the existing system and the new one; between database tables and other system components. Migration or archiving should be carried out using qualified tools and the necessary precautions taken for not losing any data during this exercise. The quality assurance department will decide the cut-off point from where the sample results data needs to be in the new system. Among the data that must be migrated are the static data which belongs to the dictionaries: material specifications, tests, calculations, for instance, as well as other data that was on the preceding system, such as database queries, report definitions, and operating system settings files, for example.

All these activities will need to be fully documented to ensure future traceability and maintenance.

Archiving of records is a business sensitive task: keeping only as many records that have to be on-line in the system prevents the system losing performance and therefore saves users' time. Also, as the database grows considerably, the risk of suffering system crash also rises considerably. It is advisable, therefore, to carry out this activity at time periods according to the company's schedule declared in a SOP. This is, technically, an activity not exempt from threats. Very powerful hardware will be needed to roll the database over and rebuild the new tables whenever deleting records from a table and rebuilding it. Failure to achieve this successfully may lead to data loss.

Today's available hardware creates options when choosing a strategy for data archiving. The prices for data storage solutions are much cheaper than in the past, thus allowing more data to be stored at lower cost. A possible strategy might consist, then, of making duplicate replicas of the system database from time to time and placing the files on an archiving storage drive, keeping them ready for connection when needed, thus minimizing the time needed to have the old data ready for either business or regulatory purposes.

Reporting and Query Tools

Reporting tools are used to retrieve and show the information stored in the database for specific purposes — tracking of in-process samples and batches, planning of an analyst's daily tasks, and at a higher level in the organization, for trend analysis, quality-based decisions on a product or process, and certificates of analysis and release. Whatever the case, the developer must make sure that the reports, whether using electronic signatures or not, respond to a precise design, in order to retrieve the information as required in each case, and make the logical decisions matching the results obtained with specified criteria. Queries shall be validated, as well as the templates used for preparing each report, since quality decisions will be made on them.

Also, when an external application is used to retrieve data from the database, it has to be made clear that the application should have read-only access to the system tables, and that the use of such information shall be documented.

It is advisable then, to use qualified and reliable tools for querying the system and producing reports, with frozen queries as much as possible and authority control for accessing these templates. If the records have to be submitted electronically, the use of electronic signatures is mandatory. In this context, if the report needs to travel across an open network (where the company does not exercise any control on the system access, such as the Internet, for instance), then encryption of that data becomes a requirement, according to the regulatory expectations.

Disaster Recovery and Business Continuity

Another aspect of the implementation and validation of a LIMS system regards disaster recovery measures to ensure business continuity. Here, the solution to be adopted depends on the nature of the risk analyzed. In case of a power supply shutdown it may be appropriate that the system will use an emergency alterative power source, such as an uninterruptible power supply system (UPS) or even by a separate mains power supply, that will allow enough time to successfully shut the system down, thus avoiding the risk of data loss or further damage to the system.

In other high complexity scenarios, the company must evaluate the potential impact of data loss, and other solutions can be adopted. In some cases the solution might be the use of two mirror servers, one running locally and other remotely, to reduce the risk of losing data to a very low level, since only the last transactions will be vulnerable.

In any case, it is up to the company to evaluate how much risk of data loss is acceptable. This assessment is made with the following elements:

- Maximum period the system can be inoperative because of automatic data loading or external access to the system (other company sites need to have access to the local LIMS).
- Time needed to upload the handwritten recorded information.
- Maintenance costs of backup or mirror systems.
- Availability of local technical support for backup systems.
- Likelihood of all given disaster scenarios to occur.

Assuming that the company has made the decision for the most cost-effective and technically sound solution, it will be necessary to test the disaster recovery plan periodically. This not only includes testing the technical system recovery, but also the existence of accurate and up-to-date procedures. Normally the related tests will be run when the system is not needed for normal operation, e.g., during an annual manufacturing shutdown period.

Maintenance

As with any other computerized system, maintenance of a LIMS comprises a series of operations destined to ensure the proper ongoing operation of the system, as specified. This is achieved by a series of activities such as change control management, procedural controls, ongoing performance evaluation (in order to detect system slowdowns or database overload), maintenance of user access controls (logical and procedural), SOP reviews, and system log reviews. All such activities are carried out in order to keep the system in a validated state. Criteria for revalidation should be based on a careful evaluation on the change to be implemented and the impact on the data accuracy, security, and integrity. This will allow for targeting of revalidation efforts.

Examples of changes to a system include hardware maintenance and upgrade, upgrade of the operating system, and evolution of the LIMS application overtime. Configuration management will ensure adequate identification, control visibility and security of any changes made to hardware, firmware, network, program source code, or any specialized equipment associated with the LIMS.

The ultimate responsibility for ensuring that the system is still under a validated state relies upon the local IS/IT and quality assurance departments: As demonstrated until now, the IS/IT department will have the primary responsibility for the technical aspects related to the system, including the execution of some revalidation work, periodic retesting of some features according to internal procedures (e.g., backup and restore), and the updating of technical documentation whenever needed. The QA department however, will monitor that all the procedures and working instructions are in place and up to date, and maintain a good liaison with IS/IT for all the user-related maintenance activities, including maintenance of user accounts and system access, assignation of system access levels, identification of new business requirements and user training.

CASE STUDY: A LIMS IN ASTRAZENECA

This case study considers the validation of a LIMS at one of AstraZeneca's manufacturing sites. The site carries out formulation and packing operations for products for the U.S.A. and other countries, and so is subject to FDA regulation. There are both chemical and microbiological laboratories, and all of the samples are managed using a common LIMS. This section deals with the project management and technical approaches adopted for the LIMS validation.

The topics discussed include:

- Background and resource issues.
- Project planning and start-up.
- Document development and management.
- Project monitoring.
- Risk assessment.
- Conclusions.

Background and Resource Issues

The site has around 450 employees and systems validation expertise is provided by a two-person systems quality group. Due to the range of systems validation and quality aspects managed across the site, this group was unable to provide sufficient resource for the preparation of lifecycle documents for the validation project. Similarly, the system administrator in the IS department, although having the technical expertise to carry out some of this task, did not have sufficient time available. It was decided to employ an external validation consultancy company to assist in this task.

Generation of Proposals

Based on the knowledge within the systems quality group and others in the factory, a shortlist of four consultancy companies was drawn up. The first step in the selection process was to meet with each consultancy company in turn to discuss AZ's requirements and expectations. Before doing this, internal meetings were held to agree these requirements and expectations, and a summary of these was provided to each company prior to the meetings. This summary was not in the form of a user requirements specification, since the contract to be awarded was not for the supply of a system but for the supply of services. Instead it included a description of the scope of the system, and statements of AZ's expectations around the scope of supply for the company. It was indicated to each consultancy company that it should recommend methods and approaches for the work as well as suitably-skilled people.

Each company was given between half and one day, depending on mutual availability, to discuss the project requirements, at the AstraZeneca site. To maximize the common understanding, AZ ensured that a cross-section of people from systems quality, IS and QC departments were available for these discussions. The agenda for each meeting was similar. The company was given time to present its background, experience, and approach to validation. AZ then presented the general scope of the project, and time was allowed for the company to ask further questions to enable it to develop a proposal for the work.

Assessment of Proposals

Within three weeks of the conclusion of these meetings, all the relevant proposals had been received by AZ, and the assessment of the proposals began. The key stakeholders from systems quality, IS, QA, and QC were invited to a meeting where a structured decision-making technique was used. After a brief review of the status of the project and the proposals, the following steps were carried out.

- A brainstorm of factors that would influence the decision (selection criteria).
- Grouping and filtering of the factors to produce a final list of criteria.
- Relative weighting of the criteria.
- Scoring of each proposal against the criteria.
- Multiplication of scores by weights and totalling of weighted scores.
- Discussion of, and conclusions from, the results.

From the first two steps, the following criteria were identified (*not* in order of importance).

- Validation expertise.
- Knowledge of LIMS in general.
- Knowledge of Beckman LIMS in particular.
- "Confidence" level in the consultant to deliver.
- Availability and location.
- Quality of presentation during proposal discussions.
- Cost.

For commercial reasons it is not possible to state the relative weights given to each criterion by AZ, in any case, these would vary from project to project, depending on constraints such as regulatory risk and budget. The criteria included measurable factors as well those requiring judgement to assess. The purpose of using the technique was to give these varying factors the correct relative weighting and therefore reach the optimum choice. The method of allocating weight was agreement on which criterion was the most important, and give it a weight of 10. All the other criteria were then judged in relative importance against this, giving a range of weights from 10 down to three.

Once weights were allocated, the proposals were judged against each criterion in turn. Again, the proposal scoring best for a particular criterion was given 10, and the other proposals were scored relative to this. In both the weighting and scoring processes, there was no constraint on giving the same weight or score more than once.

Once the scoring process was concluded, one proposal was provisionally selected, but before this decision was finally agreed, all the key stakeholders were given the opportunity to raise and discuss any concerns. In any structured decision-making process like this, it is vital that this chance is given, to ensure that buy-in has been achieved from all the people present. In this case, no concerns were raised which altered the provisional decision, and the choice of consultant was confirmed.

Project Planning and Start-Up

Once the consultancy company was chosen, the next major step was to conduct a project kick-off meeting, at which the final scope of the project would be agreed. The other major objective of this meeting was to make a positive start to the process of building the project team who would carry out the work. It was agreed with the consultancy that its resource would be based primarily on-site for the duration of the project, to maximize the integration of its people into the AZ project team.

Prior to the kick-off meeting, it was agreed with the consultancy that an initial period of a week would be used for the consultancy to perform its own assessment of the project in more detail. The aim of this was to provide further information on the time and resource planning stage, thereby reducing the risk of inaccurate estimates. During this and the succeeding stages, the availability of the system administrator and the key users from QC was vital, to ensure the consultancy was given the support it needed.

At the kick-off meeting, a team-building exercise was used to help create a sense of team unity. The consultants on the project were included in this process from the outset, as the intention was to integrate them into the working environment on-site as much as possible.

In agreeing the final scope of the project a brainstorm was held to list all the possible activities that could be included in the project. Having reviewed the primary objectives of the project, this list was then assessed and the detailed scope agreed.

One area where there were options on scope was the interface to SAP R/3. This interface is used to automatically transfer data about batches and required samples from SAP to LIMS, and to pass back the status results of the samples after completion. Since this interface uses bespoke code in both systems to carry out the data transfers, but operates and is tested as one entity, it was decided to designate the interface as a separate "system," and document and test it independently of the main LIMS. The validation of this interface was carried out in parallel with the LIMS validation but was carried out entirely by AZ personnel, with the exception of the technical code review carried out by the consultants.

The development environment for the site LIMS includes a development and test machine in addition to the production machine. It was decided that from the time of the kick-off meeting, further changes in system requirements would not be introduced, so that the documentation could be developed against a frozen version of the system requirements, implemented on the development machine.

Building on discussions during the proposal phase, the scope of supply for the consultants had to be finalized in addition to the technical scope of the project. AZ on site, in their systems quality group, have people experienced in systems validation, and so the scope of supply for the consultants was not to deliver the entire validation package as a turnkey job. Rather, their scope was to provide expertise in particular phases of the validation. Using the standard validation lifecycle described in the local validation SOP, based on GAMP, the following documents were planned, with the prime responsibility for the preparation of each indicated.

Document	*Prime responsibility*
Validation plan	AZ
Functional specification	Consultants
Hardware design specification	AZ
Software design specification	Consultants
Code review report	Consultants
Protocol (test specification)	Consultants/AZ
Validation report	AZ
Maintenance and operation procedures	AZ

Documentation Development and Management

Validation Plan

The validation plan was prepared by the systems quality group and approved internally. The validation approach documented in this plan was shared and discussed with the consultants during the revision phase of the document.

Functional Specification

The functional specification (FS) was prepared by the consultants, working primarily with the AZ system administrator and a number of key users in order to verify the functionality. Due to the use of many standard functions of the core system, the document was written with the emphasis on the structure of the configuration for AZ's use.

Hardware Design Specification

The hardware design specification (HDS) was written by AZ in line with local SOPs, following the style and level of other recent projects.

Software Design Specification

The FS included all the configuration detail for AZ's application, but excluded the design for bespoke areas of code. The main function that required further design detail was that of reporting, where fixed reports had been written in a standard report generating language (a tool provided by the system supplier). Since these reports could be said to be implemented using code rather than simple configuration of standard functions, the detail design was taken out of the FS and included in a software design specification (SDS). Again, this document was prepared by the consultants. As described earlier, the bespoke code for the SAP interface was documented and validated separately.

Protocol

The protocol document included the hardware acceptance testing (IQ), the system acceptance testing (OQ), and the performance testing (PQ). This document was primarily prepared by the consultants, although the hardware test scripts for the IQ were prepared by AZ, due to the fact that the consultants had not been involved in the preparation of the HDS. This document required the most iterations and discussion of all those produced, because of the need to reach a common understanding of the testing approach, the depth of testing, and the style of preparation of the test scripts. There were significant differences in the "normal" approaches adopted by AZ and the consultancy company. While these differences were not fundamental in the ability to qualify the system successfully, they were significant enough to cause a degree of rework to meet AZ's preferred style. It is recommended that existing protocols are used as examples and time is spent discussing in detail the structure of the test scripts with any consultant prior to the preparation of such a document, in order to reduce the leadtime for preparation.

One example of these differences was in the use of generic test scripts which could be used and re-used to test the application of a similar function with different instances or parameters. AZ preferred to adopt a generic style where possible, to minimize the size of the protocol. The alternative is to include in the protocol all the necessary steps, with instances and parameters specified therein, to allow full testing without looping back to steps previously conducted. Both approaches are equally acceptable, but they have different advantages and disadvantages.

Generic test script	*Linear test script*
One per function, execution repeated for each instance.	All instances specified sequentially in script.
Instance-specific parameters excluded from script: reference made to design specifications.	Instance-specific parameters included in script: reference to design specifications unnecessary.
Lack of specific parameters reduces the chance of discrepancy with design specifications.	Repetition of specific parameters from design specifications increases the chance of discrepancy.

Generic test script	*Linear test script*
One script for all instances can be a problem if a subset of instances have slightly different functionality.	Differences in functionality between instances can be accommodated.
Preparation and review time reduced.	Preparation and review time increased.
Execution more complex due to continual cross-referencing to design documentation.	More simple execution.
More experienced testers needed.	Less experienced testers may be sufficient.

The AZ preference was to use generic-style scripts where possible. This approach took several iterations to achieve, but as an indication of the savings made in terms of the size of the protocol, the functional specification and hardware and software design specifications totalled 167 pages; the protocol to test these was only 41 pages.

Validation Report

The documentation stage following testing was the preparation of the validation report. At the AZ site concerned, this is carried out in two steps: the first report summarizes each test and confirms the completion of the qualification. The second and final report summarizes the completion of all the steps outlined in the validation plan, and justifies any excursions from that plan.

Procedures

In parallel with the validation life cycle activities, maintenance, operating and change control procedures for the system were prepared and approved internally where appropriate.

Project Monitoring

The timescale of the project meant that close monitoring of progress against plan was required. The production schedule on the site is such that there are only two normal shutdowns of any length during the year. Although the IQ and OQ testing could be performed offline on the development or test machine, the PQ could only be performed on the production machine after the transfer of the completed application from the development environment. This meant that the project had to be completed in a little over three months to meet the next planned shutdown. The only other alternative would have been to create another shutdown later or wait a further 7 months until the following shutdown. Neither of these alternatives were desirable from a business perspective.

To this end, a detailed project plan was drawn up by the consultants with AZ's input, detailing all the activities, milestones, and responsibilities. Several review meetings were then held to monitor progress against this plan, and new versions issued when appropriate. The most important progress meeting was held just before the start of the agreed shutdown. This was a final progress review to confirm the go or no go decision to implement the validated system in the production environment during the shutdown. Based on the progress made, the decision was go.

During the shutdown, the version of the system held on the development or test machine was loaded onto the production machine and the PQ tests were conducted. The validation report, which had been drafted earlier, was finalized and made ready for approval on the first morning of start-up following the shutdown. This meant that approval of the completion of the validation exercise could be given quickly to avoid any unnecessary delay in the use of the system in the laboratories. The end result was a project which was concluded on time, within the budget, and met its regulatory objectives.

Risk Assessment

An additional activity carried out for the LIMS was a process known within AZ as threats and controls analysis (TCA). This process uses a checklist to discuss key areas of system functionality, to identify potential threats to the proper performance of the system or the integrity of its data, and to recommend controls which should be put in place to meet these threats. Such controls are normally either system controls (i.e., the system design needs to be reviewed or changed) or procedural (i.e., included in the SOPs for the system operation and maintenance). This analysis ideally takes place when the functional specification is substantially complete (caution must be used to ensure any changes to the functional specification after the original TCA do not affect the recommendations from the analysis). The closure of the actions from the TCA is then reported in the validation report, although it is recommended that a status review of the actions is undertaken prior to the formal testing and qualification phase.

The standard checklist on site, which was used for the LIMS system, is:

General aspects

1 Security and access.
2 Hardware and software alarms.
3 User or operator interfaces.
4 Interfaces with other systems.
5 System hardware.
6 Operating system hardware.

Automated equipment

17 Impact of equipment environment.
18 Interfaces with equipment and processes.

Information systems

19 Coding and identification.
20 Change of status of controlled items.
21 Traceability of information.

General aspects

7 Application software.
8 Data input (including initial data take-on).
9 Maintenance, services, and suppliers.
10 Change control (at all levels).
11 Loss of electricity.
12 Audit trail and maintenance of data.
13 Backup and restore.
14 Startup and shutdown.
15 Disaster recovery.
16 Operating procedures.

Automated equipment

22 Management of data and material parameters.
23 Allocation, reconciliation, and returns.

The analysis was led by the systems quality group, to provide experience in the use of the checklist. An open question approach was used (how, which, why, when, etc.), rather than using closed questions which only require yes or no answers. IS, technical and user representatives were present to minimize the chance of unanswered questions. As a result of the analysis, a number of improvements and changes were made to the specifications, test coverage, and the procedures.

Conclusions

At the conclusion of the validation project, it is considered that the key factors in its success have been:

- Involvement of key stakeholders at the outset.
- Close involvement of the consultant company in the scoping and estimating process.
- Involvement of the key users at an early stage.
- Detailed review of the specifications and protocol by key users as well as technical and validation staff.
- Involvement of the key users in the OQ and PQ testing.
- Use of knowledgable, experienced consultants.
- On-site presence of the consultants.
- Use of standard project management techniques.
- Freezing of change: no additional requirements were introduced during the project.
- Commitment of all people involved in the project.

The site now has a firm baseline for the validated status of its LIMS, and the experience of the project has shown that it is possible to achieve such positive results by clearly managing scope and the working relationships and responsibilities within the whole project team, including the consultants.

REFERENCES

American Society for Testing and Materials. *Standard Guide for Validation of Laboratory Information Management Systems*, ASTM Guide E-2066, 2000.

GAMP Guide for the Validation of Automated Systems, GAMP 4, ISPE 2001.

Hinton, M.D. *Laboratory Information Management Systems — Development and Implementation for a Quality Assurance Laboratory*, Marcel Dekker, 1995.

Paszko, C., Turner, E. *Laboratory Information Management Systems* — Second revision, revised and expanded, Marcel Dekker, New York, 2002).

U.S. Food and Drug Administration, Federal Register. *21CFR Part 11 — Electronic Records; Electronic Signatures; Final Rule*, 1997.

Chapter 17

Compliance and Validation in Central and Eastern Europe (CEE)

Paul Irving, Carl Turner, Wayne Duncan, and David Forrest

CONTENTS

INTRODUCTION

GAMP (Good Automated Manufacturing Practice) has been in use from the first version in Western Europe for over 10 years.

Initially supported by ISPE (International Society of Pharmaceutical Engineering) Europe, over the past few years it has been adopted by ISPE in America, with the start-up of GAMP Americas. Even more recently it has been supported by the U.S. FDA as a recognized guideline for ensuring computer systems can be validated and fit for purpose.

This chapter looks at some of the fundamentals of GAMP that are now well established and can now be used by Central and Eastern European (CEE) pharmaceutical companies to allow them to ensure compliance of IT systems, which may in turn help them to gain a competitive advantage. It also discusses the evolution of IT systems over the past 10 years, and details how systems now have more compliant functionally, and can be more easily implemented and subsequently validated.

As established compliance and validation practitioners who were involved with the creation of the initial GAMP guide, the writers of this chapter have been able to rely on many years practical knowledge and experience of the global market place in order to assist companies in the CEE marketplace by proactively enabling both cultural and business changes required in order to meet Western regulatory compliance.

The issues discussed in this chapter are based on a large-scale project in Poland between 2002 and 2004. Building on the principles laid out in GAMP and previous implementation skills, this ensured that a quality-driven system development lifecycle was enforced from the beginning. By starting with an approved validation master plan (VMP) all quality and validation tasks were clearly identified and used as the driving force behind the project and the deliverables. This example of good planning based on the GAMP guidance is the basis for future successful projects and implementations throughout Eastern Europe and beyond.

THE EUROPEAN MARKETPLACE

Pharmaceutical companies that manufacture in the CEE zone can only supply their products on a more global market if their systems are compliant and validated in accordance with U.S. and current EU (European Union) regulations.

Also, current global organizations are looking for expanding markets, with the possibility of reducing research and development, and manufacturing costs, and may consider transferring operations, or subcontracting drug manufacture to the CEE zone.

The entry of the 10 new member states, detailed below, into the EU in May 2004, opened an expanded market population of approximately 100 million and a collective EU economy close to 9.3 trillion euros (approaching the same level as the U.S.A.). There has been an increased emphasis on the subject of compliance within the pharmaceutical and biotech healthcare industry throughout all companies in the CEE, and access to these localized manufacturing, storage, and distribution facilities will only be possible if the quality and compliance standards in the CEE zone match up to current U.S. and EU regulations.

Healthcare Spending in Western Europe

Maintaining a balance between costs and income is the biggest challenge faced by all companies in any marketplace. In line with various Western European government efforts to curb rising healthcare debts and costs, the proportion of gross domestic product (GDP) allocated to healthcare spending has remained either static or has fallen in recent years. This trend is likely to continue in most Western European countries in the near to medium term.

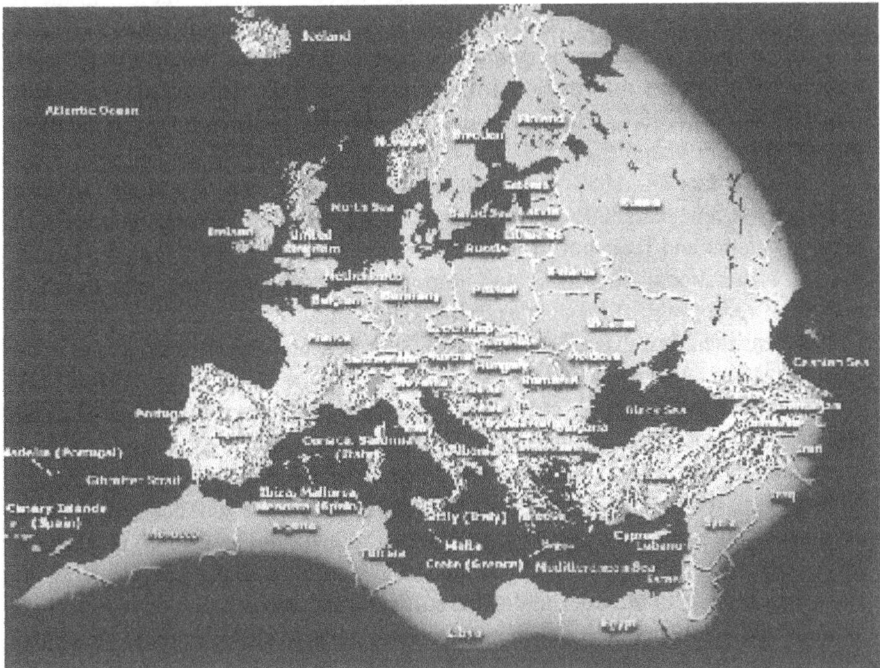

Figure 17.1 Map of Europe.

Healthcare and IT Spending in Eastern Europe

In the CEE region the trend is somewhat more optimistic, with compound annual growth rate (CAGR) of 13.5% expected in the larger countries. The following 10 countries joined the EU by signing The Treaty of Accession 2003: Czech Republic, Estonia, Cyprus, Latvia, Lithuania, Hungary, Malta, Poland, Slovenia, and Slovakia. Other countries that have applied to become members but not yet signed up are: Bulgaria, Romania, and Turkey.

CEE pharmaceutical organizations are therefore being targeted for acquisitions, mergers or involvment in partnerships with current global companies, such as GlaxoSmithKline, Pfizer, and Novartis. These global companies bring over 10 to 15 years experience in IT compliance. Existing knowledge, experience and policies and procedures, based on the GAMP principles, are available to the CEE organizations from central offices and headquarters, in the U.S.A. or Western Europe.

Those that are not acquired, and retain their independence, will need to get up to speed rapidly on their own to ensure that they are competitive in both local and wider markets.

It has been estimated that 41 billion euros will be invested by the EU in the 10 new members states between 2004 and 2006; of this it is estimated that 5–7%, i.e. 2–3 billion euros will be on IT spend. It is thought that a good deal of this IT spend will be on a secure information infrastructure, to meet general EU regulatory requirements by 2005. Within this are the specific pharmaceutical regulations discussed in this chapter.

It is also a fact that 80% of this money will be spent on new systems, whereas over the past few years, 80% of IT budgets in Western Europe have been spent on legacy systems and their interface with new systems, year 2000 upgrades (rather than new functional upgrades) and retrospective validation and assessment in respect of recent regulation such as 21 CFR Part 11.

It is clear therefore that a new wave of IT implementations will take place in the CEE in the next 3 to 5 years.

It is imperative, therefore, that these organizations embrace GAMP to establish policies and procedures as quickly as possible. They have a good opportunity to implement a brand new IT strategy based on a new and qualified IT infrastructure, with modern, functionally rich, software. These organizations will not have to spend millions of pounds on retrospective validation, and will not have to go through the 10 year learning curve. They will not have to spend time training and educating the software suppliers to provide validatable software, and encouraging them to include pharmaceutical functionality such as electronic records and electronic signatures (ERES) which comply to 21 CFR Part 11.

The following sections detail areas where we believe focus should be given to ensure an organization can increase the level of compliance and validation of IT systems, and thus conform to the Western European, U.S., and other regulations in a speedy manner.

KEY AREAS OF GAMP FOR EMERGING EUROPEAN COUNTRIES

IT and Automated Systems

The continuous development and availability of high technology systems and equipment means that organizations within CEE will be less reliant on people to manufacture and produce goods and more dependent upon IT and automated systems.

A global business system will increase efficiency by providing fully integrated and efficient processes, while not compromising quality standards. Companies that have the vision to implement such systems will become more efficient and therefore more successful, giving themselves a more competitive edge.

It is not practical or realistic to expect Eastern European companies or countries to immediately ascertain the levels of experienced Western entities, but in order to supply products in the European or global marketplace a pragmatic and realistic approach to validation and compliance must be taken.

Figure 17.2 shows the relationship of a typical system and how applied technology is intended to support and underpin it. This is particularly true for IT Infrastructure, as an unstable and nonvalidated platform effectively invalidates any system that operates upon it.

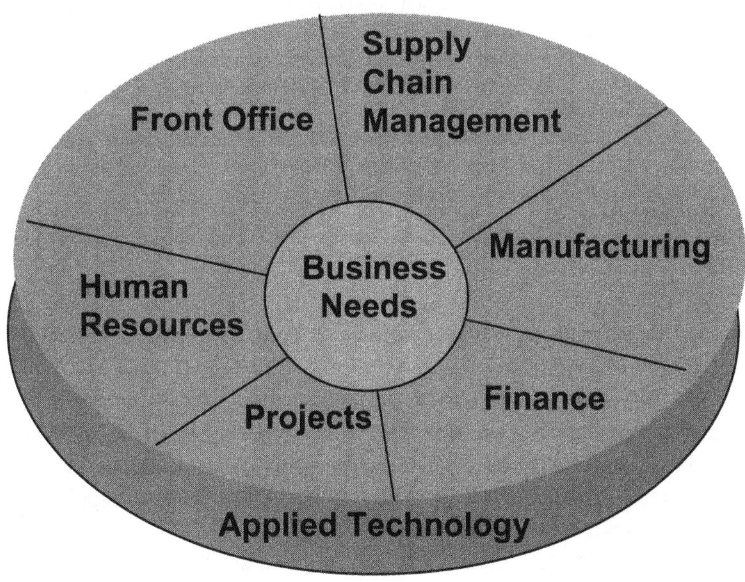

Figure 17.2 ERP system relationships and how applied technology supports the system.

In many instances the business system shown in Figure 17.2, often referred to as an enterprise resource management (ERP) system is interfaced to other business critical systems such as a laboratory information management system (LIMS), manufacturing execution system (MES), electronic document management system (EDMS), enterprise asset management system (EAMS), and also to numerous plant, equipment, and laboratory systems, such as filling and packing lines, sterilizers, coaters, granulators, etc.

Table 17.1, taken from GAMP, details a system categorization, and briefly outlines the type of validation approach that is required for each system.

Table 17.1 Software categories

Category	Software type	Validation approach
1	Operating system	Record version (including service pack). The operating system will be challenged indirectly by the functional testing of the application.
2	Firmware	For nonconfigurable firmware record revision. Calibrate instruments as necessary. Verify operation against user requirements. For configurable firmware record version and configuration. Calibrate instruments as necessary and verify operation against user requirements. Manage custom (bespoke) firmware as category 5 software.
3	Standard software packages	Record version (and configuration of environment) and verify operation against user requirements. Consider auditing the supplier for critical and complex applications.
4	Configurable software packages	Record version and configuration, and verify operation against user requirements. Normally audit the supplier for critical and complex applications. Manage any custom (bespoke) programing as category 5.
5	Custom (bespoke) software packages	Audit supplier and validate complete system.

Ten years ago most of these systems were bespoke or custom developed systems, and were specific to each client. They were classed as GAMP *category 5* systems. Not only was the supplier documentation poor, but a 100% on-site validation exercise had to take place. This was very expensive on top of the software and hardware costs. The software products contained only partial required functionality, and the functional requirements were added onto the system via bespoke code, or bespoke reports, again all requiring validation.

Over the past 10 years, focussed user groups and special interest groups have worked together with the suppliers to ensure that critical functionality, along with good software quality practices are built into the software. A key example of this is the 21 CFR Part 11 functionality. However, some companies are now stuck with older versions, as they are working and validated. They cannot be upgraded as IT budgets have been high in recent years with the year 2000 problems and retrospective validation costs. Therefore this new compliance functionality is not available to the users.

CEE countries can take advantage of all this effort by the suppliers over the past 10 years by implementing software and systems today that are more often *category*

3 or *4* Systems. This gives organizations an opportunity to have a speedy and cost-effective implementation. From our experience and involvement over this period we can now help these organizations to implement a "vanilla" system, where the system is configured to meet requirements and not tailored or customized. In this way the CEE countries will then not be caught in the trap of many existing companies where they have older software but cannot upgrade to new versions to include new functions and features which may provide financial benefits.

With new member states in the enlarged EU coming under the scrutiny of external regulators, they will effectively have to control their business growth and new systems and ensure that quality and compliance is never compromised. This will take time due to various financial, cultural, and language differences.

Such changes within the new EU mean tremendous practical changes for staff, who have been used to more labor-intensive operations with minimal automation. New regulatory initiatives from organizations such as the U.S. Food and Drug Administration (FDA) are set to minimize manual systems and encourage the use of technology in order to improve the quality and traceability of business and system processes.

Communication, Training, and Education

Regulatory awareness and training in validation processes and techniques using tools such as GAMP is essential.

Knowledge of the pharmaceutical business and good practices are vital. Continued education and training of human resources is therefore of paramount importance. This can be said for all companies, either east or west.

It is impossible to recruit a fully qualified team with local language skills, so consultants are often the prime deliverer of one-to-one and on-going training as projects progress.

Effective communication channels, good project infrastructure, and team building adds to the success of any project. It is important that project team members can work together and include developers, users, and validation staff. All team members should be aware of risks and issues that can potentially impact upon the project by carrying out daily and weekly progress updates and reviews.

Representation on technical subcommittees, and attendance at seminars and exhibitions, including those of organizations such as ISPE should be encouraged. This provides networking opportunities for staff to develop compliance and validation skills by sharing experiences.

IT Infrastructure

While each country has its own particular culture and problems, the key underlying element for each is the infrastructure, which is sometimes taken for granted in more established western countries.

This can also be true with respect to IT infrastructure, without which no system would function.

Established, documented, and tested platforms with backup processes and uninterruptible power supplies (UPS) are considered a must, as many of the new countries and markets have problems with power-cuts and have traditionally not considered validation or compliance issues which can arise around these areas.

CEE countries are often in the position to build new facilities on greenfield sites, and a key part to this is the planning and specification of the cabling and network hardware such as routers and hubs. These must be documented and tested as part of the build program, removing the need for costly and expensive rework as part of a retrospective qualification process.

If we look at the analogy of building a house, a good builder would not build a house on weak foundations.

The IT infrastructure is the foundation of all IT systems. If an ERP business system is implemented and validated on an IT infrastructure that is not documented, tested, and ultimately qualified, then the ERP system itself is not validated!

Validation Planning

Validation planning and the creation of a validation plan (VP) or VMP is a method of building quality into your implementation at an early stage. This will ultimately prevent costly rework and ensure that the system is validated in a controlled and sequenced manner.

For the recent project undertaken in Poland, policies, practices. and principles from GAMP were adopted. Effective validation planning is the key to successful compliant and validated systems. By linking this plan to the overall implementation plan, completion of tasks with predefined timescales were carried out within time and on budget.

The VP therefore becomes the key *driver* for the project.

The VP described the validation approach and activities for the project by dividing the system implementation into phases.

Key to all successful validated and compliant systems are the people involved. Roles and responsibilities assigned within the VMP are therefore vital, and the project undertaken in Poland was no different in this respect.

By carefully defining key project deliverables within the VMP and assigning responsibility, both the supplier and the user agreed on key activities and the sequence upon which they were to be conducted. While this process is well-established within existing markets in Western Europe, the application of this proved to be somewhat more difficult and required much more focus and attention.

Sufficient allocation of validation resource to projects is a key factor and there is a distinctive need for cooperation between users and suppliers at all stages of implementation using a documented and approved system development life cycle.

Misunderstanding of project tasks proved to be a major risk to the efficiency of the project timescales. When agreeing the validation project team and the definition of roles and responsibilities it is essential that key staff have the required skill sets and are competent to undertake the key validation activities.

For example, during the testing phase of the system, testing that the system worked within its normal operating limits was easily explained and understood. However, testing that the system operated as expected under certain conditions, i.e., negative or challenge testing, boundary and limit testing, was more difficult to explain and justify. Detailed documentation creation, review, update, approval, and issuing throughout the project life cycle to provide documentary evidence as required by regulatory authorities was even more of a challenge, but was accepted by all eventually.

Supplier Audit

This is a fundamental part of any new IT system implementation. The organization should follow the GAMP guidelines rigorously, *before* agreeing to buy the software product.

Historically organizations had already invested heavily, implemented systems and were committed to software suppliers, and therefore audits of the current software and of new releases were not carried out.

Over the past 10 years IT software and equipment suppliers have been encouraged to provide documented and validatable systems. There are many software products available on the market and the organization should be able to purchase a system today that meets most of the GAMP guidelines. The organization should be encouraged to use the PDA Audit Repository Centre (ARC) to check if an audit report exists for the software under review. If the package has not been audited and included in ARC, then the organization should encourage ARC to perform the audit on the organizations' behalf, as this saves time and money.

Obviously the cheapest solution may provide the organization with the most risk, whereas a more expensive system enables a less risky, more speedy, and ultimately more economical option, i.e., the system *can* be validated. This is due to the complete software development lifecycle and associated quality management system and documentation available.

Departments within companies that monitor and manage elements of quality assurance should always be included in the supplier selection process from the beginning wherever possible.

Risk Management

By using risk-based analysis and management, categorization of criticality throughout the lifetime of the project was implemented. By adopting this process, project managers are able to validate the critical areas of the business system. The result is a lower probability of noncompliance and resulting regulatory action.

Current trends in approach from the regulators, and embodied in GAMP, is that risk assessment and management is another key driver.

A traceability matrix was developed in order to map the requirements specified within the user requirements specification (URS) and functional design specification (FDS) down to the system design specification (SDS) and ultimately to software modules or units, on which the qualification testing was conducted. This ensured that all the user's requirements, including any requirements to comply with specific regulations were met and properly tested. Equally, where gaps existed, future enhancements to the core product were fed back to the supplier.

The traceability matrix can then be used as a vehicle to assist in identifying potential risks. Each risk identified can then be reviewed and extra tests or standard operating procedures or other actions can be used to mitigate or minimize the risk. Specific consideration was also given here to the U.S. FDA ruling covering ERES, often referred to as 21 CFR Part 11.

Software Engineering Techniques

There are still several software engineering techniques of a system implementation that while used in other industries, such as the defense industry, have not really been used extensively in pharmaceutical organizations.

Three such examples of this are requirements management, software configuration management, and automated testing. The adoption of these software engineering techniques would provide better traceability from logical requirements definition, through functional design and then onto mapping of test cases. Software configuration management is essential in understanding monitoring and controlling the many versions of systems and software that are part of an organization. Automated testing enables companies to create a suite of test scripts on initial implementation, so that when upgrades to operating systems, package releases, and patches or minor changes are made, the tests can be rerun automatically to ensure consistent performance and hence validation.

CEE organizations would be well advised to adopt some of these techniques as part of their IT strategy so that *all* systems can be developed, controlled and tested in a consistent manner at the very start of their IT life cycle.

CONCLUSIONS

The information in this chapter provides a summary of the past 10–15 years in the development of compliance and validation in the pharmaceutical industry and in particular in relation to the development of GAMP.

By adopting good practice and validation principles specified within GAMP, the project implementation was successful and within specified timescales. More importantly the CEE pharmaceutical organization has an IT compliance and validation platform and foundation for its staff and organization to build on.

The endorsement of GAMP by regulatory authorities such as the U.S. FDA provides the company with a high degree of assurance that by adopting this, it will be able to withstand rigorous inspections as well as having a much more robust system which will enable the organization to progress in the next 5 to 10 years.

Some key points discussed were:

- Validation planning as the driver of the project.
- Use GAMP risk management guideline to pinpoint areas of concern, where focussed validation effort can be conducted. This reduces costs and timescales, by ensuring that time and money is not spent on areas that are not seen as GMP critical.
- IT infrastructure should be planned, specified, and tested during the initial building phase of new facilities.
- Category 3 and 4 systems are now available and can be purchased and implemented in a speedy and compliant manner by ensuring the scope is limited to configuration and not customization.
- Communication, training, and education is important for the CEE countries to get their organizations to a base platform level of knowledge.
- Both suppliers and users should build quality into systems from the beginning, while conducting quality and design reviews throughout the lifecycle.
- Where possible use the ARC and encourage sharing of audits.
- Review the use of current software engineering techniques as part of the lifecycle to provide better traceability, control of software, and better test repeatability and coverage.

Chapter 18

Distribution Management Validation in Practice

Ben Gilkes

CONTENTS

THE SCENARIO

As a provider of supply chain services to the pharmaceutical, medical device, consumer (OTC) and hospital services industries, Exel (from now on referred to as the organization) recognizes the requirement to validate systems used to ensure regulatory compliance, a high level of assurance to clients and to continually improve on services provided.

Although the organization identified this as a global requirement that could potentially apply to food, cosmetics, and perishables, over time it was decided to establish the processes in one geographical area, Europe, and roll this out globally as shared best practice. This meant that the initial development of the organization's validation expertise is based on our European healthcare operations. As a supply chain service provider, the emphasis within the regulatory compliance arena had been more focused towards complying with current good distribution practice (cGDP), whereas the majority of the focus from our customers had been on the other cGxP critical processes, including cGMP, cGLP, and cGCP. There was increasing overlap as the organization expanded services into areas such as clinical trials logistics, repackaging and rework of returned goods which are essentially GMP regulated processes.

The fact that the organization's healthcare sector provides services to a large number of clients means they are potentially subject to a broader level of inspection by a wider audience of audit teams than a standard manufacturer. These consist of client QA teams in many different industry segments, as well as country regulatory authority such as FDA inspectors. This results in a considerable variance in type and depth of audit and inspection, dependent upon the local country, market, or segment regulatory requirements.

The challenge of ensuring that the organization complies with these differing requirements has historically been addressed through the sector-wide implementation of cGDP. However it was recognized that there was a need to embrace the GAMP 4 guidelines, as an international standard covering all healthcare areas, to reflect the increased reliance on IT systems to manage and control cGxP stocks.

The service-based nature of our healthcare operation compared to our customers' manufacturing-based products, has meant that when interpreting whether a system or operation has GxP impact, it is not as straightforward as we would like. An example of this ambiguity is a new building access control system for installation in a new pharmaceutical validated warehousing facility. In a manufacturing operation, the access control system would have clear GxP impact, since uncontrolled access to the manufacturing process would have obvious consequences for the guaranteed efficacy and quality of the products produced. The case is not as clear in the storage environment. Since the manufacture is complete, the opportunity to directly compromise the product is limited to flaws in the warehouse management process which could affect, for example, shelf life or batch identity. These can be said to be under control through the validation of the warehouse management or inventory systems. Of course, it can still be argued that the access control system has GxP impact because unauthorized access could result in direct tampering with the products and influence product efficacy. In this case therefore the access control system was included in the final validation master plan ensuring we erred on the side of caution.

The organization sought to build upon our existing project processes and procedures, in order to map them to the GAMP 4 guidelines. This meant that the revised processes would be a development of existing processes, which reduced the level of retraining and disruption to the existing implementation and support methodology.

Revisions were viewed much more positively as strengthening the established methods, rather than introducing a new approach. Instances of these improved processes are the improvements in the organization's system specification techniques, where increased clarity and control in project scope now results in clear tracking of project scope creep. This helped to eliminate a common source of problems for project teams.

As a result the final protocols use existing project implementation terminology and terms such as IQ, OQ, PQ, which are primarily pharmaceutical industry terms, and the 'V' Model, which was not widely used. However, for clarity at audit and inspection, this terminology is referred to when relevant, e.g., in the process mapping documentation and quality manual. Other examples where alternative models can be used to implement validated systems are the capability maturity model (CMM) and the project activity model (PAM) [2].

A dedicated validation team was established using internal resources and leveraging external consultancy firms. The recognition that systems validation is an important area for the organization has meant that there has been very high level sponsorship for this project from our global president for the sector. The validation team has been working in conjunction with operational site teams, our suppliers, and customers (blue chip pharmaceutical and medical device manufacturers) to establish a standard protocol within a dedicated quality manual, which is now complete.

This quality manual contains all the procedures to be followed by the project, the site support and the validation teams when producing documentation for new system implementations. These procedures also cover legacy system validations and the maintenance of existing validated systems. They also contain all the process maps, which link all the procedures and explain how the validation protocol functions in terms of the inputs and outputs of each process step.

The quality manual also contains a breakdown of the process steps using the IDEF0 process-modelling tool, an integration definition tool, developed by the U.S. Air Force and released by the National Institute of Standards and Technology as a standard function model in 1993. The organization found IDEF0 useful, not only in mapping out the process steps involved, but also in educating project and site teams. Consequently, at each step the inputs, outputs, restraining controls, and mechanisms are explained, and team members can clearly see the process transition from one step to the next. In our experience, communicating the functional purpose of a system in clear graphical terms is probably the greatest strength of this technique. Figure 18.1 shows the basis for the IDEF0 function box and interface arrows followed by an example in our healthcare quality manual.

DEVELOPING THE PROTOCOL

The team made a conscious decision not to directly follow the "V" model, outlined in detail in the GAMP 4 guidelines. Although the "V" model is a sound and entirely logical process model, it was accepted early on that disruption to the teams who were implementing and running our computer systems should be minimal. Consequently

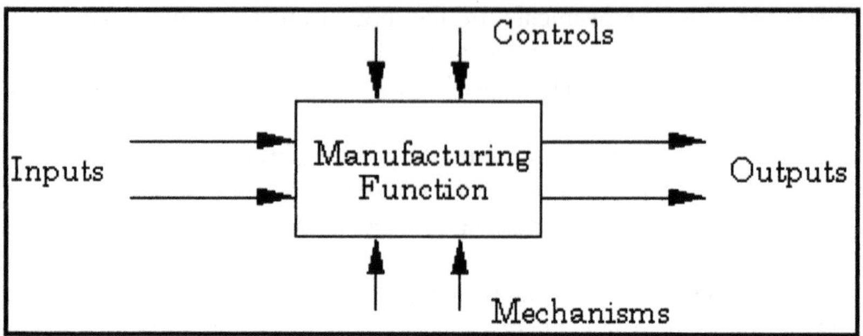

Figure 18.1 Example taken from Exel's healthcare quality manual.

the decision was taken to utilize existing project methodology, already of a high standard. This enabled the teams to refer to terminology already well understood within the business.

During successive brainstorming sessions with various members of the project delivery teams the existing project lifecycle were mapped to the key phases.

Using the process flows detailed in Figure 18.2 [4] and Figure 18.3 [5] of the GAMP 4 guide, the team analyzed the existing life cycle in terms of the key validation phases and process steps. As a result, the implementation lifecycle was broken down into four distinct project phases:

1 Planning and specification.
2 Design.
3 Construction and testing.
4 Final testing and operation.

Each phase was then broken down (as illustrated in the figures) to represent the activities and documents required by the project and validation teams, the software houses and the organization's quality assurance team in order to produce a fully validated system. The results are illustrated in Figure 18.2.

The swimming lanes highlight the ownership of each document or process step. This schematic illustrates how the business development team finalize the requirements for the system solution (e.g., a new warehouse management system) to be implemented. In tandem, the project team will create implementation and project plans, along with a project definition document (PDD) as a general reference for project information. These three high-level project documents will all be inputs into the first project document that is reviewed by the validation team, the high level business processes (HLBP) (in some cases the HLBP document may be included as part of the user requirements specification.). The planning documents also feed into

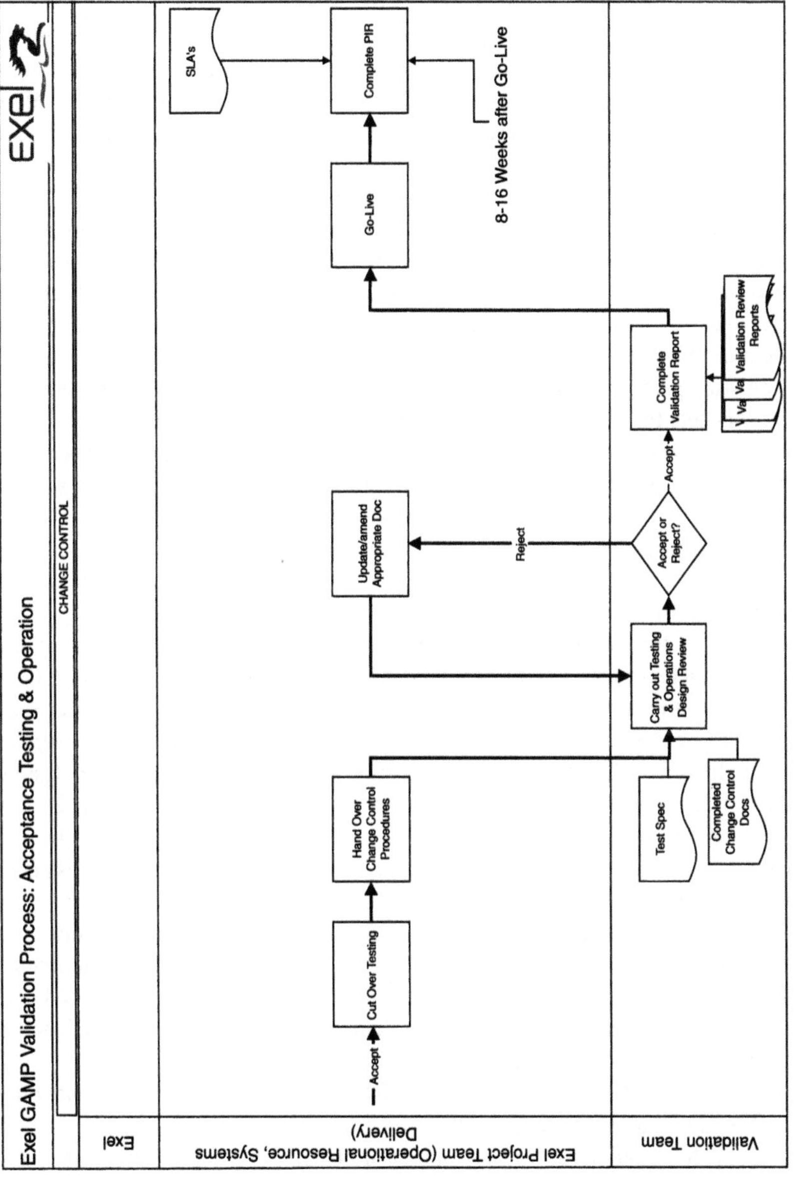

Figure 18.2 Planning and Specification.

the first documents produced by the validation team, the validation master plan (VMP) and the individual validation plans (VP).

The distinction between the VMP and VP is key to the way that the organization approaches validation of its systems. The VMP will lay out the general approach to validation of all systems as part of an overall project implementation or site activity whereas the VP will describe in detail the activities to be undertaken in validating a particular instance of a system for a particular client. The organization will therefore not say that it has validated one particular system but instead, in most cases, will state that it has validated a system as it is used by a specific customer. This is because of the differences in configuration, network requirements, and hardware that occur between multiple users of the same system. This approach is a direct consequence of operating sites on a multiuser basis in order to make best use of key areas of expertise across a number of clients. Operating multi-user facilities is another key factor in the approach that the organization has taken to computer system validation. Where a manufacturer validates a computer system used for a specific task, the organization, as the logistics partner for several manufacturers, will be operating a system that contains data sets for all the manufacturers using the same set of programs.

Although not explicitly using the "V" model, many of the principles are derived from it. Ensuring that every activity or step laid out in the VP is referred to in the final Validation Report guarantees that each activity is verified.

For a new supplier, a supplier assessment is conducted to gauge quality processes and procedures in place before detailed project and validation planning documents are put together. In the model shown in Figure 18.2 this occurs at a later stage. This is a key step in the validation process for the organization. One reason for the importance attached to the assessment is that Exel's healthcare sector division does not design any of its software solutions itself. Consequently any system that is to be validated will be designed and constructed by a third-party supplier. The supplier assessment therefore has to thoroughly ensure that the process of code design, construction and testing is sound. (This also explains why the model lacks any process steps for software design reviews, as they are not carried out by the organization.) The procedure or template for carrying out a supplier assessment reflects these needs.

Following the production of the VMP, VP, and HLBP by the validation and project teams respectively, the project team then constructs its user requirements specification, following a set procedure or template. This URS is reviewed and signed off internally and by client before it is submitted to the supplier (subject to a successful supplier assessment).

The supplier will then respond to the URS by providing a formal functional specification document, which is fully referenced to the URS and details how each requirement is to be satisfied. One key output of the GAMP 4 guide is a quality plan. During initial validation exercises the validation team did produce a quality plan with the QA staff in conjunction with the VMP. However, as the process evolved, the quality plans for each system were so similar in content that the decision was taken to produce a single high-level quality plan. This could be applied to any system implementation. It states the commitment to quality in certain defined areas and describes how the organization would achieve its aims in the area of quality through the quality manual.

Though not represented in Figure 18.3, the validation team also establish an ongoing risk, threat, and issue log which tracks all issues considered to have a potentially detrimental impact on the ultimate validation of the system.

Once these documents have been produced, all the deliverables for the planning and specification stage are in place and the first formal validation review can take place. Following a set procedure the validation team will meet with the project team and a representative of the QA team to review each document against the procedures laid out in the quality manual. During this review each document will be checked for adherence to the quality plan, consistency and completeness, and against all the checklisted points of the review procedure. At this point the review members can make a decision, based on the review checklist, as to whether to accept the documents in their current state and proceed to the design phase or to recommend necessary amendments before progressing. A formal report detailing the results of the review process forms an input into the final validation report.

Upon successful review of the planning and specification stage, the system implementation then moves into the "design" phase. Having established the key specification documents, the project team now create a new series of documents, which detail the configuration of the system. Existing and well-established procedures are followed to produce specifications for hardware, network and software configurations. (The latter only applies where there will be interfaces between different software modules.) There will also be a master data definition document outlining which static data needs to be set up on the system prior to full testing and operation. An example of such data are the locations of defined pick faces or customer and supplier address details. This is a document that is not included in the GAMP guidance. However, the characteristics of the multiuser environment not only necessitate this, but mean that it becomes a key specification. As the validation and project teams handle individual instances of the same system with data sets for each client, the static data, which needs to be configured prior to live operations for a client, becomes a vital area when maintaining close control over the system for each client. Similar issues can be seen in the software configuration specification required for modular computer systems.

Other documents produced by the project team during this phase are the disaster recovery and business continuity plan. The testing specification document defines the approach to testing from the philosophy to the structure of the scripts, their acceptance criteria and the testing scripts themselves.

The project team will also at this stage compile a traceability matrix linking all the key system documentation and the functional areas within them. This allows an external reader such as an inspector, to follow any functional requirement, from the initial specification or business process document through to the eventual testing of

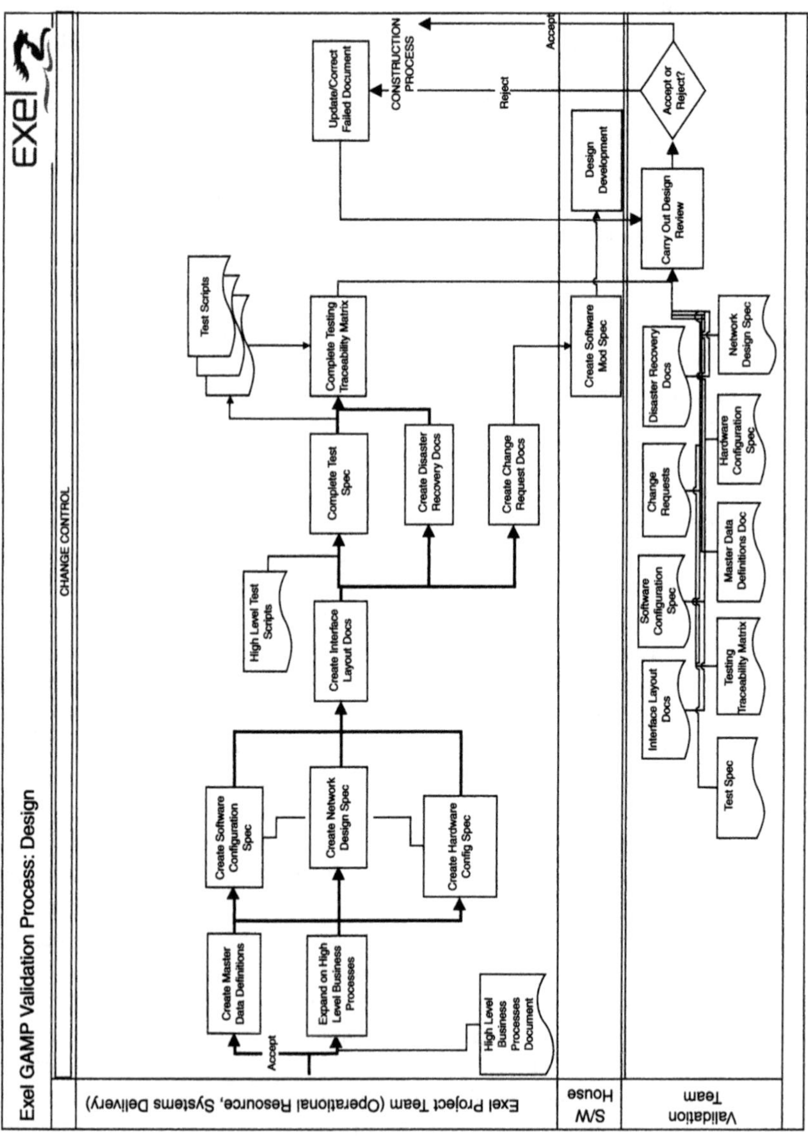

Figure 18.3 Validation process: design.

that function in the delivered system. This matrix is updated throughout the system's life by the site support teams reflecting any changes resulting from change requests. These are recorded and retain full traceability for the URS, the FS, and the testing scripts. Using such a matrix has also been an incidental benefit of implementing GAMP methodology, since tracking areas of functionality through documentation had occasionally been a problem area. This is now much improved in terms of speed and reliability

Again, when the deliverables are in place, the validation, project, and quality team members will carry out a formal review of the project phase before deciding whether to proceed to the construction and testing phase (Figure 18.4).

Moving into the third project implementation phase, the initial versions of the software were installed. The testing strategy laid out previously in the testing specification can now be implemented. The schematic for this project phase lays out all the possible areas of testing, and also bridges the terminology gap between GAMP and the existing project terminology. The IQ, OQ, and PQ steps are identified without creating extra process steps for the testing teams.

The testing specification is included in this phase as well as the previous one. Here it is used as a reference to ensure that the test scripts have been produced according to the testing plan.

If the business processes are to be expanded then they should be included in this section. The other key deliverable here is the structured training material that is produced to support users of the finally implemented system. This may include project training material. As before, once all the deliverables are in place, a formal review will determine whether the project team can progress to the final phase of the implementation (Figure 18.5).

The final project phase involves completing the system testing (as per the testing specification) so cutover testing documentation is included. All of the change control documentation is also collated for future reference. This involves making sure that all the specification and testing documents, as well as the traceability matrix, are current prior to the handover from the project to the site support team. This will also be documented, following a predefined procedure or template. Upon completion, the final review can take place. Once all the project deliverables have been satisfactorily completed, then the final validation report can be written. This report will be written by the validation team, reflecting the results of all the activities planned, in light of the original validation plan.

Once the validation team is satisfied that the system has been implemented in line with all the processes and procedures as set out in the quality manual and all risk and issue logs are closed out, then a validation certificate will be issued and the systems or validation register is updated. This will then reflect that the system implemented in this particular instance is considered validated and inspection ready.

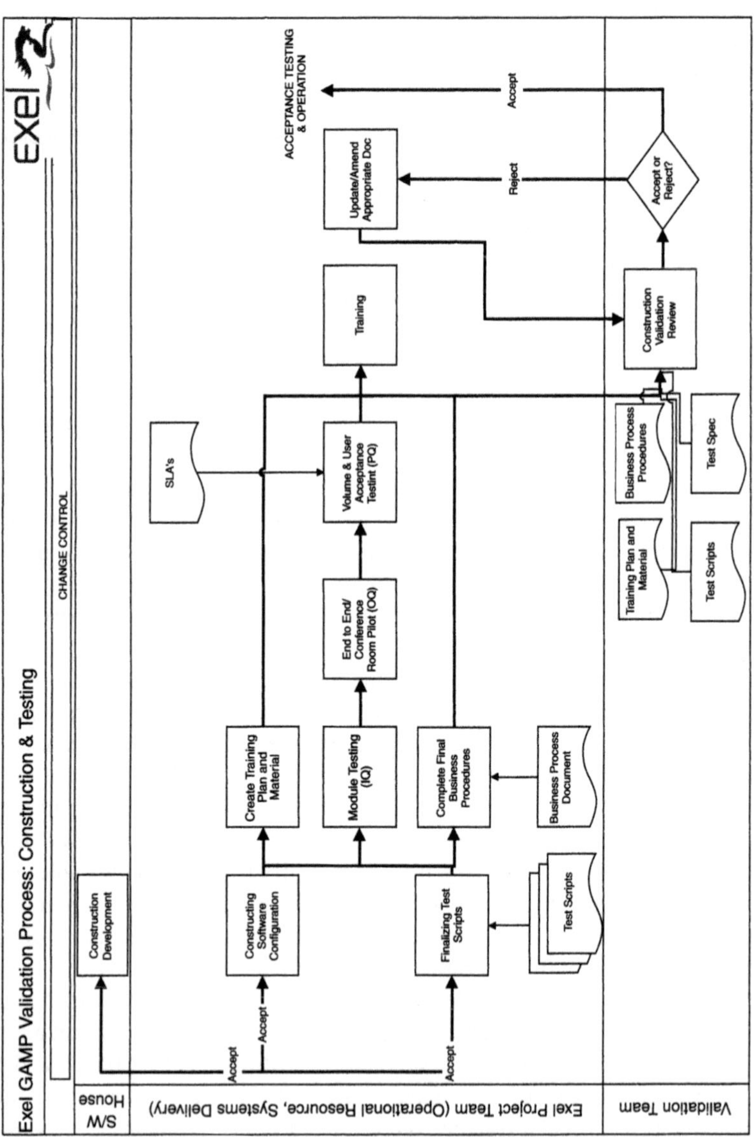

Figure 18.4 Validation process: construction and testing.

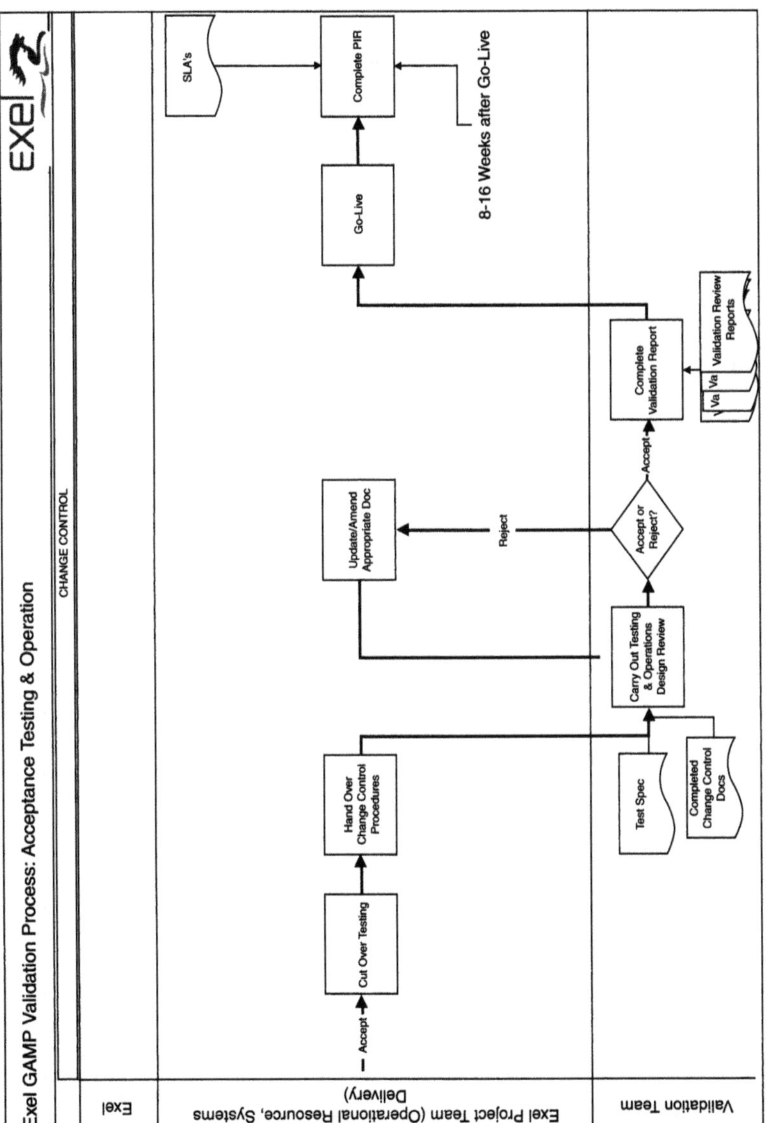

Figure 18.5 Validation process: acceptance testing and operation.

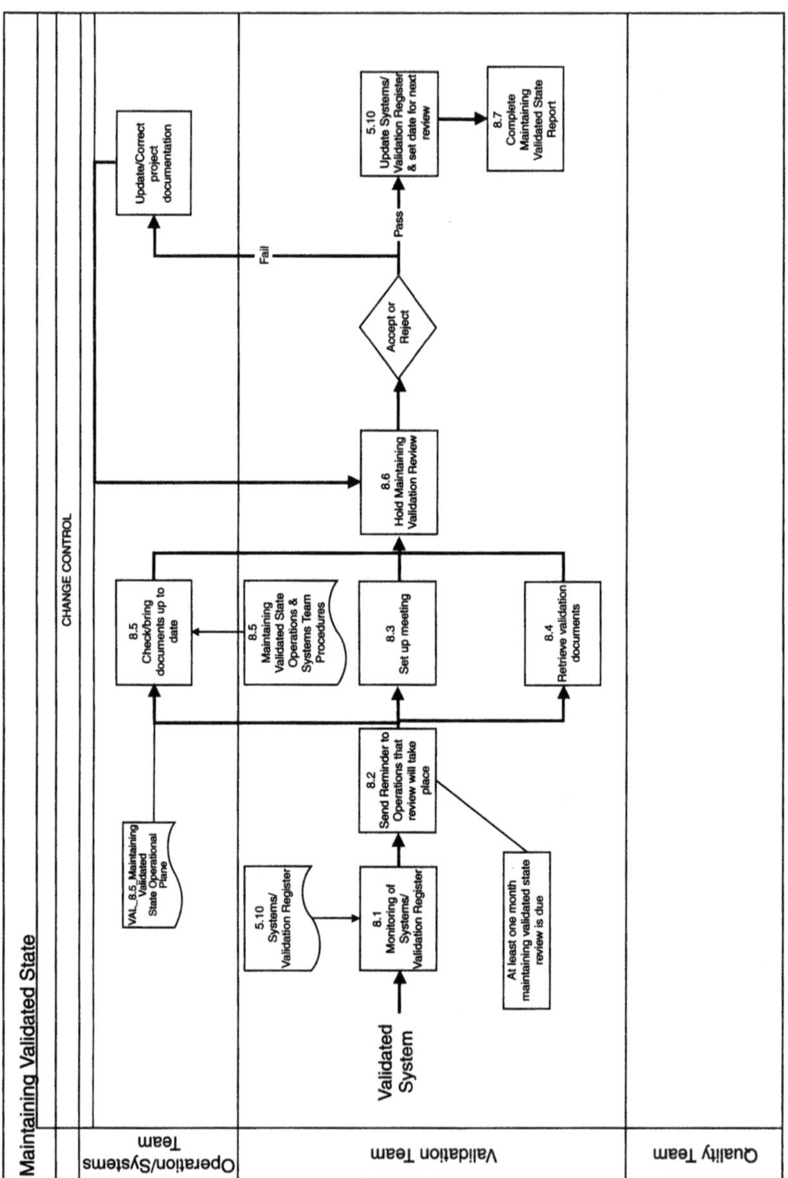

Figure 18.6 Maintaining validated state.

MAINTAINING THE VALIDATED STATE

One of the biggest misconceptions that we encountered within the organization was that once we had implemented a validated system all the work is done!

Using MS Visio Process models and IDEF0 charts we also constructed detailed mechanisms for maintaining the validated state, which were held within the quality manual.

The emphasis here is on the work to be done by the site support team who provide live support to the individual clients once the system has been implemented. Typically there will be one analyst or super user per client who will have support from the validation team in maintaining the validated state.

The overall process is represented in Figure 18.6.

This time the starting point is the systems or validation register, which shows the validation status of each system, and reflects the work required to achieve and maintain this status. The work flow for the site team begins by following the operational plan as laid out in the quality manual. This details how the system must be maintained in terms of:

- Training.
- Problem management,.
- Service level agreements (SLA).
- System backups.
- Business continuity planning.
- Performance monitoring.
- System security.
- System retirement.

It is through adherence to the operational plan, associated procedures, and regular document reviews that the validation team assure adequate system maintenance.

LEGACY SYSTEM REVIEW

The retrospective process therefore forms the third plank of this approach to validating all systems with GxP implications (e.g., after new systems and maintaining the validated state).

This is still very much based on the processes already discussed. However the emphasis here is on ensuring that the key deliverables are already in place. This involves carrying out "gap analysis" and then performing any necessary remedial work. In this sense the organization's approach as a distributor does not differ significantly from a manufacturer, although the deliverables do, of course.

As in a prospective implementation, validation plans are created. Once all the documents have been collated then a series of validation reviews will determine if the system meets the required standards prior to production of a final report, and update of the systems or validation register.

Electronic Records and Signatures

The area of electronic records and signatures is no easier for those working to cGDP than it is for those working to cGMP, cGCP, or cGLP. Also the recent withdrawal of guidelines and recent interpretations of the CFR 21 Part 11 legislation makes this a very difficult area in which to achieve full compliance.

The Approach

The organization has incorporated the ER/ES requirements within the overall validation approach. There is no separate plan to achieve Part 11 compliance per system. There is a policy document that states how to achieve compliance published within the quality manual, detailing the requirements of each section of the regulation and sets out how compliance is achieved.

This approach is illustrated by the extract from the quality manual shown in Figure 18.7.

Part 11 Ref.	Ref.	Challenge	Challenge Met (Yes, No)	Comments/Recommendations (including reference to supporting evidence)
	A1	POLICIES AND TRAINING		
	A1.1	Policies and Training	ANSWER ALL QUESTIONS	
§11.10 [i]	A1.1.2	Do policies exist to ensure that personnel have the necessary experience or training to carry their assigned roles and responsibilities?	Yes	See VAL_3.4_Training Plans and Materials-Procedures.
§11.10 [j]	A1.1.3	Do policies exist to ensure that personnel understand that their electronic signature is legally equivalent to their hand-written signature and that records be established to document their understanding?	Yes	See above, also mentioned during induction and systems specific training
§11.10 [a]	A1.1.5	Do policies exist to ensure that computerised systems are validated?	Yes	See Healthcare IS Library/Quality Manual for Validating Systems.

Figure 18.7 Extract from quality manual.

Emphasis has been placed on the following areas:

- Policies.
- Protection of records.
- Security (system and logical).
- Sequential checks.
- Training.
- Documentation.

The approach achieves compliance through a combination of internal policies and procedures and the organization's software suppliers' technical controls (assessed during supplier assessments and reviews). The three main areas considered necessary to achieve compliance are graphically represented in the Venn diagram in Figure 18.8.

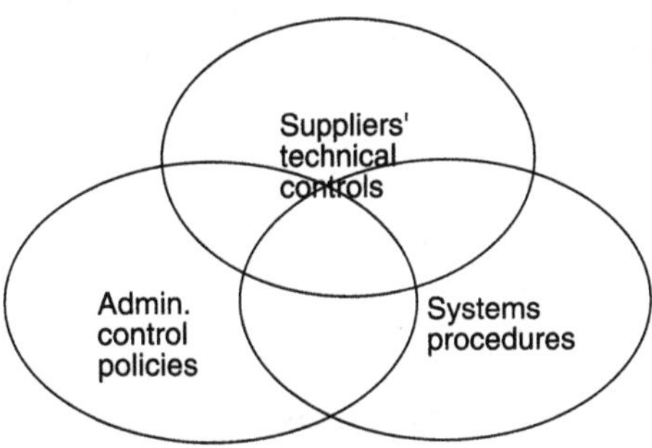

Figure 18.8 Venn diagram representation of areas necessary to achieve compliance.

SPECIFIC VALIDATION WORK

The quality manual was first launched in the final quarter of 2002 as the validation and project team members used the new processes and procedures to retrospectively validate the core versions of the key healthcare warehousing solutions. These are the warehouse management system (WMS), task management system and the integration solution that links the WMS with our clients own ERP and MRP systems. This exercise was termed the validation of generic versions of the systems.

Identification of core functionality through the high-level business processes was followed by the creation of a URS, supplied to our software suppliers in conjunction with supplier audits. As previously illustrated this assessment is vital to ensure the software design quality, achieved through rigorously challenging the potential supplier's design methods.

We experienced some issues with our suppliers because they supply systems that are not used exclusively in a healthcare environment. They also wanted to know afterwards if they were then "GAMP compliant." (The answer was that there is no such thing as being "GAMP compliant," however vendors could be technically compliant with the guidance but this is heavily dependant on the administrative and procedural controls applied by their customers as illustrated in Figure 18.8.) Another benefit of doing the work was that we were able to improve, or suggest potential improvements, for some of their procedures with regard to future software development.

We have also found that audited and potential suppliers with previous experience of applying the GAMP principles were much further ahead in areas such as QMS, continuous improvement, code design and review, in comparison to their uninitiated counterparts.

We were then able to follow through the rest of the validation processes, holding formal reviews at predefined stages of the implementation lifecycle to ensure that the key documents had been produced to satisfactory standards and in line with the established procedures, for example, the user requirements specification, the functional specification and the testing specification and attendant scripts. This culminated in the production of final validation reports for each of the systems, which summarized the results of each of the validation reviews and the creation of a systems or validation register, updated with the results as well as any actions, which remained outstanding.

Since the completion of the generic validation project the validation protocol has been fully deployed to validate specific instances of the WMS and several other systems such as those used for clinical trials logistics and temperature monitoring.

THE REGULATORY ENVIRONMENT

The regulatory environment has changed while the validation protocol has been developed, the merger between the MCA and the MDA to form the MHRA in the UK demonstrates how it is vital to constantly review the environment that we as a business operate in. Regular housekeeping tasks now include reviewing the main regulatory communications channels for white papers and new draft guidance documents. This is increasingly done in partnership with our colleagues in the U.S. and APAC regions.

More specifically, recent guidance issued by the FDA, following on from the ISPE's white paper has led to a different, narrower interpretation of the scope and application of 21 CFR Part 11 [6]. This has meant that we have reviewed our approach to the issues of electronic records and signatures, and revised the documentation within the quality manual where necessary to do so.

MOVING FORWARD

The validation protocol is rolled out as a standard implementation methodology for all healthcare systems projects as a matter of policy and has become a well-established and ingrained operating mode amongst all members of the organization's healthcare community.

The European validation team has also begun to develop a common approach based on the work done for the generic exercise in the U.S. and the Asia Pacific regions (the latter taking into account the requirements of the Australian regulatory body, the TGA, which borrows from the MCA and PICS literature).

The global arena offers us further validation challenges as the organization deals with several major pharmaceutical companies in different areas. A consequence of this is that care must be taken when dealing with a client who may have a validated warehouse management system in its U.K. operation and therefore assumes that an instance of a different or even the same system in Australia or the U.S.A. is also validated. This may be especially true if global system brands are used. This issue is particularly relevant when discussing global branding of computer systems.

TACKLING AND SOLVING PROBLEMS

There has been some organizational resistance by parts of the business community who have viewed validation as a commercial option rather than a necessity. It was viewed as adding to the paper workload and being an "IT" cost rather than adding any value, so a lot of education and communication has been required. This communication has taken the form of internal presentations at different levels of the business and production of information packs for project, site support, and business development teams. The validation team has tried to remove the perception that validation is something which the IT community come and do to the operations and encourage the philosophy that the organization builds validation into our way of doing things such that it becomes part of good project and support practice.

There has also been a presumption that operations more concerned with medical devices have a lesser regulatory onus than for pharmaceuticals. The recent merger of the MCA and MDA to form the MHRA in the U.K., and the inevitable harmonization of regulatory requirements, is evidence that this will no longer be the case. Again, by building the validation protocol into standard project practice this problem is gradually being eliminated.

Misconceptions in some European locations have included varying interpretations of the stringency of country regulations when compared to the U.K. and U.S. Also a different perception existed in some countries of what validation involves. The organization has addressed this issue at the highest level by building validated systems into our healthcare sector brand through an insistence that all new system implementations will be validated.

Another misconception has been by the third party software suppliers that has ISO900x accreditation can act as a substitute for following GAMP! The challenge here was enforcement of any noncompliance since we do not have any direct power to enforce changes without resorting to the commercial arrangement. Through our existing excellent supplier relationships we have worked together to reach a point where we are happy that our suppliers fulfil their obligations to us and our requirements.

There was also a feeling early on that only the warehouse management systems required validation, little regard was given to other software or even process control systems. Subsequently Exel's healthcare sector having recently built a new UK pharmaceutical export warehouse facility has extended validation to the building itself as part of the process of gaining MCA license approval, including the temperature monitoring system, the access control system, and the chilled goods storage areas.

As has already been seen, perceptions like this would be a one-off exercise that the IT community would perform. However, as part of the education and communication process, emphasis has been placed on the importance of maintaining the validated state following initial implementation and this is a message that has gradually been accepted by the business and is now owned by the various support functions.

Members of the validation team are now often present at early stage meetings or presentations to potential clients or where we are trying to extend the scope of our business with existing customers. Senior management have recognized that many pharmaceutical and medical devices manufacturers will not consider us as a third party logistics partner if we cannot offer validated systems to them. It is now recognized as an important tool by which we can differentiate itself from its peer group and provide us with a distinct competitive advantage.

REFERENCES

1 Figures taken from www.the organization.com figures for financial year ending 01/04/02.
2 Foote, L. Quality Systems in the Pharmaceutical Industry, *CMM — Pharmaceutical Engineering,* Vol. 23, no. 2.
3 Christoffersen, B.C., Jespersen, J.B. Documentation as Part of the Project Management Tool. *PAM — Pharmaceutical Engineering*, Vol.23, no. 4.
4 Taken from www.idef.com/idef0.html
5 GAMP Guide for Validation of Automated Systems, p. 23.
6 GAMP Guide for Validation of Automated Systems, p. 38.
7 FDA Guidance docket 03D0060.

Rules and Guidance for Pharmaceutical Manufacturers and Distributors, 2002 (The Orange Guide), The Stationery Office, 2002.

Chapter 19

Good Testing Practice: Part 2

David Stokes

CONTENTS

INTRODUCTION

As discussed in Chapter 9, a successful program of testing in the life sciences industry starts with a risk-based test strategy and test plans based upon pragmatic experience.

The need for pragmatism extends into the execution of the test program, the review of the results and the associated reporting (typically in the form of an operational qualification or performance qualification report, although these may use other titles such as "test summary report").

This chapter discusses some of the practical issues relating to conducting cost effective and compliant test execution, review, and reporting in the life sciences industries.

MORE SPEED, LESS HASTE

As outlined in Chapter 9, using trained staff to execute tests that have been appropriately scoped and properly planned pays dividends. This is true in all industries, but the additional constraints of testing a validated system in a regulated environment means that the benefits of not rushing into test execution may be even greater.

Key Roles

Most important is a test manager (or equivalent) who is intimately familiar with testing in such an environment. A good test manager will understand the balance between meeting important project milestones and delivering a quality product or application. Fundamentally this means understanding where attention to detail will pay dividends later in the test program.

Equally, lead testers will be very familiar with the execution of test cases in the life sciences sector and the requirements for producing documented proof that test objectives have been met. These should be formatted in such a way that aids third-party review of the executed test cases.

Another important role is that of test incident manager (responsible for resolving issues associated with "failed" test cases). A good test incident manager will quickly be able to identify patterns associated with failed test cases, identify root causes and work with the test manager and leads testers to ensure that any systematic problems are rectified as early as possible in the test program.

This knowledge only comes with experience gained from previous projects. While testers and developers responsible for resolving problems with software or test cases may have limited experience, these three key individuals should ideally have experience testing similar systems in a similar environment.

While large organizations may choose to retain a core of experienced testers, smaller organizations may benefit from the experience of third parties such as contractors or consultants in these key roles. As with any other key role in a validation project, user organizations should, of course, review the training, qualifications, or experience of any third party resource, but this is especially important in these central test roles.

Where experienced and trusted resources are used, such insight on the preparation and timing of a test program will prove invaluable. While to the inexperienced eye the preparation and planning may take longer than appears desirable, this will usually pay benefits later in the program.

Scalability

Although these roles are crucial to the effective execution of test program, it should be recognized that the testing of small or relatively simple systems will support the creation of each of these roles cost effectively.

These roles may of course be combined, but where this is the case it is perhaps even more important that the persons fulfilling these multiple roles are capable. If there is any doubt as to the capability of individuals involved, additional support or reviews may be called for.

MANAGING THE PAPERWORK

Most importantly, the time taken in preparing the document management aspects of the test program is seldom wasted.

Test programs in a regulated environment generate a great deal of information. Newcomers will often be daunted by the volume of paperwork generated before and during the execution of the test cases.

Despite the availability of some excellent automated test tools, many organizations still choose to use paper as their preferred medium for managing and documenting test activities. If this is the case, the paper management is important for two main reasons:

- Efficient management of the paper leads to more efficient testing. This saves time and money.
- The loss of important test evidence may require complex tests to be repeated. Where the volume of repeats is sufficiently high, this may call the quality of the whole test process into question in the eyes of a third party auditor (or regulatory inspector).

An experienced test nanager will usually establish a clear method for managing the documentation. In some cases even finding critical documents can be a problem.

The use of brightly coloured folders or binders can ease this problem and is a common solution.

Another eye-catching solution (used by at least one test manager in the industry) is to tie different coloured helium filled balloons to the binders so that test team members could quickly identify key documents in a busy room (especially useful when testing in a closed-cubicle type environment).

Documentation should be structured in such a way as to survive "the drop test." Hopefully test scripts and specifications, user requirement documents and so on will not be dropped on the floor, but it is quite usual for individual sheets to be separated during testing.

There is nothing more frustrating that having to repeat a test because a sheet of paper with a necessary result or signature has been lost. Ensuring each sheet of paper has a document reference, version or iteration number and page number, and that each test binder or folder has an index will ensure that missing sheets can be returned to the appropriate document.

In the worst case, when a binder is dropped and all of the sheets explode over the test floor, it should be possible to reconstruct the binder with every sheet in the correct order and continue testing from the point of the unforeseen interruption.

On large projects the appointment of a test document coordinator can be cost effective. The test document coordinator is basically responsible for checking documentation in and out at the start and end of a day (or test session) and for tracking the documentation. This is especially important when a complex test case may require multiple testers to each execute part of the test case and document part of the results.

One other key role the test document administrator can perform is to ensure that all test cases issued to the test teams are approved for execution and are the most current version. Although a test document administrator will generally not be sufficiently trained, experienced or qualified to review executed test cases, they can also ensure that the basic document management process has been followed (all test results entered, stated test evidence attached, and executed test cases have been signed).

AUTOMATED TEST TOOLS

Because of the volume of regression tests, more and more projects in the life sciences industry are now turning towards the use of automated test tools. This is often brought about by the frequent issue of new software releases or "patches" for software errors.

The best of these automated test tools provide excellent functionality, can enforce configurable test processes through the use of workflow and can provide adequate security, audit trail functionality and electronic review and approval functionality. There are even a few that are technically compliant with the regulatory requirements for the use of electronic records and electronic signatures (such as 21CFR Part 11).

Where test processes are complex, perhaps using many individuals on multiple sites to execute tests or review test results, the use of automated test tools allows testing to continue seamlessly in an electronic environment.

Any organization thinking of undertaking the testing of a large system or application would be advised to investigate the use of an automated test tool. Where such applications or systems are likely to be subject to multiple rounds of regression testing the use of automated test cases would also be advised.

The typical return on investment of the most functional of these test tools is around three rounds of regression testing. This means that the investment in such tools can pay for itself after the third round of software development, or after the receipt of the third major upgrade or patch.

This is typically well within the expected lifetime of most large or complex systems, and most large life science organizations would benefit from the use of such tools. The return on investment is even greater when such tools are used as part of an enterprise-wide initiative (as opposed to just a single project) and even a medium sized organization would benefit if such tools were used to test a wide variety of systems and applications (ERP, LIMS, desktop images and so on).

While the need to appropriately validate such test tools increases the initial implementation and support costs (compared to testing in a nonregulated environment), there is additional benefit because the savings are greater in a more complex test environment.

FOCUS ON THE PROCESSES

Even the best automated test tool will deliver little benefit if it is used to automate poor test execution processes. Maximum benefit cannot be gained if such tools are used simply to automate inefficient processes or those that do not meet the minimum expectations of the regulatory agencies.

Organizations implementing such systems should question their existing test processes. Even those who are not looking at such systems but feel they could improve their testing efficiency may benefit from a review of their processes.

Such a review should focus on two main questions:

- Do our processes meet the expectations of the various regulatory agencies?
- Are our test processes as efficient as they could (should) be?

There is obviously a trade-off between these two issues. Processes can be streamlined to the extent that they provide insufficient evidence that the test program has met all of its objectives. Likewise, going overboard in witnesses, signatures, and reviews can slow down the test program to a nonsensical level.

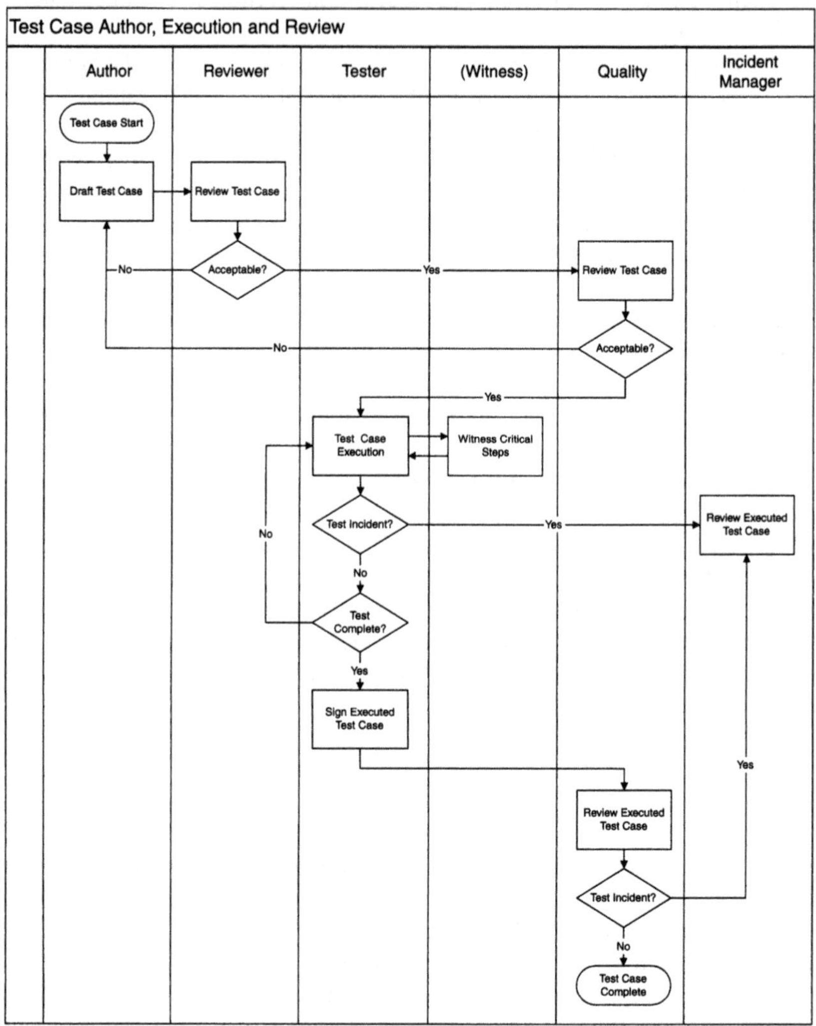

Figure 19.1 Example of role-based testing process.

The best way to do this is to map out the processes, identify the various test roles against these processes and the key checkpoints that support the validation of the system. Appropriate controls can be established at these points, and the surrounding processes can then be streamlined around these points.

Key processes that should be focused on are:

- Test management: including the monitoring of the test program and the collection, collation, and reporting of test statistics.
- Test case execution: including the issue of test cases, execution of test cases, and the collection and collation of executed cases.
- Incident management: including how a test incident is raised, categorized, assessed, resolved, and closed.
- Test reporting: including the review of individual test cases and the preparation of test summary reports.

How such processes may be streamlined will depend on whether they are paper based or leverage automated test tools, and the size and complexity of the test programs to be executed.

It is useful to document standard test processes in high-level policy documents, but to leave the detailed testing procedures to be defined on a department by department or project by project basis.

An example of a testing process flow (and associated roles) is shown in Figure 19.1.

Any standard operating procedures (SOPs) governing test activities should be proscriptive with respect to the key checkpoints and the inclusion of associated activities. For instance, in the example process included in Figure 19.1, the final QA approval of the test case prior to execution and the post execution signature by the tester may be defined as mandatory within all testing procedures (although these may not be required for strict regulatory reasons).

Specific procedures should however be more flexible with respect to the remainder of the test processes to allow test programs of all sizes and complexity to be supported by the same high-level policies. For example, the nature of certain systems may require the use of test witnesses while others may not.

It is often useful for test managers to define how such SOPs will be used on any given test program and to define project specific work instructions defining the specific roles and workflow that will be used to implement compliant test processes.

FUNDAMENTAL UNDERSTANDING

In order to define and streamline such SOPs and work instructions, organizations need to understand the fundamentals of testing within the life sciences industry. There is plenty of guidance available on the subject software testing best practice, and there is also industry specific best practice guidance available from organizations such as GAMP and ISPE (see bibliography). These are generally not written in proscriptive language and still rely upon individuals to interpret them in their own organization or on their own projects.

Unfortunately there are a number of common misconceptions (and in some organizations a good deal of "urban myth") surrounding testing in the life sciences sector. These often lead to many companies continuing to implement inefficient testing processes and even automating them using computer-based tools. Other organizations may of course implement processes that are noncompliant in the extreme.

While this may appear to lead to a conclusion that there is a “right” level of testing, the reality that although an appropriate level of testing lies between the two, there is still a “band” of appropriate testing. In some cases, belief in the “urban myths” of testing GxP critical systems takes over from common sense, and pragmatic testing is done away with for the sake of “compliance” with nonexistent “regulations.”

Although a requirement to test and retain test records can be inferred from certain regulations (21CFR Part 820 for instance, and the testing of software contained in medical devices), this is not widespread. Regulations certainly do not tell us what or how to test. This is left up to the individual organization to decide, and the latest regulatory guidance suggests that this should be determined by a justification based on a risk assessment.

We should therefore challenge some of the urban myths, and explore the underlying rationale further.

“Test Everything”

As discussed in Chapter 9, there is no need to test everything. In a large or complex system this is impossible, since there may be multiple paths through the software in any customized or configurable system. Add in the multiple different types of tests that could be performed and the number of tests approaches the infinite.

The scope and nature of testing should therefore be determined by documented risk assessment, use of sound judgement in determining the GxP impact, risk probability and likelihood of detection.

“Ensure Complete Traceability”

There are usually some requirements that cannot be tested, and can only be verified by other means. Examples of such verification may include visual inspection or post go-live performance monitoring.

It is unusual to be able to provide complete traceability between executed test cases and *all* requirements. Depending upon the nature of the requirement, traceability to a specific act of verification rather than a test may be required. Although there should be complete traceability (to demonstrate that all requirements have been fulfilled) this may not be achieved by testing alone, and the requirements traceability process (or procedure) and any requirements traceability matrix should allow for this.

"Sign Every Step"

The testing culture in some organizations require testers to sign for every test in the script. This is often time-consuming and unnecessary. In other organizations testers may sign only at the foot of each page of test script.

The key requirement for "signing" test scripts is to have a documented record of who conducted the test. This provides a record that only appropriately trained, qualified, or experienced staff have been used to conduct tests. It also allows any post-test reviewer to discuss any salient points with the tester.

It is appropriate therefore for a tester only to sign at the completion of the executed test in order to document who conducted the test. Some tests will, however, require multiple testers to conduct different steps, in which case signing for the individual steps executed may be required. An alternative may be to divide the test script into multiple sections, with each section conducted by a different tester, and each signed by the appropriate tester.

In automated test systems with a secure audit trail, signatures are not needed for these purposes because a secure log-in and audit trail will provide evidence of who conducted each stage in the test. Additional signatures may, however, be required for reasons explained below.

Because of the likelihood of test sheets going missing (see "Managing the Paperwork" above) some organizations like a signature on each sheet to differentiate between completed and incomplete pages within the test script. However, if each line is annotated with an expected result it will be obvious whether a page as been completed or not.

The important point about testing is to ensure that test objectives are met (thereby demonstrating that the associated requirement has been met, and that the system is therefore fit for its intended purpose). Many steps in a test script are there solely to instruct the tester how to setup the system to conduct the important step that demonstrates that the test objective has been met.

In some cases the system enforces a series of actions and there is only one way to reach the critical step. Such set-up steps should not need signing, although some organizations require a tester's signature on the step where the objective is demonstrably met.

In systems where the set-up may follow multiple paths to achieve the demonstrable objective, and where the sequence of such set-up steps and the entry of data is critical to demonstrating the test objective has been met, signatures are required for each set-up step.

This should not be required where the context of the signature (against the step that proves that the test objective has been met) clearly states that the set-up steps have been followed and the testers signature attests to this.

The need for tester signatures should therefore be determined based upon:

- Clearly defining the context and scope of the signature.

- Understanding the nature of the test, including the importance of set-up steps and data entry.
- Supporting evidence.

This should be borne in mind when designing the test case and test script and testers should be trained to understand the context of their signatures rather than sign everything by rote.

"Everything Should Be Witnessed"

In the early days of testing real-time control systems (and some computer systems) it was often difficult to take evidence of a test result. Capturing a fleeting screen image was difficult, and screen prints were unheard of on most systems. Test witnesses were used to observe such tests and provide independent, informed corroboration that the expected result was the one that was actually observed.

In cases where it is difficult or impossible to capture evidence, the use of a test witness may still be useful in providing independent, informed corroboration. However, the efficient and pragmatic testing of systems and the widespread capability to capture test evidence should require an extremely limited use of test witnesses.

Such test witnesses should be suitably trained, qualified or experienced, and should understand what they expect to see, specifically in the context of the test objective.

Because of the resource constraints imposed by large testing programs, the widespread "need" to use test witnesses often results in the "recruitment" of test witnesses who do not understand what they are seeing and who rely solely upon the tester's explanation of what is happening and what they have observed. This undermined the principle of independent, informed corroboration because the test witness is only "informed" by the tester, thereby undermining any element of independence.

Some organizations use test witnesses to confirm that the test process (test script) was followed by the tester (rather that to confirm the test objective had been met). While this does provide independent verification of the test process, it is an inefficient use of resources and certainly not a regulatory requirement.

In production areas and laboratories, trained staff are expected to follow SOPs without constant supervision. Although key parameters and results may be independently checked by supervisors or qualified persons, such staff are trusted to perform their everyday job in accordance with the procedures they have been trained in. This principle should be applied to all testing roles. This usually represents a much lower risk to patient safety than manufacturing or testing a pharmaceutical product.

"Record Everything"

Minimizing the use of test witnesses can be justified where there is verifiable evidence that the test has been conducted in accordance with the test script and of the observed results.

Test evidence can be produced by a number of methods. These may include printouts from databases updated by the test, report outputs, by screen shots generated from within the application under test, or by the use of specialist data capture or screen image software.

As stated above, some systems enforce a series of actions between one critical step and the next. Where this is known to be the case (usually with GAMP software category 3 and 4 software in widespread commercial use) it is not necessary to produce evidence of the steps taken to progress from one critical step to the next. In such systems it is sufficient to capture evidence associated with demonstrating that the test objective has been met.

Even in such systems the expected test objective will be resultant upon input data. This may, of course, be generated from a controlled and approved set of test data (details of which should of course be recorded). Where the tester enters data manually it is usually necessary to capture evidence of the input data.

In determining the nature, scope, and detail of test evidence required the fundamental underlying principle should be to ask whether a copy of the executed test script and the associated test evidence will allow an independent reviewer to confirm whether the objectives of the test have been met.

Assuming that testers are trained and trusted to execute testing in accordance with established test procedures, test evidence should only be required to confirm that a particular sequence of steps was followed (when not enforced by the system under test), that the stated test data was entered and that the actual results match (or otherwise) the expected results. It should not be necessary to capture test evidence for every set-up step in a test.

Test evidence should also be capable of standing "the drop test." Pages of test evidence should be annotated with the test case reference, version and test iteration number. Where it aids independent review of the test, evidence should be referenced to a specific test step and pages should be numbered.

"Use Only Black Ink"

Other organizations have "rules" covering the recording of manual entries during testing. These were often based upon original pragmatic considerations, but time moves on and these "rules" become urban myths with no understanding of the original reasons.

In some organizations, only black ink may be used. This was because early photocopiers did not photocopy blue ink very well. In other organizations, blue ink is a requirement. This may be because of perceived “regulatory” reasons (for instance, the Danish Medicines Control Board continue a tradition of blue ink for “official” documents that originally began with the church and government).

Other organizations understand that black and white photocopiers now copy blue ink, but the use of blue ink quickly shows the difference between an original document and a photocopy. Other organizations “ban” the use of fluorescent highlighter pens, because the colours change and fade over time.

The use of pencil is universally “banned” because it allows testers or reviewers to change results after the test execution.

Rather than make rules around the recording “technology” (which changes over time), it is important to have an understanding of the fundamental requirements for recording test results, and make project specific “rules” at any given time, based upon the recording “technology” to be used.

These fundamentals include:

- Entries should be “permanent.” Although some change in color or tone may occur over time, entries should still be legible for the lifetime of the document. A minor change in color is not a problem (unless multiple colors are used for different purposes, such as green for “pass” and pink for “fail” and it becomes impossible to distinguish between the two).

  The “permanence” may need confirmation by inspection over time and if entries change unexpectedly it may be necessary to make verified copies.
- Changes should have an audit trail. Any corrections should be made in a way that does not obscure previous entries or original data. Significant changes should be explained in appropriate notes recorded in a “comments” column or in the margin.
- It should be possible to make copies of documents, including all entries and annotations. Ideally it should be possible to distinguish between originals and copies (but copies can always be marked as such, by use of rubber stamp).

Designing good documents can do away with many of these problems. For instance, where a simple “pass” or “fail” indication is appropriate (where there is independent test evidence of the actual results) colored highlighters may be used for speed and convenience to provide an easily reviewed status. Test scripts can be designed with a “pass” box to be filled in with green highlighter pen and a separate “fail” box to be filled in with a pink highlighter pen. Even if the colors fade over 15 years it should still be clear which box was filled in.

These same principles apply to the use of automated test tools, with the use of secure audit trails as a fundamental requirement.

“Review Everything”

Tests should be independently reviewed to ensure that test objectives have indeed been met, and it is traditional that every test is subject to independent review by a quality unit or validation group.

While this might be appropriate for highly critical systems or functional areas in a system it may not be necessary for systems of lower criticality. As long as the executed test script and test evidence is capable of supporting independent post-execution verification that the test objective has been met, it may not be necessary to do this at the time.

It may be appropriate for quality units or validation groups to review a percentage of tests to ensure that testing is conducted in accordance with established procedures, that test results are recorded properly, that test evidence is properly managed, and test failures are managed objectively.

This may be done on a percentage basis, and as with any other statistical review there should be a sound basis for determining the sample size. Factors used to determine an appropriate sample size will include the numbers of different test types, testers, and expected errors.

To support such a regime it is important that accurate test statistics are maintained. Where test statistics demonstrate that the likelihood of test errors is low a larger sample size may be required to confirm the error rate, but such reviews may be conducted on a less frequent basis.

Higher error rates (or a deteriorating trend) may require more frequent sampling or a stricter regime (such as reviewing every test for functions of high GxP priority). The use of test statistics in this manner can be used as part of an overall approach that uses statistics collated throughout the validation lifecycle to determine which verification activities contribute most to assuring software quality. This can be done by monitoring the number of errors identified by different verification activities, such as requirements traceability monitoring, source code walkthrough, design qualification, unit testing, integration testing, and acceptance testing.

Recognizing the fundamental difference between manufacturing operations and computer software testing, statistical techniques and risk assessment can nevertheless be used to justify the premise that not every test needs independent review. It is accepted, however, that this may only be appropriate in a culture where testing is conducted by a trained and experienced test team and where there is no pressure to inappropriately accelerate the testing process, cut corners, or falsify results.

TESTING

Testing is, of course, where things either go well, or in some cases disastrously wrong. There have been a number of examples where a poorly planned and managed test program has led to projects running significantly over budget, timescales and cost, and in some instances led to the cancellation of a project.

The Test Team

As stated above, the principles of testing in the life sciences sector is no different from other industries, with the exception of the level of documentation usually produced. Also as discussed earlier, the use of an experienced core of individuals will make a significant difference to whether or not a program of testing is successful or not.

Some life sciences organizations are now setting up dedicated test teams, who move from system to system, allowing multiple projects to benefit from their collective experience. In smaller organizations similar benefit can be gained from the use of specialist service providers who can help set-up and execute a testing program.

If either of these approaches are taken, it is important that the experienced team of testers pass on their experience and knowledge to those individuals who will be responsible for the ongoing regression testing of the system during its operational life. This usually means that the most effective test teams will be made up of a combination of experienced testers, systems owners and those who will be responsible for the long-term system support.

Test Execution

Test execution should be well planned in advance, and as discussed in Chapter 9 the test team should be appropriately trained.

Unless the system under test is small or particularly simple, test cases are usually grouped into test sets and allocated to testers. When appraising the sequence of testing test managers need to consider:

- The number of tests to be conducted and the number of testers available.
- The anticipated duration of each test case.
- The sequencing of interdependent tests (for example, test cases that rely on the data created by previous test cases as input data).
- An allowance for a percentage of test cases to fail, and require re-execution.

Consideration should also be given to complex test cases that may require several testers (or users) to conduct part of the test. In large or complex systems this may even involve testers or users on different sites or in different time zones.

Tests should be executed in a calm manner, by individuals with a clear understanding of the test objective and what is happening "behind-the-scenes." Less experienced testers should be aware of issues or problems to look out for, and if they have any doubts as to whether to proceed with a test or abort it they should seek the advice of the test lead or a quality reviewer.

Should any unusual events occur it is useful to capture as much information as possible, including taking screen shots, hard copy output or additional notes of what happened leading up to the event, during the event, and the final end state.

Test Review and Incident Analysis

Any tests that do not clearly demonstrate that the test objective has been met (i.e., those that "fail"), should be analyzed to determine the nature and underlying cause of the failure.

Testers should be trained to identify tests that fall into this category and these should be subject to independent review. Any tests that "pass," but which are queried by a post-execution review should also be subject to the same analysis process.

An initial analysis will usually confirm that the test objective has not been met (although in some cases the test incident analysis may conclude that the test objective *has* been met and that the tester was over-zealous in raising a test incident).

Test incidents are usually further categorized according to the nature of the incident (or reason for the "failure"). Different organizations or projects may categorize incidents in different ways, but common reasons for test incidents include:

- Problems with test data.
- Problems in test execution (tester error during set-up, data entry, or execution).
- Problems with the test environment.
- Problems with the test script.
- Problems with the specification under test.
- Software or hardware errors in the system under test.

Only the latter of these is a genuine system failure under test, but in most test programs these represent a minority of the test failures.

Test Metrics and Statistics

Test statistics should be maintained during the test program and retained for long-term analyses.

Certain statistics provide a useful overview of how testing is proceeding and are a useful way of managing the test program. Useful test statistics for the test manager to capture and monitor include:

- The number of tests (percentage) executed (a useful indicator of overall test progress).
- The number of tests (percentage) passed after a single execution or the distribution of tests passed after one, two, three, etc. executions (a useful indicator of the "quality" of the test program).
- A breakdown of statistics by test team or functional area (to identify potential bottlenecks or problems).

In addition, statistics from the analysis of test incidents can also highlight problems with the quality of test data, test scripts or the test environment, or problems with the teams conducting the actual testing. These may need to be addressed by additional training.

It is often useful to compare the statistics from similar test programs, but this is only useful if identical statistics (defined in the same way) are captured for each program. This can be a useful indicator of testing "quality" on any given project.

As discussed, such long-term statistics can be used to justify the sample size of certain checks and reviews. A deviation from an accepted standard may highlight a need for more rigorous (or relaxed) independent review.

It should, however, be noted that where the nature and scope of the test program is determined by a risk-based test strategy, the comparison of statistics from dissimilar projects will be a little benefit.

It may therefore be useful for organizations to define standard approaches to test programs. A risk-based test strategy may be used to determine the relevant approach to testing, which will include the nature and scope of tests to be conducted. This will include the categorization of tests and associated test metrics, allowing test statistics for different types of tests to be collated and compared between projects.

SUMMARY

To conclude, testing in the life science sector is very similar to the testing of computer based systems and software in other industries and a great deal of good practice can be leveraged.

There are, however, additional documentation requirements that need to be considered when executing a test program in such a regulated industry. Unless this is approached in a thoughtful and pragmatic manner many of the benefits of a risk-based test strategy and test plan may be lost.

The use of experienced personnel is a key to success. While a good test background will be of some practical use, there is no substitute for industry specific experience. Where this experience has been gained in a proscriptive test regime, care should be taken not to fall prey to some of the "urban myths" associated with testing in the life sciences industry. There is no substitute for a thorough understanding of the underlying reasons for, and the principles of, testing, and how these relate to the practical testing of the system being validated.

Chapter 20

Practical Applications of GAMP Version 4

Siegfried Schmitt

CONTENTS

INTRODUCTION

The following case studies have been written from an information management department perspective. Most articles and presentations on practical applications of GAMP 4 seem to either cover computerized systems within the manufacturing or the laboratory area, either from the perspective of the user, the vendor, or the validation consultant. It is rare to come across the information technology (IT) or information systems (IS) perspective. Information management (IM), which encompasses IT and IS, plays a dual role, as the user and as the provider.

IM acts as a service provider, managing and owning the infrastructure, the operating systems and some major applications. Furthermore, IM assists in the entire software and hardware life cycle, providing specialist knowledge for the business users. As IM operates in a regulated pharmaceutical industry environment, compliance with rules and regulations and in particular European Union (E.U.) and U.S. requirements is mandatory. Within the company these regulations are reflected and adopted via the Quality Assurance (QA) departments' standards, which are also compulsory for IM.

Only a limited number of QA staff are up to date with the regulations and are in a position to competently interpret them, mainly because this is not a traditional field of QA activities. It is advantageous, as in the case presented here, where this expertise sits within the IM department with a strong link and reporting line into QA. A QA function within IM is probably the most efficient way for implementing a quality management system (QMS) that assures compliance with the predicate rules, 21 CFR 11 and most importantly, integrates with and reflects the specific ways of working of an IM department. GAMP 4 is one important tool available to the IM QA manager for implementing adequate and well documented processes and procedures. It is also a valuable training resource.

The case studies have been selected for interest and show where we found GAMP 4 beneficial, and where its limitations lie. It is worthwhile mentioning some of the shortcomings of the electronic version of GAMP 4, which were much disliked by our user community. The screen size is fixed to fill about a quarter of the screen, which makes reading the contents somewhat awkward. In addition, the disk contents can not be installed on the hard drive, thus necessitating the availability of a CD drive, something not all laptops are equipped with. Lastly, copy and paste is disabled, a much used functionality by those preparing presentations and wishing to quote from the original. Unsurprisingly, the paper copy remains the preferred format.

VENDOR AUDITING USING GAMP 4 GUIDANCE AND TEMPLATES

Vendor audits are carried out for a variety of reasons and by a diverse number of departments on systems that often have automated features as part of the system. Traditionally engineering would conduct most audits as part of the vendor evaluation phase, or as part of factory acceptance testing (FAT) during commissioning. Other audits would be conducted by the QA function to review and assess a vendor's quality system. In most cases these audits would not comprehensively address compliance issues for the computerized system.

It is within the IM QA function where staff has many years of in-depth experience in performing and assisting in vendor audits for compliance with GXPs and the widely accepted principles of GAMP. For critical applications, either from a business or a regulatory perspective, it is highly advisable to include such an expert in the auditing team. GAMP 4 has become a popular source for information on how to conduct a vendor audit (Appendix M2), and its vendor assessment form templates are a suitable starting point for the development of company specific forms. Immediately the question arises whether these forms should be used as is, or should they be modified, and if so, to what extent? It is our experience that it is always necessary to modify the original GAMP 4 template in order to capture the specifics of an audit. However, one thing we never change is the original numbering system. We amend or add to the existing entries and extend the existing lists, using consecutive numbers.

Although specialists may be aware of it, many others are not, that GAMP 4 does *not* address 21 CFR 11, the U.S. FDA's rule on electronic records and electronic signatures. This chapter is not on 21 CFR 11. It is sufficient to note here that it is good practice to add the company specific detailed assessment checklist to the audit questionnaire. In the absence of a specifically developed version, it is possible to insert the rule itself, without any interpretation.

The following is an example of an extended audit questionnaire, with additional entries taken from a wide variety of questionnaires the author has come across over the years. Again, it has to be stressed that for each audit this list is revised, amended or extended, as necessary. This checklist should be used when auditing suppliers of automated systems. It is intended as a guide only, and there may be other factors which require consideration when auditing suppliers. All headers are as in GAMP 4, and any original text entries from GAMP 4 are in italics, for easy reference.

A. Company Overview

A.1 Audit details
Company name, company *address* and contact numbers, contact names, titles and roles of *audit team* members, qualifications of the auditors, titles and roles of (key) *supplier representatives*, date of the audit, initial or follow-up audit.

A.2 Company information
Size, name of parent company, *structure* (include organizational diagrams) and *summary of history (number of sites, staff, organizational charts, company history*, how long has the company been in business, what are the future business plans, financial basis (consult annual report, etc.). Complement verbal information from vendor with that publicly available, e.g., brochures, Internet information, etc.

A.3 Product and service history
Main markets, numbers sold, systems (differentiate between beta versions and the present version, and between systems effectively sold and installed from those ordered) in *use in healthcare sector* (how many current installations are there and what is the current growth or reduction in installed bases), etc. Support verbal information with sales material for the services or products.

Request references that can be contacted post-audit. Have they been cited for good work? Is the company in any litigation? Does the company hold a recognized quality certification (check carefully to what parts of the company these apply)?

What is the company's experience in the pharmaceutical area (ask for white papers, article reprints, presentation slides, etc.). Is the pharmaceutical and healthcare related business profitable?

A.4 Summary of product/service under audit

Request *product literature*. How important is this product to the company?

A.5 Product or service development plans

What is the long term pharmaceutical and healthcare related business plan?

A.6 Tour of facility

To verify housekeeping, general working environment, working conditions. It is worth noting how tidy and well organized the computer room is to get an idea about its actual usage.

B. Organization and Quality Management

B.1 Management *structure*

Roles and responsibilities.

Are there QA and project management structures?

B.2 Method of assuring quality in product/service.

Has a *quality system* been established?

Is it documented? Who is *responsible for quality*?

Are project work practices documented?

B.3 Use of documented QMS

For example, *quality policy and objectives, quality manual, process definitions/procedures, standards* (which ones? IEEE, GAMP, ISO, ITIL).

B.4 Maturity of QMS *(relevance to product/service under audit)*

Are there SOPs covering:

- Software development life cycle
- System specification
- System testing
- Development environment
- Product release
- Programing standard
- Document control
- Use of electronic/digital signatures (if relevant)
- Record retention
- Source code management
- Security
- Maintenance

- Change control
- Problem resolution
- Back-up
- Disaster recovery
- Customer installation
- Complaint handling, bug fixing
- Quality assurance
- Internal training
- SOP management

B.5 Control of QMS documentation (*reviews, approvals, distribution, updates*)

B.6 Maintenance of QMS documentation (*regularly updated and updated when appropriate*).

B.7 QMS certified to a recognized standard
For example, *ISO 9001*. Is certification current and still valid?

B.8 Method of checking compliance with QMS
Regular *internal audits* or *management reviews*.

B.9 Qualification and suitability of staff

B.10 Independence of auditors, inspectors, testers, reviewers

B.11 Staff training
How many permanent, contract or temporary staff does the company employ?
How long on average do employees stay with the company?
What is the company's training policy (*general, QMS, product/service related, new staff, changes to QMS*, use of methodologies, *regulatory (GxP) issues*)?
Are there any job descriptions and *training records*?
Do these conform to the SOP and are they current?
What are the training requirements for new employees prior to involving them in the development, testing, or maintenance of a product?

B.12 Use of subcontractors
Method of selection (individuals, companies)
Subcontractor qualifications and training records (general, QMS, product/service related, new staff, changes to QMS, regulatory (GxP) issues).
Specification of technical and quality requirements in orders placed.
Method of accepting product delivered by sub-contractor.

B.13 Experience of validation process
With other customers, previous supplier audits, services provided by supplier, involvement in regulatory inspections.

B.14 Awareness of healthcare regulatory requirements
Knowledge of regulations, subscription to publications, attendance at relevant events, involvement in industry groups.

B.15 Continuous improvement program
Use of metrics to evaluate and improve effectiveness of QMS.

C. Planning and Product/Project Management

C.1 Use of quality and project plans
Are plans produced *per project/product*?
Who approves these?
What are the *defining activities, process definitions*/controlling *procedures, responsibilities and timescales*?
Does planning include contract review?
If the project is executed at more than one site, how are the project and the project documentation coordinated?
What are the responsibilities and reporting mechanisms?
Where is the information/data kept, and if copies are kept on various sites, how is completeness and management assured?

C.2 Status of planning documentation
Reviews, approvals, distribution, maintenance, and update.
Where is documentation kept?
What is the retention period for documentation?
Is the systems development life cycle documentation in a mutually acceptable language (preferably English)?

C.3 Documentation of user/supplier responsibilities

C.4 Use of validation plan where supplied by user company

C.5 Project management and monitoring
Mechanism, tools, progress reports.
Are subcontractors audited?
How are they managed?
Are subcontractor standards audited?
Are signatoree lists up to date and complete with names, initials, and signatures for ready reference and are CVs or job descriptions available for those persons?
When did the development of this software first begin?
What is the release history of this product?

C.6 Accuracy of, and conformance to, planning and management process definitions/procedures

C.7 Use of formal development life cycle
Is there a defined project life cycle?
What is it and what is it based on?

C.8 Evidence of formal contract reviews where applicable

D. Specifications

D.1 User Requirements Specifications
Is there a documented list of the user requirements used as a basis for the

design of the system and how are customer specific user requirements incorporated into this list?

D.2 Functional Specifications
Are there any narrative descriptions of the system functions?

D.3 Software Design Specifications
Do design considerations cover reliability, maintainability, security, and safety?
Do they cover standardization or interchangeability?
Do they account for 21 CFR Part 11 requirements?

D.4 Hardware Design Specifications
Do design considerations cover reliability, maintainability, security, and safety?
Do they cover standardization or interchangeability?

D.5 Relationship between specifications
Together forming a complete specification of the system, which can be tested objectively.
Were there any minimum performance targets documented in the system design?

D.6 Traceability through specifications
For example, for a given requirement, can these be traced (preferably using a matrix) and are these indexed in a controlled manner?
Are design changes proposed, approved, implemented, and properly controlled (SOP, master index for work requests/punch list)?

D.7 Status of specifications
Reviews (documented, minuted, are users invited to attend design review meetings?), *approvals, distribution, maintenance, and update.*

D.8 Accuracy of, and conformance to, relevant process definitions/procedures

D.9 Use and control of design methodologies
CASE tools.

E. Implementation

E.1 Specification of standards covering use of programming languages
For example., naming and coding conventions, commenting rules.
Does the source code contain explanatory remarks throughout the code?
How does the company ensure these conform to current industry requirements?

E.2 Standards for software identification and traceability
For example, for each software item — unique name/reference, version, project/ product reference, module description, list of build files, change history, traceability to design document.

E.3 Standards for file and directory naming

E.4 Use of build files to compile and link individual software configuration items into a formal release of the software product
Guidelines or standards for hardware assembly
What third party hardware or software is used?
Is software and hardware supplied by reputable firms?
How would changes to third party products affect the user's end product?

E.5 Use and version logging of development tools
For example, compilers, linkers, debuggers used for each software configuration item and the formal build and release of the software product.

E.6 Evidence of source code reviews prior to formal testing
Checking design, adherence to coding standards, logic, redundant code, identification of critical algorithms.
Is there documented evidence that code walk-throughs have been done on each module (including information on the outcome)?

E.7 Independence and qualifications of reviewers

E.8 Source code reviews recorded, indexed, followed-up, and closed off (with supporting evidence)
Evidence of timely management action for reviews which remain open or where reviews were not closed off satisfactorily.

E.9 Listings and other documents used during source code reviews identified, controlled, and retained with review reports

F. Testing

F.1 Explanation of test strategy employed at each level of development
For example, module testing, integration testing, system acceptance testing or alpha/beta testing, predelivery testing.
Is there a formal test plan?
Are test specifications produced?
Are expected results defined?
Is there a specific testing environment?

F.2 Software test specifications

F.3 Hardware test specifications
Are all drawings, specifications, and related documents available, current, correctly signed, and in the right format?

F.4 Integration test specifications

F.5 System acceptance test specifications
Is there documented testing of the system to check that mathematical functions, audit trails, and other system functions work correctly?
How are printouts and datasets cross-referenced to the tests?
Does this allow the tests to be reproduced?

F.6 Structure and content of each test script

Unique reference, unambiguous description of test, acceptance criteria/ expected results, cross-reference to controlling specification.
Are test scripts executed as paper or electronic copies?
If test scripts are executed electronically, are these signed in wet ink or with electronic signatures?

F.7 Relationship between test specifications and controlling specifications
Demonstrating system has been thoroughly tested with traceability between specifications and test.

F.8 Evidence that test specifications cover:
Both structural (white box) *and functional* (black box) *testing, all requirements, each function of the system, stress testing (repeat testing under different conditions*, including values above and below the valid range as well as things like input of characters in a numeric field), alarm message testing, performance testing *(e.g., adequacy of system performance), abnormal conditions.*
Is testing rigorous?
Are versions of hardware and software inspected?

F.9 Status of test specifications
Reviews, approvals, distribution, maintenance, and update.

F.10 Formal testing procedure to execute test specifications
Method of recording test results (signing and dating), *use of pass/fail, retaining raw data, reviewing test results.*
Documenting, *progressing*, correcting *and resolving test failures.*
Are all failures analyzed?
Are corrective actions promptly taken?
Are responsibilities for change control assigned?
Are these records maintained?
Who signs for overall acceptance of testing?

F.11 Status of test results and associated review records
Indexed, organized, maintained, followed-up on failure.
Are obsolete documents withdrawn?
Are changes notified to the user (these may be published on the Web, mailed to a select user group, available on request only or admitted upon detection by the user only)?

F.12 Involvement of QA function
As witnesses and/or reviewers, conducted by individuals who do not have direct responsibility for matters being audited?
Are periodic audits planned and auditing procedures documented?
Are responsibilities for documentation review assigned?
Are audit results reviewed by management having responsibility for the matters audited?
Does the company have a copy of the last audit report on file?
Is follow-up corrective action, including re-audit of deficient areas, taken when indicated?

Is there evidence that the system documentation has been reviewed throughout the system life cycle?

F.13 Independence and qualifications of testers and reviewers
Who performs the tests?
How is testing organized?

F.14 Accuracy of, and conformance to, relevant test process definitions/procedures.
Does the QMS provide for prompt detection of failures?

F.15 Control of test software, test data, simulators

F.16 Use of testing tools
Documented, controlled, and versions recorded in the test results.

F.17 Traceability of test results back to the appropriate specifications/test scripts
Does the vendor supply an official software test package for validating the system?

G. Completion and Release

G.1 Documented responsibility for release of product
Such as certificate of conformity, authorization to ship (including evidence that testing has been accepted with/without reservations).

G.2 Handover of project material in accordance with quality plan/contract
For example, release notes, hardware, copies of documentation/software.
Is there a listing of recommended critical and non-critical spare parts for the product(s)?

G.3 Provision of user documentation
User manuals, administration/technical (installation, operation, maintenance) *manuals* (when and how are these being delivered/released in relation to system delivery?
What on-going documentation is supplied with the product(s)?
How are these kept current with regards to functionality changes?
For how long will on-going documentation be supplied?
Are manuals version controlled? What language are they in?, *update notice with each release.*
Is there documentation on what terminals, clients and printers are supported by the system?
Is there documentation which describes how to migrate data from one system version to another?
Data migration: what data can be migrated between what versions? Is it necessary to migrate data via a specific release or can releases be "jumped?"
What is the expected downtime for data migration?
Which vintage of data files can be processed using the most recent software release?

G.4 Records of releases
For example, which customers have which version of system/software?
Are project documents handed over to the user?
Is there configuration and version control within projects?

G.5 Warranties and guarantees
Is there a certificate of conformity?

G.6 Archiving of release
Software, build files, supporting tools, documentation.

G.7 Availability of source code and documentation for regulatory inspection
Is there an access agreement for regulatory inspections, e.g., *an ESCROW account? If so, for which releases?*
Will the company provide information to the regulatory authorities if requested?
Where is the source code archived?
Is a periodic check of data integrity ensured?

G.8 Customer training
Summary of courses, given by staff or third parties.
Is training available on how to use this system?
Where will the training sessions be held, i.e., is on-site training available?
Does this include modern interactive tools for training?
What is the frequency of training events?
Is there documented evidence relating to the trainers' qualifications?

G.9 Accuracy of, and conformance to, release process definitions/procedures
What is the mechanism for deciding a project is complete?

H. Support and Maintenance

H.1 Explanation of support services
Agreements, scope, procedures (response mechanisms and timings for user problems), support organization, responsibilities, provision locally/internationally.
How many software support staff work in development on the system being audited?
How many work to support the product here and worldwide?
Use of third parties, maintenance of support agreements.
Is staff used to support the system trained or experienced in the product?
How long have they been working for the company on this product?
Is there a list of users provided with a similar service/product that is the subject of this audit?
Is there a support fee?
Does your company provide consulting and validation services? E.g., IQ, OQ for equipment hardware and software?

Is the service compliant to an international standard, e.g., ISO 9002?

H.2 Duration of guaranteed support

Number of versions, minimum periods.

How long or for how many versions will old releases be supported? Is there a SOP/procedure, which addresses support for existing system versions?

Who is responsible for ongoing user support?

H.3 Provision of help desk

Levels of service, hours of operation.

Do the support staff speak a mutually acceptable language (preferably English) well enough to offer support over the phone?

What remote support sites do you have and where are they situated?

What method of communication is used to contact remote support sites (routine and emergency communications)?

How do the remote sites know the status of error reports as well as new bugs, fixes, and patches?

How are remote site employees trained on new revisions, procedures, and policies?

Do your remote sites perform local modifications/configuration of the system?

If local sites do modify the system locally what procedures do they follow and how is the original development documentation updated?

How is this enforced?

H.4 Fault reporting mechanism

Logging (unique identifier, global system?), *analyzing, categorizing, resolving* (is there a procedure on how a fault is escalated depending on the severity and the time it is outstanding?), *informing, closing* (how often does management review outstanding error reports from the helpdesk?), *documenting, distribution, notification of other customers with/without support agreement.*

Are faults (detected by the company or other users) notified to the user (these may be published on the Web, mailed to a select user group, available on request only or admitted upon detection by the user only)?

Are users solicited for feedback?

How are user responses folded into development plans?

Do you provide information on why a change has been made and how this affects any other functionality?

Is there documentation on known current system faults and any workarounds?

H.5 Link between fault reporting mechanism and change control

H.6 Method of handling of customer complaints

Preferably have an example from someone in Amersham who has contacted the company with a problem and see if the records can be found.

H.7 Accuracy of, and conformance to, support process definitions/procedures

I. Supporting Procedures and Activities

I.1 Documentation management
Covering QMS and product/project documents, *in accordance with QMS/ quality plan, following documentation standards, indexed, organized, reviews carried out prior to approval and issue, reviews recorded, indexed, followed-up and closed off (with supporting evidence), evidence of management action for reviews which remain open* or where reviews not closed off satisfactorily, *formal approvals recorded, meaning of approvals defined, distribution controlled, document history maintained, removal of superseded/obsolete documents.*

I.2 Software configuration management:
System for identifying, controlling and tracking every version of each software item, system for recording the configuration of each release (i.e., which software configuration items and versions are used), identification of point at which change control is applied to each software item, control of build tools and layered software products, including introduction of new versions (e.g., addition of new functions/modules, alteration of existing function/module logic, deletion of existing functions/modules, addition of new data items, creation of new data stores/tables, alteration of system defaults, alteration of internal calculations, new/altered error messages, alteration of range check values).

I.3 Change control covering software, hardware, and documentation
All change requests formally logged, indexed, assessed, rejected requests identified as such, reasons documented, signed by those responsible and the originator informed, changes authorized, documented, tested and approved prior to implementation (except emergencies), emergency process definitions/procedure documented, covering reviewing, testing, approving, recording, impact of each change (on other items and on requirements for re-test) assessed and documented.

I.4 Security process definitions/procedures
Physical access, logical access to accounts/software/hardware (prevention of unauthorized or accidental modification, destruction or disclosure), *virus controls.*
Source code security (including previous versions).
Is there a disaster recovery plan?

I.5 Backup and recovery process definitions/procedures
Secure storage and handling of media, on-site, off-site, recovery procedure exercised.

I.6 Disaster recovery process definitions/procedure
Tried and documented evidence of disaster recovery testing.

I.7 Control of purchased items bought on behalf of customer
For example, computer hardware, layered software products, including associated packaging, user documentation, warranties.

I.8 Accuracy of, and conformance to, relevant process definitions/procedures

When conducting an audit using the above questionnaire, it is advantageous to relate at least some of the questions to the specific product you wish to or have already committed to purchase. Typically, custom support, change control and adherence to the lifecycle model can be tested identifying a serious bug in the software. If procedures are followed correctly, the vendor should have an entry in the relevant logs of your fault report. Following from there one expects appropriate change control procedures to be followed, which can result either in the bug not being fixed (maybe postponed for a later release), a procedural workaround suggested, or a bug fix initiated. Where new code has to be written or existing code has to be corrected, there must be appropriate documentation, with the changes reflected in the amended test scripts, and possibly revised user manuals. Also, there should be the correct patch release notes and any other form of client update.

Where it is not possible or feasible for a company to conduct an audit, alternatives are available, such as audits by independent consultants or audit reports from repositories. Only in the first case has the company any control over the audit scope and contents. One well-advertised example for an audit repository is the Parenteral Drug Association's Audit Repository Center (www.pda.org). These audits are carried out to a predetermined specification and are conducted by specially qualified, certified, and trained auditors. These audit reports provide a good insight into a company's quality system, with large parts of the audit strategy following GAMP 4 requirements.

This concept of sharing audit reports does not come cheap, and at $5,000 a piece they are not necessarily within everybody's reach. Before a company decides on the purchase of such a report, it is important to consider whether the scope of the repository's report will cover the very specific issues the purchaser is interested in. For example, if the healthcare company is interested in the vendor's capability to deliver a system that would satisfy the requirements of 21 CFR 11, it would be unwise to rely on such a report that only covers the supplier's quality system.

It is understandable when some vendors limit the number of customer audits, as they need to strike a balance between customer service and efficient operation. It has, however, become a nasty habit in recent times for some vendors to charge would-be customers exorbitant amounts for the permission to audit. In one case $2,500 per day was quoted by a leading laboratory automation supplier. It is hoped that market forces will rectify this unhealthy development.

TRAINING IN GAMP 4

Adopting the principles of GAMP 4 makes good business sense. It does then require the company to train staff in the correct use and interpretation of the book. It is good practice to provide this training to all involved in projects concerning automated systems. We found that project managers are particularly interested in the topic and we now run special training sessions for this specific group. When putting together the training material, it was convenient to use the historic review on the GAMP history in *Pharmaceutical Engineering*'s November/December 2001 issue. The redesign of the GAMP website offers an incentive to regularly review the links in the presentation for ongoing correctness.

Especially for those operating outside the U.S. it is recommended that background information is provided on other (interest) groups, such as PDA, IEEE, NAMUR, APV, DIN, ISO, and others.

Participation in the special interest groups (SIG) is not only encouraged, it also provides a good opportunity to link GAMP to current issues within the company, such as infrastructure validation, electronic data archival, to name just a few. The audience will not only be able to relate better to GAMP, it will also provide them with a more lasting impression of the presented material.

If the electronic version of GAMP 4 was more user-friendly, it would have been possible to make good use of it when preparing the presentations. However this is not supported and much of the information has to be retyped.

Project managers deal with systems that have to comply with all areas of GXP. GAMP 4 is strongly biased towards good manufacturing practice (GMP), which has to be stressed and the presenters must be aware of. Where appropriate, the presentation can be extended by including specific guidance on medical devices, clinical trial systems, etc. Some of the terminology is unclear or unfamiliar to some in the audience as a result of the basis in GMP. It is helpful to pull together a glossary of terms, as used in the company for explanation and to point out where they fit into the lifecycle model. As an example, user acceptance testing is often synonymous with performance qualification.

Most companies base their methodology on the V-model as promoted by GAMP 4. It is not helpful to have seemingly contradictory presentations of this model in the guide. It is suggested that a firm's methodology is explained using the V-model as described in the quality management guide, rather than simply copy the GAMP 4 presentation.

A software classification guide is helpful and generally useful. It can become an issue when applied rigidly. Most systems are a mix of various classes of software and it requires expert knowledge to decide on the appropriate level of validation, depending on the type of software encountered.

Lastly, it is beneficial to outline which parts of GAMP 4 have been incorporated into the company's quality system and how they are being interpreted. For example, GAMP 4 is not designed for legacy systems, and it is up to the company's experts to establish how these systems need to be treated, making best use of the elements in GAMP 4. This will not be limited to the GAMP recommendations, as the healthcare industry also has to adopt the ever-changing interpretations on computer systems validation given by the regulators, such as the U.S. FDA.

WHO ARE YOU TALKING TO?

Whereas the former versions of GAMP may have overstressed which part of the validation activities had to be the user's responsibility and which the vendor's, by having two separate chapters, GAMP 4 still offers this distinction. For many simple systems this may be the correct approach, which can, and indeed should, be followed by both parties, the user, and the vendor. This is no longer true for complex systems or projects. As mentioned in the introduction, IM acts in both capacities, often dealing with one internal customer and several external vendors and consultants. It is not unusual to find ratios of external to internal staff in IM departments ranging from 1 to 1, up to 5 external to 1 internal staff. To complicate matters, the contracts with the external parties are generally drawn up and managed by the user, not by IM.

As a consequence, vendors may not be contractually obliged to adopt or follow GAMP 4 guidance. Their documentation may not have to be aligned with established IM formats and procedures may not satisfy the requirements for fully validated systems, as defined by IM's QA. Thus, even if a company's IM and user function have established a validation framework, which is based on the lifecycle model and follows GAMP 4 recommendations, validation success may be jeopardized through inadequate, or inappropriate third-party contracts and working practices.

Figure 20.1 helps to illustrate the situation.

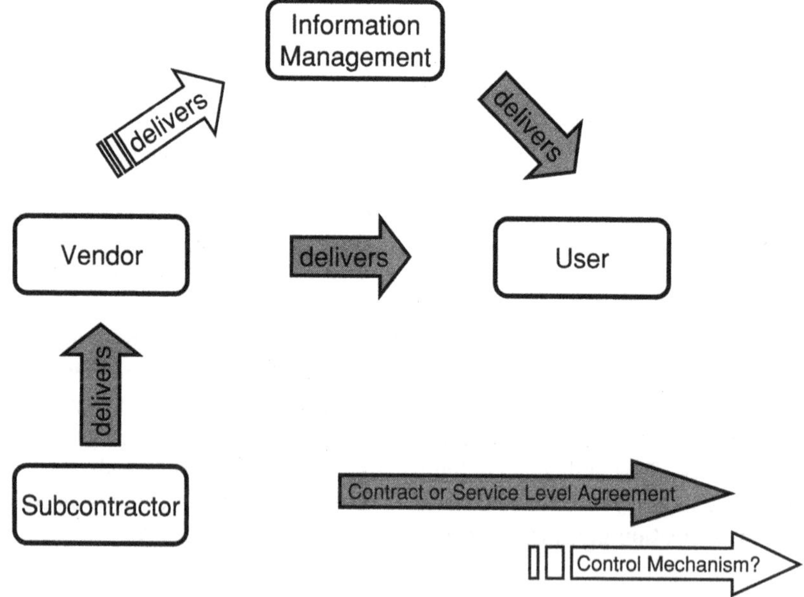

Figure 20.1 Contractual relationships.

When this relationship model is properly understood by all parties involved, the first step towards a successful implementation and associated validation activity is made.

In summary, GAMP 4 is indeed a most welcome and versatile guide, which is likely to become much more of a global standard over the coming years. It is however, necessary to understand its limitations and it is imperative to interpret and adapt its contents and spirit to reap optimum benefit for each company's specific circumstance.

REFERENCES

GAMP 4, www.ispe.org

U.S. Food and Drug Administration — Center for Devices and Radiological Health, Quality Systems Audits, http://www.fda.gov/cdrh/qsr/17audit.html

Wingate, G. *Audit Preparation for Suppliers*, www.suehorwoodpubltd.com.

1028-1997 IEEE Standard for Software Reviews, www.ieee.org

Chapter 21

Glossary and Abbreviations

Orlando Lopez

For additional terms, refer to the *Glossary of Computerized System and Software Development Terminology* and *A Globally Harmonized Glossary of Terms for Communicating Computer Validation Key Practices*.

Abstraction This is a basic principle of software engineering, and enables an understanding of an application and its design, and the management of complexity.

Acceptance Criteria The criteria that a system or component must satisfy to be accepted by a user, customer, or other authorized entity (IEEE).

Acceptance Test Testing conducted to determine whether a system satisfies its acceptance criteria and to enable the customer to determine whether to accept the system (IEEE).

Access The ability or opportunity to gain knowledge of stored information (DOD 5015.2–STD).

Application A group of computer instructions that is used to accomplish a business function, control a process, or facilitate decision-making. Refer to **Application Software** in *Glossary of Computerized System and Software Development Terminology*, August 1995.

Approver(s) In the context of configuration management, the approver is the person(s) responsible for evaluating the recommendations of the reviewers of deliverable documentation, and for making a decision on whether to proceed with a proposed change, and for initiating the change request implementation.

Auditor In the context of configuration management, the auditor is the person responsible for reviewing the steps taken during a development or change management process, to ensure that the appropriate procedures have been followed.

Audit Trail An electronic means of auditing the interactions between records within an electronic system, so that any access to the system can be documented as it occurs, to identify unauthorized actions in relation to the records, e.g., modification, deletion, or addition (DOD 5015.2–STD).

Authentication The process used to confirm the identity of a person, or to prove the integrity of specific information. In the case of a message, authentication involves determining the message source, and providing assurance that the message has not been modified or replaced in transit (ABA).

Authenticity A condition that proves a record is authentic and/or genuine, based on its mode (the method by which a record is communicated over space or time); on its form (format and/or media that a record takes when received); state of transmission (the primitiveness, completeness, and effectiveness of a record when initially set aside after being made or received); and manner of preservation and custody (DOD 5015.2–STD).

Automated systems Include a broad range of systems including, but not limited to, automated manufacturing equipment, automated laboratory equipment, process control, manufacturing execution, clinical trials data management, and document management systems. The automated system consists of the hardware, software, and network components, together with the controlled functions and associated documentation (GAMP).

Certification authority The authority (part of the public-key infrastructure) in a network that issues and manages security credentials and public key for message encryption and decryption from a certificate server (NARA).

Change Any variation or alteration in form, state, or quality. It includes additions, deletions, or modifications impacting the hardware or software components used affecting operational integrity, service level agreements, or the validated status of applications on the system.

Cipher Series of transformations that converts plaintext to ciphertext using the Cipher key.

Cipher key Secret cryptography key that is used by the Key Expansion routine to generate a set of round keys.

Cipher text Data output from the Cipher or input to the Inverse Cipher.

Code audit An independent review of source code by a person, team, or tool to verify compliance with software design documentation and programming standards. Correctness and efficiency may also be evaluated (IEEE).

Code inspection A manual (formal) testing (error detection) technique where the programmer reads source code, statement by statement, to a body that can ask questions; for example, when analyzing the program logic, analyzing the code with respect to a checklist of historically common programming errors, and analyzing its compliance with coding standards. This technique can also be applied to other software and configuration items (Myers/NBS).

Code review A meeting at which software code is presented to project personnel, managers, users, customers, or other interested parties for comment or approval (IEEE).

Code walkthrough A manual testing (error detection) technique where program (source code) logic (structure) is traced manually (mentally) by a group or body with a small set of test cases; the state of program variables is simultaneously manually monitored, to analyze the programmer's logic and assumptions (Myers/NBS).

Complexity In the context of this book, complexity means the degree to which a system or component has a design or implementation that is difficult to understand and verify. Sample factors for establishing the complexity of a system or a component can be reviewed in Appendix D.

Compliance Compliance covers the adherence to application-related standards or conventions or regulations in laws and similar prescriptions.

Configurable software Application software, sometimes general purpose, written for a variety of industries or users in a manner that permits users to modify the program to meet their individual needs (FDA).

Computer A functional unit that can perform substantial computations, including numerous arithmetic operations and logical operations without human intervention.

Computer System (1) A system including the input of data, electronic processing, and the output of information to be used either for reporting or automatic control (EU PIC/S). (2) A functional unit, consisting of one or more computers and associated peripheral input and output devices, and associated software, that uses common storage for all or part of a program and also for all or part of the data necessary for the execution of the program; executes user-written or user-designated programs; performs user-designated data manipulation, including arithmetic operations and logic operations; and execute programs that modify themselves during their execution. A computer system may be a standalone unit or may consist of several interconnected units (ANSI).

Computer Systems Validation (CSV) The formal assessment and reporting of quality and performance measures for all the life-cycle stages of software and system development, its implementation, qualification and acceptance, operation, modification, requalification, maintenance, and retirement, such that the user has a high level of confidence in the integrity of both the processes executed within the controlling computer system(s), and in those processes controlled by and/or linked to the computer system(s), within the prescribed operating environment(s) (MCA).

Concurrent Validation In some cases, a drug product or medical device may be manufactured individually or on a one-time basis. The concept of prospective or retrospective validation as it relates to those situations may have limited applicability. The data obtained during the manufacturing and assembly process may be used in conjunction with product testing, to demonstrate that the instant run yielded a finished product meeting all of its specifications and quality characteristics (FDA).

Control System Included in this classification are Supervisory Control and Data

Acquisition Systems (SCADA), Distributed Control Systems (DCS), Statistical Process Control systems (SPC), Programmable Logic Controllers (PLCs), intelligent electronic devices, and computer systems that control manufacturing equipment or receive data directly from manufacturing equipment PLCs.

Criticality In the context of this book, criticality means the regulatory impact to a system or component. Sample factors that establish the criticality of a system or a component can be reviewed in Appendix D.

Custom-built software Also known as a Bespoke System, Custom-Built Software is software produced for a customer, specifically to order, to meet a defined set of user requirements (GAMP).

Digital certificate A credential issued by a trusted authority. An entity can present a digital certificate to prove its identity or its right to access information. It links a public-key value to information that identifies the entity, associated with the use of the corresponding private key. Certificates are authenticated, issued, and managed by a trusted third party called a CA.

Documentation Manuals, written procedures or policies, records, or reports that provide information concerning the use, maintenance, or validation of a process or system involving either hardware or software. This material may be presented from electronic media. Documents include, but are not limited to, Standard Operating Procedures (SOPs), Technical Operating Procedures (TOPs), manuals, logs, system development documents, test plans, scripts and results, plans, protocols, and reports. Refer to **Documentation** and **Documentation, level of** in the *Glossary of Computerized System and Software Development Terminology*, August 1995.

Emergency change A change to a validated system determined necessary to eliminate an error condition that prevents the use of the system and interrupts business function.

Emulation The process of mimicking, in software, a piece of hardware or software so that other processes 'think' that the original equipment/function is still available in its original form. Emulation is essentially a way of preserving the functionality of, and access to, digital information that might otherwise be lost due to technological obsolescence.

Encryption The process of converting information into a code or cipher. A secret key, or password, is required to decrypt (decode) the information, which would otherwise be unreadable.

Entity A software or hardware product that can be individually qualified or validated.

Establish Establish is defined in this book as meaning to define, document, and implement.

Factory Acceptance Test (FAT) An acceptance test in the supplier's factory, usually involving the customer (IEEE).

Field Devices Hardware devices typically located in the field at or near the process, necessary for bringing information to the computer or implementing a computer-driven control action. Devices include sensors, analytical instruments, transducers, and valves.

GxP A global abbreviation intended to cover GMP, GCP, GLP, and other regulated applications in context.

GxP Computerized Systems A computerized system that performs regulated operations that are required to be formally controlled under the Federal Food, Drug, and Cosmetic Act, the Public Health Service, and/or an applicable regulation.

Hybrid systems In the context of Part 11, hybrid computer systems save required data from a regulated operation to magnetic media. However, the electronic records are not electronically signed. In summary, in hybrid systems some portions of a record are paper and some are electronic.

Impact of change The impact of change is the effect of change on the GxP computerized system. The components by which the impact of change is evaluated may include, but not be limited to, business considerations, resource requirements and availability, application of appropriate regulatory agency requirements, and criticality of the system.

Inspection A manual testing technique in which program documents [specifications (requirements, design), source code or user's manuals] are examined in a very formal and disciplined manner to discover any errors, violations of standards or other problems. Checklists are typical vehicles used in accomplishing this process.

Installation qualification Establishing confidence that process equipment and ancillary systems are capable of consistently operating within established limits and tolerances (FDA).

Key practices Processes essential for computer validation that consists of tools, workflow, and people (PDA).

Legacy systems Production computer systems that are operating on older computer hardware or are based on older software applications. In some cases, the vendor may no longer support the hardware or software.

Logically secure and controlled environment A computing environment, controlled by policies, procedures, and technology, which deters direct or remote unauthorized access that could damage computer components, production applications, and/or data.

Major change A change to a validated system that is determined by reviewers to require the execution of extensive validation activities.

Metadata Data describing stored data; that is, data describing the structure, data elements, interrelationships, and other characteristics of electronic records (DOD 5015.2–STD).

Migration Periodic transfer of digital materials from one hardware/software configuration to another, or from one generation of computer technology to a subsequent generation.

Minor change A change to a validated system that is determined by reviewers to require the execution of only targeted qualification and validation activities.

Model A model is an abstract representation of a given object.

Module testing Refer to **Testing, Unit** in the *Glossary of Computerized System and Software Development Terminology*, August 1995.

NEMA enclosure Hardware enclosure (usually a cabinet) that provides different levels of mechanical and environmental protection to the devices installed within it.

Noncustom Purchased Software Package A generally available, marketed software product that performs specific data collection, manipulation, output, or archiving functions. Refer to **Configurable, off-the-shelf software** in the *Glossary of Computerized System and Software Development Terminology*, August 1995.

Operating environment All outside influences that interface with the computer system (GAMP).

Ongoing evaluation A term used to describe the dynamic process employed after a system's initial validation that can assist in maintaining a computer system in a validated state.

Operational testing Refer to **Operational Qualification** in the *Glossary of Computerized System and Software Development Terminology*, August 1995.

Operating system Software controlling the execution of programs and providing services such as resource allocation, scheduling, input/output control, and data management. Usually, operating systems are predominantly software, but partial or complete hardware implementations are possible (ISO).

Password A character string used to authenticate an identity. Knowledge of the password that is associated with a userID is considered proof of authorization to use the capabilities associated with that userID (CSC-STD-002–85).

Packaged software Software provided and maintained by a vendor/supplier that can provide general business functionality or system services. Refer to **Configurable, off-the-shelf software** in the *Glossary of Computerized System and Software Development Terminology*, August 1995.

Periodic review A documented assessment of the documentation, procedures, records, and performance of a computer system to determine whether it is still in a validated state and what actions, if any, are necessary to restore its validated state (PDA).

Personal Identification Number A PIN is an alphanumeric code or password used to authenticate the identity of an individual.

Physical environment The physical environment of a computer system comprising the physical location and the environmental parameters in which the system physically functions.

Planned change An intentional change to a validated system for which an implementation and evaluation program is predetermined.

Policy A directive that usually specifies what is to be accomplished.

Predicate regulations Federal Food, Drug, and Cosmetic Act, the Public Health Service Act, or any FDA Regulation, with the exception of 21 CFR Part 11.

Predicate regulations address the research, production, and control of FDA regulated articles.

Procedural controls (1) Measures taken to ensure the trustworthiness of records and signatures established through the implementation of standard operating procedures (SOPs). (2) Written and approved procedures providing appropriate instructions for each aspect of the development, operations, maintenance, and security applicable to computer technologies. In the context of regulated operations, procedural controls should have QA/QC controls equivalent to the applicable predicate regulations.

Process system The combination of the process equipment, support systems (such as utilities), and procedures used to execute a process.

Production environment The operational environment in which the system is being used for its intended purpose, i.e., not in a test or development environment.

Production verification (PV) Documented verification that the integrated system performs as intended in its production environment. PV is the execution of selected Performance Qualification (PQ) tests in the production environment using production data.

Prospective validation Validation conducted prior to the distribution of either a new product, or product made under a revised manufacturing process, where the revisions may affect the product's characteristics. (FDA)

Qualification (1) Action of proving that any equipment works correctly and actually leads to the expected results. The word *validation* is sometimes widened to incorporate the concept of qualification (EU PIC/S). (2) Qualification is the process of demonstrating whether a computer system and associated controlled process/operation, procedural controls, and documentation are capable of fulfilling specified requirements.

Qualification protocol A prospective experimental plan stating how qualification will be conducted, (including test parameters, product characteristics, production equipment, etc.) and decision points on what constitutes an acceptable test. When executed, a protocol is expected to produce documented evidence that a system or subsystem performs as required.

Qualification reports These are test reports that evaluate the conduct and results of the qualification carried out on a computer system.

Raw data The original data that has not been manipulated or data that cannot be easily derived or recalculated from other information.

Record A record consists of information, regardless of medium, detailing the transaction of business. Records include all books, papers, maps, photographs, machine-readable materials, and other documentary materials, regardless of physical form or characteristics, made or received by an Agency of the United States Government under Federal law; or in connection with the transaction of public business and preserved or appropriate for preservation by that Agency or its legitimate successor as evidence of the organization, functions, policies, decisions, procedures, operations, or other activities of the Government or because of the value of data in the record (44 U.S.C. 3301, reference (bb)).

Record owner 'Record owner' means a person or organization who can determine the contents and use of the data collected, stored, processed, or disseminated by that party regardless of whether or not the data was acquired from another owner or collected directly from the provider.

Record reliability A reliable record provides contents that can be trusted as a full and accurate representation of the transactions, activities, or facts to which they attest, and can be depended upon in the course of subsequent transactions or activities (NARA).

Regulated operations Process/business operations carried out on an FDA-regulated product covered in a predicated rule.

Replacement The implementation of a new Part 11-compliant system after the retirement of an existing system.

Requalification Repetition of the qualification process or a specific portion thereof.

Remediate software hardware and/or procedural changes employed to bring a system into compliance with 21 CFR Part 11.

Retirement phase The period in the SLC in which plans are made and executed to decommission or remove a computer technology from operational use.

Retrospective evaluation Establishing documented evidence that a system does what it purports to do, based on an analysis of historical information. The process of evaluating a computer system currently in operation against standard validation practices and procedures. The evaluation determines the reliability, accuracy, and completeness of a system.

Retrospective validation See Retrospective evaluation.

Site Acceptance Test (SAT) An acceptance test at the customer's site, usually involving the customer (IEEE).

Software development standards Written policies or procedures that describe practices a programmer or software developer should follow in creating, debugging, and verifying software.

Source Code The human readable version of the list of instructions (programs) that enable a computer to perform a task.

Specification A document that specifies, in a complete, precise, and verifiable manner, the requirements, design, behaviour, or other characteristics of a system or component; and often the procedures for determining whether such provisions have been satisfied (IEEE).

Static analysis (1) Analysis of a program performed without executing the program (NBS). (2) The process of evaluating a system or component based on its form, structure, content, documentation (IEEE).

Standard instrument software Software driven by non-user-programmable firmware, which is configurable (GAMP).

Standard software packages A complete and documented set of programs supplied to several users for a generic application or function (ISO/IEC 2382–20:1990).

System (1) People, machines, and methods organized to accomplish a set of specific functions (ANSI). (2) A composite entity, at any level of complexity, of personnel, procedures, materials, tools, equipment, facilities, and software. The elements of this composite entity are used together within the intended operational or support environment, to perform a given task or achieve a specific purpose, support, or mission requirement (DOD).

System backup The storage of data and programs on a separate media, and stored separately from the originating system.

System Life Cycle (SLC) The period of time commencing from when the system product is recommended, until the system is no longer available for use or is retired.

System owner The person(s) who have responsibility for the operational system, and bear the ultimate responsibility for ensuring a positive outcome of any regulatory inspection or quality audit of the system.

System retirement The removal of a system from operational usage. The system may be replaced by another system or may be removed without being replaced.

System software See Operating System.

Technical controls Measures taken to ensure the trustworthiness of records and signatures established through the application of computer technologies.

Test report Document presenting test results and other information relevant to a test (ISO/IEC Guide 2:1991).

Test script A detailed set of instructions for execution of the test. This typically includes the following:

- Specific identification of the test
- Prerequisites or dependencies
- Test objective
- Test steps or actions
- Requirements or instructions for capturing data (e.g., screen prints, report printing)
- Pass/fail criteria for the entire script
- Instructions to follow in the event that a nonconformance is encountered
- Test execution date
- Person(s) executing the test
- Review date
- Person reviewing the test results

For each step of the test script, the item tested, the input to that step, and the expected result, are indicated prior to execution of the test. The actual results obtained during these steps of the test are recorded on (or attached to) the test script. Test scripts and results may be managed through computer-based electronic tools. Refer to **Test case** in the *Glossary of Computerized System and Software Development Terminology*, August 1995.

Test Nonconformance A test nonconformance occurs when the actual test result does not equal the expected result or an unexpected event (such as a loss of power) is encountered.

Training plan Documentation describing the training required for an individual based on his or her job title or description.

Training record Documentation (electronic or paper) of the training received by an individual that includes, but is not limited to, the individual's name or identifier; the type of training received; the date the training occurred; the trainer's name or identifier; and an indication of the effectiveness of the training (if applicable).

Trustworthy Reliability, authenticity, integrity, and usability are the characteristics used to describe trustworthy records from a record management perspective (NARA).

Transient memory Memory that must have a constant supply of power or the stored data will be lost.

Unplanned (emergency) change An unanticipated necessary change to a validated system requiring rapid implementation.

User back-up/alternative procedures Procedure describing steps to be taken for the continued recording and control of the raw data in the event of a computer system interruption or failure.

Unit A separately testable element specified in the design of a computer software element. Synonymous to component, module (IEEE).

UserID A sequence of characters that is recognized by the computer and that uniquely identifies one person. The UserID is the first form of identification. UserID is also known as a PIN or identification code.

Validated The term 'validated' is used to indicate a status that designates that a system and/or software is compliant with all regulatory requirements.

Validation Action of proving, in accordance with the principles of Good Manufacturing Practice, that any procedure, process, equipment, material, activity, or system actually leads to the expected results (see also qualification) (EU PIC/S).

Validation coordinator A person or designee responsible for coordinating the validation activities for a specific project or task.

Validation protocol A written plan stating how validation will be conducted, including test parameters, product characteristics, production equipment, and decision points on what constitutes acceptable test results (FDA).

Validation plan A multidisciplinary strategy from which each phase of a validation process is planned, implemented, and documented to ensure that a facility, process, equipment, or system does what it is designed to do. May also be known as a system or software Quality Plan.

Validation Summary Report (VSR) Documents confirming that the entire project planned activities have been completed. On acceptance of the Validation Summary Report, the user releases the system for use, possibly with a requirement that continuing monitoring should take place for a certain time (GAMP).

Verification The process of determining whether or not the products of a given phase of the SLC fulfill the requirements established during the previous phase.

Work products The intended result of activities or processes (PDA).

Worst case A set of conditions encompassing upper and lower processing limits and circumstances, including those within standard operating procedures, which pose the greatest chance of process or product failure when compared to ideal conditions. Such conditions do not necessarily induce product or process failure (FDA).

Index

Milton Keynes UK
Ingram Content Group UK Ltd.
UKHW021928071024
449327UK00022B/1734